Innovation in Healthcare Technology and Management

Edited by

Arun Kumar Rana
Department of Electronics and Communication Engineering
Galgotias College of Engineering and Technology
Greater Noida, Uttar Pradesh, India

Mandeep Kaur
Mittal School of Business
Lovely Professional University
Punjab, India

&

Sumit Kumar Rana
Department of Computer Science and Engineering
Chandigarh University, Punjab
India

Innovation in Healthcare Technology and Management

Editors: Arun Kumar Rana, Mandeep Kaur and Sumit Kumar Rana

ISBN (Online): 979-8-89881-537-0

ISBN (Print): 979-8-89881-538-7

ISBN (Paperback): 979-8-89881-539-4

Published by Bentham Science Publishers Pte. Ltd. Singapore, in collaboration with Eureka Conferences, USA.

First published in 2026.

Bentham Science Publishers Pte. Ltd.
No. 9 Raffles Place
Office No. 26-01
Singapore 048619
Singapore
Email: subscriptions@benthamscience.net

BENTHAM SCIENCE

CONTENTS

PREFACE i

LIST OF CONTRIBUTORS ii

CHAPTER 1 MOBILE TECHNOLOGY FOR HEALTH MANAGEMENT 1
Saptarshi Kumar Sarkar and *Anupama Sen*
INTRODUCTION 2
Overview of Mobile Technology in Health 2
Importance of Mobile Technology in Modern Healthcare 3
Objectives of the Chapter 3
EVOLUTION OF MOBILE TECHNOLOGY IN HEALTHCARE 4
Early Uses of Mobile Technology in Health 4
The Rise of Smartphones and Health Apps 5
Current Trends in Mobile Health Technology 6
KEY APPLICATIONS OF MOBILE TECHNOLOGY IN HEALTH MANAGEMENT 7
Telemedicine and Remote Consultations 7
Health Monitoring and Wearable Devices 8
Mobile Health Apps for Chronic Disease Management 9
Mobile Technology in Mental Health Support 10
BENEFITS OF MOBILE TECHNOLOGY IN HEALTH MANAGEMENT 11
Improved Access to Healthcare Services 11
Enhanced Patient Engagement and Empowerment 12
Real-time Data Collection and Analysis 13
Cost-Effectiveness and Efficiency 14
CHALLENGES AND LIMITATIONS 14
Privacy and Security Concerns 15
Digital Divide and Accessibility Issues 16
Regulatory and Compliance Challenges 17
Data Accuracy and Reliability 18
CASE STUDIES AND REAL-WORLD EXAMPLES 19
Successful Implementation of Mobile Health Solutions 19
Lessons Learned from Mobile Health Initiatives 20
Future Prospects of Mobile Technology in Healthcare 20
FUTURE DIRECTIONS AND INNOVATIONS 21
CONCLUSION 23
REFERENCES 23

CHAPTER 2 TRANSFORMING HEALTHCARE THROUGH AI: ADOPTION TRENDS AND CHALLENGES IN MODERN MEDICINE 27
Sangeeta Patil and *Reshma K.P.*
INTRODUCTION 28
AI IN PHARMACEUTICAL RESEARCH AND ADVANCEMENT 28
PROTEIN STRUCTURE PREDICTION 28
AI IN DRUG DESIGN 29
AI IN DRUG SCREENING, ACTIVITY SCORING, PHARMACOKINETIC PARAMETERS, TOXICITY (ADME/T) ATTRIBUTES, AND TOXICITY ASSESSMENT 30
CLINICAL TRIAL STRATEGY AND ANALYSIS 32
DRUG REPURPOSING AND SAFETY 32
AI ADAPTATION IN NANOMEDICINE 33
FUTURE AND CHALLENGES 34
CONCLUSION 35

ACKNOWLEDGEMENTS ... 35
REFERENCES ... 35

CHAPTER 3 ADVANCEMENTS IN WEARABLE HEALTH TECH: APPLICATIONS, CHALLENGES, AND FUTURE DIRECTIONS ... 39
Muhammad Thesa Ghozali and *Anita Agustina Styawan*
INTRODUCTION ... 39
THE TECHNOLOGICAL FOUNDATIONS OF WEARABLE DEVICES ... 41
Key Components and Architecture ... 41
Types of Wearable Medical Devices ... 41
Integration with IoT and Data Analytics ... 41
Applications in Healthcare ... 42
Remote Monitoring and Diagnostics ... 42
Therapeutic Devices for Rehabilitation ... 43
Disease Prevention and Early Detection ... 43
Post-Surgical Care and Elderly Assistance ... 43
CHALLENGES AND LIMITATIONS ... 44
Technical Challenges ... 44
Regulatory and Ethical Issues ... 44
User Acceptance and Usability ... 45
NEW DEVELOPMENTS AND EMERGING TRENDS ... 45
Integration of AI and ML ... 45
Future Wearables ... 46
Wearable Sensors for COVID-19 and Future Pandemics ... 46
FUTURE DIRECTIONS AND RESEARCH PROSPECTS ... 46
Multidisciplinary Research Projects ... 46
Models of Patient-Centered Healthcare ... 46
Wearables in Public Health ... 46
CONCLUDING REMARKS ... 47
REFERENCES ... 47

CHAPTER 4 BLOCKCHAIN TECHNOLOGY IN HEALTHCARE ... 51
Kajal Jain and *Sanjeev Rana*
INTRODUCTION ... 51
Definition of Blockchain Technology ... 51
Brief Overview of Healthcare Industry Challenges ... 52
CURRENT CHALLENGES IN HEALTHCARE THAT BLOCKCHAIN COULD ADDRESS ... 54
Data Security and Privacy Issues ... 54
Issues of Interoperability between Healthcare Systems ... 55
Drug Supply Chain Integrity ... 55
Claims and Billing Inefficiencies ... 55
POTENTIAL OF BLOCKCHAIN TO ADDRESS HEALTHCARE CHALLENGES ... 56
BLOCKCHAIN APPLICATIONS IN HEALTHCARE ... 58
Electronic Health Record Management ... 58
Enhancing Interoperability ... 58
Enhancing Data Security and Privacy ... 58
Empower Patient Control ... 59
Data Integrity ... 59
Challenges and Considerations ... 59
Supply Chain Management for Pharmaceuticals ... 61
Enhanced Efficiency in Recall ... 61

Maintaining Compliance with Legislation ... 61
Supply Chain Efficiency Enhancement ... 62
Challenges and Considerations ... 62
Clinical Trial Data Management ... 62
More Granular Data Integrity and Transparency ... 63
Strengthening Patient Privacy and Consent Management ... 63
Improve Recruitment and Retention ... 63
Challenges and Considerations ... 64
KEY BENEFITS OF IMPLEMENTING BLOCKCHAIN TECHNOLOGY IN HEALTHCARE ... 64
More Security Regarding Data and Privacy ... 64
Improved Interoperability ... 65
Drug Traceability ... 65
Clinical Trial Management ... 65
Claims and Billing Processing ... 65
CHALLENGES AND LIMITATIONS OF BLOCKCHAIN ADOPTION IN HEALTHCARE ... 66
Technical Challenges ... 66
Scalability ... 66
Energy Use ... 66
Interoperability ... 67
Regulatory and Compliance Issues ... 67
Adoption Barriers and Resistance to Change ... 67
FUTURE OUTLOOK FOR BLOCKCHAIN IN HEALTHCARE ... 68
Trends and Innovations Coming Up ... 68
Potential Impact on Healthcare Delivery and Patient Outcomes ... 68
ETHICAL CONSIDERATIONS ... 69
Data Ownership and Control ... 70
Equity and Access Issues ... 70
CONCLUSION ... 71
REFERENCES ... 72

CHAPTER 5 AUTOMATION AND ROBOTICS IN HEALTHCARE: TRANSFORMING PATIENT CARE ... 76
Vinod Kumar, Kanupriya Singh, Mandeep Kaur, Vikas Verma and *Olivier Niyompuhwe*
INTRODUCTION ... 77
Workflow Automation in Healthcare ... 78
LITERATURE REVIEW ... 78
Robotics in Healthcare ... 79
Societal Drivers ... 79
Technological Drivers ... 80
Advanced Imaging Systems ... 80
METHODOLOGY ... 81
Objectives of the Study ... 82
APPLICATIONS OF ROBOTICS IN HEALTHCARE ... 82
Public Safety ... 82
Clinical Care ... 82
Continuity of Work and Education ... 83
CLASSIFICATION OF ROBOTS IN HEALTHCARE ... 84
Nurse Robots in Hospitals ... 84

Ambulance Robots 84
Assistive Robots 85
Rehabilitation Robots 85
Walking Assisting Robots 86
Cleaning Robots 87
Surgical Robots 87
CHALLENGES AND OPPORTUNITIES 87
Usability and Acceptability 87
Safety and Reliability 88
Capability and Function 88
Cost Effectiveness 89
Clinical Effectiveness 89
LIMITATIONS 89
IMPLICATIONS 90
CONCLUSION 90
REFERENCES 91

CHAPTER 6 ENHANCING HEALTHCARE DATA SECURITY AND PRIVACY USING BLOCKCHAIN TECHNOLOGY 94
Liz George and *Jubilant J. Kizhakkethottam*
INTRODUCTION 94
Overview of Technological Advancements in Healthcare 95
Importance of Data Management in Modern Healthcare 96
Enhancing Patient Outcome 96
Improving Operational Efficiency 96
Ensuring Compliance and Security 96
Facilitating Research and Innovation 96
TECHNOLOGIES TRANSFORMING HEALTHCARE 97
Wearable Devices and IoT 98
Artificial Intelligence in Patient Care 98
The Role of the Metaverse in Healthcare 99
Medical Training and Education 99
Telemedicine 100
Smart Surgery 100
Medical Research 100
CHALLENGES IN HEALTHCARE DATA MANAGEMENT 101
Security Concerns 101
Privacy of Sensitive Patient Data 102
Issues with Data Interoperability 102
Data Source Heterogeneity 102
Absence of Standardization 103
Challenges with Scalability and Flexibility 103
Concerns Regarding Privacy and Security 104
Separation of Technology and Operations 104
Limitations in Financial and Resource Availability 104
Matters of Regulation and Compliance 104
BLOCKCHAIN TECHNOLOGY 104
Fundamental Attributes of Blockchain 105
Node 105
Transaction 105
Block 105

Chain 105
Miners 105
Merkle Tree 105
Smart Contract 106
Cryptographic Security Mechanisms 106
Hashing Algorithms for Data Integrity 106
Public-Key Cryptography for Authentication and Privacy 107
Decentralization and Its Advantages 107
APPLICATION OF BLOCKCHAIN IN HEALTHCARE 108
Impact on Telemedicine and Remote Monitoring 108
Monitoring Drug Supply Chain Management 109
Improving Diagnosis and Treatment 110
Effective Handling of Medical Billing and Insurance Claims 111
BENEFITS OF BLOCKCHAIN INTEGRATION 113
Enhancing Privacy and Security 113
Streamlining Data Sharing and Accessibility 113
Fostering Trust and Transparency 114
BLOCKCHAIN IN THE HEALTH CARE SECTOR- CHALLENGES 115
FUTURE PROSPECTS AND CONCLUSION 116
REFERENCES 116
CHAPTER 7 WEARABLE TECHNOLOGY AND SMART MEDICAL DEVICES 124
Heena Dhiman, Sachin Dhiman, Gurpreet Singh and *Arun Kumar Rana*
INTRODUCTION 124
Role of Wearable Technology in Healthcare 126
SMART WEARABLE DEVICES IN KEY AREAS OF HEALTHCARE 127
Physical Fitness and Health Prevention 128
Remote Patient Monitoring (RPM) 130
Chronic Disease Management 131
Precision in Disease Diagnostics 132
Personalized Examinations 133
IMPACT OF AI AND DATA ANALYTICS IN WEARABLES 133
BENEFITS OF WEARABLE SMART MEDICAL DEVICES 135
POTENTIAL RISKS 136
CONCLUSION 137
REFERENCES 137
CHAPTER 8 AI IN HEALTHCARE: ANALYZING ADOPTION DRIVERS USING FUZZY AHP 139
Ashwarya Kapoor and *Rajiv Sindwani*
INTRODUCTION 139
IDENTIFICATION OF CRITICAL DRIVERS TO AI ADOPTION IN HEALTHCARE SERVICES 141
Performance Expectancy (PE) 143
Effort Expectancy (EE) 143
Social Influence (SI) 144
Perceived Trust (PT) 144
Personal Innovativeness (PI) 144
RESEARCH METHODOLOGY 145
Fuzzy AHP 145
ANALYSIS 148
DISCUSSION AND IMPLICATIONS 149

CONCLUSION 150
LIMITATIONS AND FUTURE SCOPE 150
REFERENCES 151

CHAPTER 9 MULTIDISCIPLINARY ADVANCES IN HEALTHCARE 155
Srinjoy Chatterjee and *Shouvik Das*
INTRODUCTION 156
KEY AREAS OF MULTIDISCIPLINARY ADVANCES 157
Medical Technology and Engineering 157
Role of Biomedical Engineering in Diagnostics and Treatment 157
Integration of Artificial Intelligence and Machine Learning in Clinical Decision-making 157
Pharmaceutical and Life Sciences 158
Collaboration Between Pharmacists, Biochemists, and Healthcare Providers 158
Advances in Personalized Medicine and Drug Discovery 158
Public Health and Policy 159
Influence of Epidemiologists, Social Workers, and Policymakers in Managing Global Health Crises 159
Impact of Multidisciplinary Teams in Health Policy Development 159
Dentistry, Oral Health, and General Medicine 160
Contributions of dentistry to oVerall Health (e.g., Systemic Diseases and Oral Health Connections) 160
Role of Dental Professionals in Multidisciplinary Care Teams 163
TECHNOLOGICAL INNOVATIONS DRIVING MULTIDISCIPLINARY CARE 166
Telemedicine and Remote Care 166
Robotics and Minimally Invasive Surgery 167
Genomic Medicine and Bioinformatics 168
CHALLENGES IN MULTIDISCIPLINARY HEALTHCARE 169
FUTURE TRENDS 170
CONCLUSION 171
DECLARATION 173
ACKNOWLEDGEMENTS 173
REFERENCES 173

CHAPTER 10 MOBILE HEALTH APPS: IMPROVING HEALTHCARE DELIVERY AND PATIENT OUTCOMES 179
Sanjay Kumar, Vivek Agrawal and *Kuldeep Singh Kaswan*
INTRODUCTION 179
Background 179
Overview of Mobile Technology Evolution 179
Importance of Health Management in the Modern Era 180
Scope and Objectives 181
Purpose of the Chapter 181
Key Questions the Chapter Will Address 181
HISTORICAL PERSPECTIVE OF MOBILE TECHNOLOGY IN HEALTH 182
Early Applications of Mobile Technology in Healthcare 182
Initial Uses of Mobile Devices in Health Management 182
Case Studies of Early Implementations 183
Evolution of Mobile Health (mHealth) 183
Development from Basic Mobile Tools to Advanced Applications 183
The Role of Mobile Networks in Health Management Growth 184
MOBILE HEALTH TECHNOLOGIES 186

Types of Mobile Health Applications ... 186
Health Monitoring Apps ... 186
Telemedicine and Remote Consultation Platforms ... 187
Fitness and Wellness Tracking Apps ... 187
Mobile Health Devices ... 188
Wearable Technology ... 188
Sensors and IoT Devices in Health Management ... 189
Key Aspects of IoT in Health Management ... 189
Integration with Other Technologies ... 189
Integration with AI, IoT, and Big Data ... 189
Cloud Computing in Mobile Health Management ... 190
IMPACT OF MOBILE TECHNOLOGY ON HEALTH MANAGEMENT ... 191
Enhancing Patient Engagement ... 191
Improved Communication between Patients and Healthcare Providers ... 191
Role of Mobile Apps in Patient Education ... 192
Data Collection and Analysis ... 192
How Mobile Devices Facilitate Health Data Collection ... 193
Use of Analytics in Personalizing Healthcare ... 193
Reducing Healthcare Costs ... 194
Efficiency Gains from Mobile Health Management ... 194
Cost-Benefit Analysis of Mobile Technology in Healthcare ... 195
CHALLENGES IN MOBILE HEALTH MANAGEMENT ... 195
Technical Challenges ... 195
Data Security and Privacy Concerns ... 196
Device Compatibility and Connectivity Issues ... 196
Ethical and Legal Issues ... 197
Patient Consent and Data Ownership ... 197
Regulatory Challenges in mHealth Applications ... 197
User Adoption Barriers ... 198
Accessibility and Usability Challenges ... 198
Digital Literacy and Patient Trust ... 199
CASE STUDIES AND REAL-WORLD APPLICATIONS ... 199
Successful Implementations ... 199
Case Study 1: Management of Diabetes via Mobile Apps ... 200
Case Study 2: Remote Monitoring of Patients with Heart Failure ... 200
Case Study 3: Mobile Apps for Treating Mental Health Conditions ... 200
Comparative Studies ... 200
Comparative Study 1: Health vs. mHealth – Traditional Care for Chronic Diseases 200
Comparative Study 2: Telemedicine vs. In-person Consultation ... 201
Comparative Study 3: Patient Education through Mobile Applications ... 201
Comparative Study 4: mHealth in Urban vs. Rural Settings ... 201
FUTURE TRENDS IN MOBILE HEALTH MANAGEMENT ... 201
Emerging Technologies ... 201
Artificial Intelligence and Machine Learning ... 202
Health Parameter Measurement ... 202
Blockchain for Secure Health Data ... 202
AR and VR Applications ... 202
International Perspectives ... 202
Developed Countries ... 203
Developing Nations ... 203
Global Health Initiatives ... 203

CONCLUSION 204
ACKNOWLEDGEMENTS 205
REFERENCES 205

CHAPTER 11 A PHASE-BASED HEALTH RECOMMENDATION AND PREDICTION SYSTEM FOR WOMEN 208
Gurjot Kaur, Kushagra Agrawal and *Shaveta Jain*
INTRODUCTION 208
Existing Menstrual Tracking Applications and Methodologies 210
Major Drawbacks in Existing Menstrual Tracking Applications 213
Proposed Solution 214
LITERATURE REVIEW 216
METHODOLOGY 221
Datasets 221
Recommendation System Architecture 222
RESULTS 224
DISCUSSION 224
FUTURE WORK 226
CONCLUSION 227
REFERENCES 227

SUBJECT INDEX 231

PREFACE

The landscape of healthcare is undergoing a paradigm shift with rapid advancements in technology and management strategies. The integration of artificial intelligence, wearable technology, mobile health applications, blockchain, and automation has reshaped the way healthcare services are delivered and managed. These innovations not only enhance the efficiency of healthcare systems but also improve patient outcomes, data security, and overall accessibility.

This edited volume, Innovation in Healthcare Technology and Management, brings together insights from researchers and practitioners across various domains to explore the transformative impact of emerging technologies in healthcare. The chapters cover a broad spectrum of topics, from AI-driven decision-making and smart medical devices to blockchain-based security solutions and the role of automation in patient care.

By compiling the latest research and developments, this book aims to serve as a comprehensive resource for academics, healthcare professionals, policymakers, and technology developers. It provides a foundation for understanding the current landscape of healthcare innovation and offers a glimpse into future possibilities.

We hope that this book will inspire further research, innovation, and collaboration in the field, ultimately contributing to a more efficient, secure, and patient-centered healthcare system.

Arun Kumar Rana
Department of Electronics and Communication Engineering
Galgotias College of Engineering and Technology
Greater Noida, Uttar Pradesh, India

Mandeep Kaur
Mittal School of Business
Lovely Professional University
Punjab, India

&

Sumit Kumar Rana
Department of Computer Science and Engineering
Chandigarh University, Punjab
India

List of Contributors

Anita Agustina Styawan	Faculty of Health and Technology, Universitas Muhammadiyah Klaten, Central Java, Indonesia
Anupama Sen	Department of Computer Science & Engineering-AI, Brainware University, Kolkata, West Bengal, India
Arun Kumar Rana	Department of Electronics and Communication Engineering, Galgotias College of Engineering and Technology, Greater Noida, Uttar Pradesh, India
Ashwarya Kapoor	School of Commerce, Manav Rachna International Institute of Research and Studies, Faridabad, Haryana, India
Gurjot Kaur	Apex Institute of Technology (CSE), Chandigarh University, Mohali, Punjab, India
Gurpreet Singh	MM Engineering College, Maharishi Markandeshwar (Deemed to be University), Mullana, Haryana, India
Heena Dhiman	MM Engineering College, Maharishi Markandeshwar (Deemed to be University), Mullana, Haryana, India
Jubilant J. Kizhakkethottam	Saintgits College of Engineering, APJ Abdul Kalam University, Indore, Madhya Pradesh, India
Kajal Jain	CSE Department, Maharishi Markandeshwar (Deemed to be University), Mullana, Haryana, India
Kanupriya Singh	Seth Jai Parkash Mukand Lal Institutions of Knowledge & Service, Radaur, Haryana, India
Kuldeep Singh Kaswan	School of Computer Science & Engineering, Galgotias University, Greater Noida, Uttar Pradesh, India
Kushagra Agrawal	Department of Computer Science and Engineering, Manav Rachna International Institute of Research and Studies, Faridabad, Haryana, India
Liz George	Saintgits College of Engineering, APJ Abdul Kalam University, Indore, Madhya Pradesh, India
Mandeep Kaur	Mittal School of Business, Lovely Professional University, Phagwara, Punjab, India
Muhammad Thesa Ghozali	School of Pharmacy, Faculty of Medicine and Health Sciences, Universitas Muhammadiyah Yogyakarta, Yogyakarta, Indonesia
Olivier Niyompuhwe	Department of Forestry and Landscape Management, University of Rwanda, Kigali, Rwanda
Rajiv Sindwani	Department of Management Studies, J.C. Bose University of Science and Technology, YMCA, Faridabad, Haryana, India
Reshma K.P.	Department of Chemistry, Rungta College of Engineering and Technology, Bhilai, Chhattisgarh, India
Sachin Dhiman	Chitkara College of Pharmacy, Chitkara University, Rajpura, Punjab, India
Sangeeta Patil	Department of Chemistry, Rungta College of Engineering and Technology, Bhilai, Chhattisgarh, India

Sanjay Kumar	Department of Electronics and Communication Engineering, Galgotias College of Engineering and Technology, Greater Noida, Uttar Pradesh, India
Sanjeev Rana	CSE Department, Maharishi Markandeshwar (Deemed to be University), Mullana, Haryana, India
Saptarshi Kumar Sarkar	Department of Computer Science & Engineering-AI, Brainware University, Kolkata, West Bengal, India
Shaveta Jain	Department of Computer Science and Engineering, Manav Rachna International Institute of Research and Studies, Faridabad, Haryana, India
Shouvik Das	Department of Animal Biology and Biotechnology, University of Hyderabad, Hyderabad, Telangana, India
Srinjoy Chatterjee	Department of Dentistry, The West Bengal University of Health Sciences, Kolkata, West Bengal, India
Vikas Verma	MM Engineering College, Maharishi Markandeshwar (Deemed to be University), Mullana, Haryana, India
Vinod Kumar	Department of Management, Gurugram University, Gurugram, Haryana, India
Vivek Agrawal	School of Computer Science & Engineering, Galgotias University, Greater Noida, Uttar Pradesh, India

CHAPTER 1

Mobile Technology for Health Management

Saptarshi Kumar Sarkar[1,*] and **Anupama Sen**[1]

[1] *Department of Computer Science & Engineering-AI, Brainware University, Kolkata, West Bengal, India*

Abstract: Mobile health (mHealth) has profoundly transformed healthcare delivery by harnessing portable devices and digital applications to extend access, enhance patient engagement, and streamline health management processes. This chapter critically reviews the evolution and current state of mHealth, tracing its progression from basic SMS-based interventions to sophisticated smartphone applications, wearables, and AI-driven tools. Emphasis is placed on how mobile technology has addressed—though not fully eliminated—systemic inequities in healthcare access, notably by reducing geographic barriers and offering remote consultations through telemedicine platforms. Yet, persistent challenges remain, including the digital divide, issues of data reliability, regulatory complexity, and vulnerabilities in privacy and security, all of which constrain equitable benefits across populations.

By examining major domains of application—telemedicine, chronic disease management, health monitoring, and mental health support—the chapter synthesizes evidence of outcome improvements, particularly in underserved settings. Case studies demonstrate tangible benefits such as improved chronic disease control and early detection, but also reveal lessons on low adoption rates among marginalized groups. The critical analysis highlights that while mHealth solutions have expanded access and engagement, their effectiveness depends on robust implementation strategies for inclusivity, data integrity, and cultural adaptation. The reference list follows standardized citation formatting throughout for consistency.

Key Contributions:

- Synthesis of mHealth's evolution and current technological landscape.

- Evaluation of mHealth's effectiveness in reducing healthcare inequities and barriers across diverse populations.

- Critical appraisal of challenges—digital divide, privacy, regulatory compliance—and their impact on real-world equity.

- Recommendations for improving inclusivity, adoption, and data reliability in future mHealth innovations.

[*] **Corresponding author Saptarshi Kumar Sarkar:** Department of Computer Science & Engineering-AI, Brainware University, Kolkata, West Bengal, India; E-mail: surjo.sarkar8013@gmail.com

Arun Kumar Rana, Mandeep Kaur & Sumit Kumar Rana (Eds.)

Keywords: Accessibility, AI (Artificial Intelligence), Analytics, Applications, Augmented reality, Blockchain, Diagnostic accuracy, Healthcare, Management, Mental health, Mobile health, Monitoring, Patient outcome, Predictive analytics, Privacy, Proactive health, Regulation, Telemedicine, Wearable technology, Real-time.

INTRODUCTION

One of the factors in health management that is changing in light of mobile technological improvement is the delivery and acquisition of healthcare services. Any portable device, such as a tablet, smartphone, or other wearable technology, that is now regarded as a contemporary and necessary gadget that is an inseparable part of modern society, should be used as a means of advancing the delivery of health care in order to reduce costs and increase efficiency. Therefore, this chapter is a synthesis of the foregoing discussion insofar as the state of patient involvement is concerned in the health care fraternity, with the aim of explicating the process of development, utilization, possibility, and drawback in the efficient management and governance of the health quasi-sector.

Overview of Mobile Technology in Health

Mobile technology entails the movement of technology that can be carried or taken from one place to another, which is empowered with an internet connection and is functional through applications or apps. In healthcare management, the devices allow the use of real-time interaction, information gathering, and supervision. The tools used in health management using mobile technology have started from simple calling and texting to the current complex features. The initially used Mobile technology in healthcare was limited to short message service, where mobiles were used to remind clients of their medication and appointments. With evolution over time, when mobile phones were invented and became smart with Internet connectivity, along with better sensors, the way for more complicated use was prepared. In the present day, Mobile health or mHealth has expanded its features to the areas of Health data tracking, tele-consultations, and Remote patient monitoring [1 - 3]. Today, there are many health apps developed for mobile technology that can meet different need levels, including physical activity, diet, mental health, and chronic illness. These apps use the sensors and the analytical data gathered to personalize the health information and advice, which greatly increases a person's capacity to prevent adverse health occurrences.

Importance of Mobile Technology in Modern Healthcare

The critical role that mobile technology plays in today's healthcare is immeasurable. It covers multiple primary areas of the healthcare system, such as access to the healthcare delivery system, patient participation, and proper handling of patient data.

Firstly, mobile technology enhances the delivery of health services since it brings healthcare services closer to individuals, especially those situated in rural areas. In the case of telemedicine, commonly referred to as telemedicine, an individual has been able to get a doctor's consultation without having to travel long distances [4]. This proves helpful for disabled persons or those who reside in remote areas. Secondly, mobile technology helps increase patient participation due to tools that include both the management of the disease and the education process. With the help of health applications, users set goals, input their personal health parameters, and receive feedback, thereby increasing the compliance of individuals with health applications to recommended treatment options and healthier behaviors in everyday life. For instance, applications that enable one to practice some level of exercise and monitor diet can assist the person in understanding what changes to make concerning his or her well-being [5]. Moreover, the use of mobile technology results in effective management of health data. Smartwatches and health applications record real-time health data related to heart rate, blood glucose level, and sleep, among other aspects. These metrics can be utilized for the development of hypotheses, which would in turn help healthcare providers make precise decisions and personalize therapies based on the patient's specifics.

Summing up, it can be stated that mobile technology is a must-have solution for tackling issues in the sphere of healthcare, the availability of opportunities, people's interactivity, and data collection. The impact is immense as it alters the traditional perception of healthcare delivery and the process that attends it from the patients' perspective.

Objectives of the Chapter

The objectives of this chapter are to:

- Provide an overview of the evolution and current state of mobile technology in health management.
- Examine the key applications of mobile technology and their impact on healthcare delivery and patient outcomes.
- Analyze the benefits and challenges associated with the use of mobile technology in health management.

- Explore case studies and real-world examples to illustrate the practical implications of mobile health solutions.
- Discuss future directions and innovations in mobile technology and their potential impact on healthcare.

Lastly, by achieving these objectives, the chapter's intention is to give readers a comprehensive picture of the possibilities and limitations of using mobile technology in healthcare delivery. In light of the conclusions derived from this study, a more informed approach to understanding how mobile technological devices may serve to enhance patients' quality of life and healthcare services will be achieved.

EVOLUTION OF MOBILE TECHNOLOGY IN HEALTHCARE

It is a fascinating process of the ascent of such a fundamental tool as a mobile in the context of healthcare, moving from being a simple, effective instrument to an unprecedented system that changes the entire picture of the approach to patients and health [6]. It also sheds light on the evolution of mobile technology in the healthcare field, from the early days and the era of smart mobile phones and health applications to the current trend towards the future of mobile health or mHealth technology.

Early Uses of Mobile Technology in Health

At the beginning of mobile technology adoption in the healthcare system, the adoption was aimed at increasing communication and associated clerical functions, rather than patient healthcare functions [7]. While the first years saw rather straightforward applications, they set the stage for future, more complex ones in the healthcare industry. It was only at the end of the 1990s and in the first years of the new millennium that the use of mobile phones began to prove their worth as instruments to enhance patient care by performing the simplest of functions. Some of the initial applications were for appointment reminders and mere text messages to patients regarding compliance with their medication [8]. These text message-based interventions were some of the earliest uses of mobile technology for health behavior modifications and chronic illnesses. For example, in some programs, a Short Message Service (SMS) was employed to remind patients of the need to take their medication or attend follow-up appointments in a bid to enhance levels of compliance and appointment attendance, respectively. Also, the initial mobile health interventions were mainly condition-specific, including diabetes and hypertension [9]. For instance, using mobile phones to relay blood glucose concentrations for diabetes control offered an opportunity through which patients could convey their information to carers, thus enabling subsequent examinations and treatment. In the same way, with the use of mobile technology, remote monitoring of blood pressure in hypertensive patients became possible, which was important in tweaking treatment management plans according to actual findings. Even though these early applications were narrow in terms of the services they offered and indeed more of experiments, they were the beginning of a revolution [10]. They illustrated the possibility of developing good mobile technology applications in the management of patients and created room for better developments.

The Rise of Smartphones and Health Apps

The introduction of smartphones revolutionized the field of mobile health by offering advanced capabilities and greater flexibility for health management. With the advent of smartphones in the late 2000s, mobile technology expanded beyond simple text messaging and phone calls to include a wide range of applications and features that could support various aspects of health management. Smartphones, equipped with internet connectivity, high-resolution screens, and a range of sensors, facilitated the development of diverse health applications (apps). These apps leveraged the capabilities of smartphones to provide users with tools for tracking health metrics, accessing health information, and engaging with healthcare providers. Health apps emerged as a significant component of mobile health, offering users personalized tools for managing their health. For instance, fitness tracking apps allowed users to monitor physical activity, dietary intake, and weight, providing real-time feedback and goal-setting features. Similarly, apps designed for chronic disease management enabled patients to track symptoms, medication adherence, and other relevant health data, facilitating better communication with healthcare providers and more informed decision-making. The rise of app stores for smartphones, such as Apple's App Store and Google Play, further accelerated the proliferation of health apps. These platforms provided a marketplace for developers to create and distribute a wide range of health-related apps, catering to various needs and preferences [11]. As a result, the availability of health apps grew exponentially, offering users an unprecedented level of access to health management tools. Furthermore, smartphones enabled the integration of advanced features such as GPS, accelerometers, and heart rate monitors, which enhanced the functionality of health apps. For example, GPS tracking allowed users to map their exercise routes, while accelerometers provided insights into physical activity levels. The combination of these features contributed to the development of more comprehensive and user-friendly health management solutions.

Current Trends in Mobile Health Technology

As mobile technology continues to evolve, several key trends are shaping the current landscape of mobile health (mHealth). These trends reflect the ongoing advancements in technology and the increasing integration of mobile solutions into healthcare systems.

- Integration of Wearable Devices: Wearable technology, such as fitness trackers and smartwatches, has become a prominent trend in mHealth. These devices collect real-time data on various health metrics, including physical activity, heart rate, and sleep patterns. The data collected by wearables can be synchronized with health apps on smartphones, providing users with comprehensive insights into their health and enabling continuous monitoring [12].
- Telemedicine and Virtual Care: The rise of telemedicine has been a significant trend in mobile health, particularly in response to the COVID-19 pandemic. Telemedicine platforms enable remote consultations between patients and healthcare providers, reducing the need for in-person visits and expanding access to care [13]. Mobile technology plays a crucial role in telemedicine, facilitating video consultations, secure messaging, and remote monitoring.
- Artificial Intelligence and Machine Learning: The integration of Artificial Intelligence (AI) and Machine Learning (ML) into mobile health apps is transforming the way health data is analyzed and utilized. AI algorithms can analyze large volumes of health data to identify patterns, predict outcomes, and provide personalized recommendations [14]. This trend is enhancing the capabilities of health apps and enabling more sophisticated decision-making support.
- Personalized Health and Precision Medicine: Mobile technology is increasingly being used to support personalized health and precision medicine approaches. By leveraging data from wearables, health apps, and Electronic Health Records (EHRs), mobile solutions can provide personalized health recommendations and tailor interventions to individual needs [15]. This trend is moving towards a more individualized approach to health management.
- Data Privacy and Security: As mobile health technology continues to advance, concerns about data privacy and security remain a critical issue. Protecting sensitive health information is essential to maintaining user trust and ensuring compliance with regulations such as the Health Insurance Portability and Accountability Act (HIPAA) [16]. Addressing these concerns is vital for the continued growth and adoption of mobile health solutions.

In conclusion, the evolution of mobile technology in healthcare has been marked by significant milestones, from early uses of basic mobile phones to the rise of smartphones and sophisticated health apps. Current trends highlight the ongoing advancements in mobile health technology and its potential to further transform healthcare delivery and management.

KEY APPLICATIONS OF MOBILE TECHNOLOGY IN HEALTH MANAGEMENT

Health management, without doubt, has benefited from the introduction of a host of mobile applications that redefine the provision and delivery of healthcare. This section examines the major niche that has been adopted by mobile technology in the global healthcare systems, such as telemedicine/ remote consultation, health monitoring and wearable devices, Mobile health (mHealth) for chronic ailments, and Mobile technology for mental health. In each case, a great improvement in the overall outcome in the sphere of healthcare and patients' lives is portrayed as possible through the use of mobile technologies.

Telemedicine and Remote Consultations

Telemedicine, therefore, refers to the delivery of clinical health care over a distance through Information and Telecommunication technologies. It was identified as one of the major uses of mobile technology, and this helps the healthcare givers to do consultations with the patient through the phone. This approach has gained a lot of support, especially in recent years, with the COVID-19 outbreak, which highlighted the importance of telemedicine solutions.

Telemedicine Platforms: Telecommunication platforms of practice include Telco and Amwell, where patient-physician interfaces are arranged through video calls, telephone calls, or direct messages [17]. It provides medical advice, diagnosis, and prescriptions straight to the patient, and all from the comfort of their homes or other locations. It can be especially helpful for people who live in remote zones or zones with low density, with limited possibilities to attend in-person consultations.

Benefits: The major advantages of this model include the improvement of patients' attendance to receive medical aid, decreased time and money spent on traveling, convenience, and the opportunity for physicians to establish contacts with clients more often to monitor the results of administered therapy [18]. Telemedicine also assists the management of healthcare resources as it is not limited to physical health facilities, thereby extending the reach and impact of healthcare service providers.

Challenges: Yet, telemedicine has some barriers: Telemedicine HCS 326 Week 3 Technology Paper. Telemedicine is the practice of using telecommunications and information technologies to provide healthcare services at a distance. These are data security and privacy concerns, consistent dependable internet access, and regulatory compliance [19]. Preservation of the patient information confidentiality and equality of Internet connection are the two most important aspects of telemedicine.

Case Study: One of the most stressed benefits of telemedicine is its application in the rural regions of the United States. Telemedicine has been found to increase the availability of specialists' care and decrease the number of people who attend the emergency room in these areas [20]. This has, in turn, helped to record reasonable levels of healthcare and more satisfied clients.

Health Monitoring and Wearable Devices

Smart and wearable devices are part of the mobile health technology, in which users can have access to different health parameters in real-time. These devices start out from simple activity monitors all the way up to smart watches, up to medically prescribed monitoring devices, all for the purpose of health management.

Types of Wearable Devices: Smart wearables are smart bands (Fitbit, Garmin), smart watches (Apple Watch, Samsung Galaxy Watch), and medical wearables (CGM devices and ECG monitors) [21]. These devices have the functionality of attending to different parameters, including physical activity, heart rate, sleep, and blood glucose level.

Applications: Wearable devices are used for a variety of health management purposes. Fitness trackers and smartwatches provide users with insights into their physical activity, helping them set and achieve fitness goals. Medical wearables, such as continuous glucose monitors, are used to manage chronic conditions by providing real-time data on health metrics [22].

Benefits: Some of the advantages associated with wearable technology are constant tracking and monitoring of health, provision of customized feedback, and identification of incubating medical complications [23]. As wearable devices give users instant information regarding their health, such devices help people make the right choices.

Challenges: Wearable devices are subjected to several factors whereby the data captured is inaccurate, users of the device do not adhere to wearing it regularly, and the device integration into the healthcare system is a challenge, as pointed out in [24]. This is particularly important because to be effective, data collected from wearable technology has to be accurate, and questions on privacy and security of such data have to be effectively dealt with.

Case Study: Non-pharmacological approaches, such as the use of wearable technology, have been seen to be helpful in managing diabetes. For example, pairing of continuous glucose monitoring devices with smartphones helps the patients to monitor their blood glucose levels and adjust the magnitudes of the insulin doses appropriately [25]. This has helped to cause better control of glycemia and a decrease in complications of diabetes.

Mobile Health Apps for Chronic Disease Management

Smartphone applications have also been widely recommended for chronic illnesses, as they enable patients to have various options for managing their health status, treatment routines, and providers' instructions. They are designed to support different chronic illnesses or diseases such as diabetes, hypertension, and asthma, among others.

Diabetes Management: Mobile health applications used for the management of diabetes include blood glucose monitoring, the calculator of the dose of insulin, and the educational tool [26]. Some mobile applications include MySugr and Glucose Buddy, which assist the users in recording their blood glucose levels, diet, and exercise regimen, as well as giving the user tips on how to manage the disease.

Hypertension Management: Hypertension-related applications include specific features that enable the individual to record both blood pressure data and medication compliance, in addition to changes in lifestyle [27]. Some of these are Blood Pressure Companion and Smart BP; they help the user to track their BP levels, take reminders on their medications, as well as other hypertensive-related information.

Asthma Management: Asthma management apps have functionalities for any symptoms, medication administration, and triggers [28]. Other applications include AsthmaMD and Propeller Health, where users can record their symptoms, monitor their peak flow, and get alerts on potential triggers to their condition.

Benefits: The benefits of mobile health apps for chronic disease management include improved self-management, better adherence to treatment plans, and enhanced communication with healthcare providers [29]. By providing users with personalized tools and resources, these apps support proactive management of chronic conditions and contribute to better health outcomes.

Challenges: Some of the concerns that were highlighted include the accuracy of information, the adoption of mobile health apps, and compatibility with health care organizations [30]. The validity of the data collected and the involvement of the users signify the extent to which the Chronic Disease Management Apps are useful.

Case Study: The available information about the use of mobile health apps in managing diabetes has indicated positive results in managing diabetes. For instance, the analysis on the impact of diabetes management apps revealed that patients who used these apps had better glycemic control and higher retention rates compared to patients who did not use the apps [31].

Mobile Technology in Mental Health Support

It has also positively impacted mental health by offering gadgets to help in the management of mental conditions as well as enhancing well-being among people. Consumer mobile applications and online sites provide several services for mental health.

Mental Health Apps: The capabilities of mental health apps are extensive, with functionalities such as mood monitoring, CBT, and mindfulness. It is possible to use such applications as Headspace and Calm, which provide methods of meditation, ways of relaxation, and methods of dealing with stress and anxiety.

Online Therapy Platforms: Online therapy platforms, such as BetterHelp and Talkspace, link people with licensed therapists for regular video sessions. These platforms allow a person to seek therapy from their homes, increasing the chances of people receiving therapy [18].

Benefits: Mobile technology for mental health support also came with several advantages of expanded access to mental health supports, improved convenience, and reduced embarrassment for asking for assistance. Mobile technology allows a person to seek help and use resources without delay, helping a person with mental health issues to take charge of the situation.

Challenges: Concerns associated with IMHS include: the lack of randomized control trials, issues of data privacy, and what might be considered 'low intensity' services offered [19]. To tackle these challenges, it is crucial to enhance the efficiency and security of MH interventions delivered *via* mobile technologies.

Case Study: One of the areas of mobile technology application is the implementation of CBT in the treatment of anxiety and depression. Research using CBT-based apps has found that using these apps to deliver intervention may reduce symptoms of anxiety and depression and enhance general mental health [20]. Such apps provide people with CBT and other therapy approaches, which makes them helpful in improving people's mental health.

BENEFITS OF MOBILE TECHNOLOGY IN HEALTH MANAGEMENT

Mobile technology has brought the following opportunities in the management of health, thus changing the course of delivering healthcare services. This section focuses on the goal of m-health, benefits in health management, access to healthcare, patient involvement and control, real-time data, and cost and time factors. Mobile technology is then defined, and in the case of each benefit, elaborated on about how it contributes to improved health and the delivery of healthcare.

Improved Access to Healthcare Services

The best advancement of using mobile technology in the management of health is the creation of opportunities to access health services. Mobile technology eliminates geographical and logistical constraints often associated with accessing healthcare in the current society, especially in rural areas.

Telemedicine: Mobile technology gives a good example in the telemedicine platform as a way of improving access to healthcare. Through telecommunication, the patient does not need to attend other places of diagnosis, treatment, and care, which is difficult for those in rural areas, solitary places, among others [32]. It offers people the convenience of consulting or even being diagnosed and treated in the comfort of their homes, which increases the chances of seeking medical attention.

Mobile Health Apps: Another positive impact of mobile health apps is that they also help to address the issue of access to health care. These apps offer the users information on different ailments, educational material, and other health-related paraphernalia. For example, applications that provide a possibility to check the symptoms and receive information about some diseases can assist users in making the decision about their condition and whether they should consult a doctor. Also, applications that help physicians schedule appointments and send patients' reminders improve the overall accessibility by coordinating and minimizing the chances of rescheduling cases.

Benefits: Accessibility of health care through the use of mobile technology is one way through which imbalances in the provision of health care are reduced, especially for confined groups. It leads to early and appropriate medical treatments, minimizes distances and expenses of transport, and affords follow-up care. The access and early health conditions enable early detection and management of health status, hence improving health.

Challenges: However, it is not without challenges, and some of these include problems associated with the digital divide, where special groups of people who cannot afford to own a smartphone or have access to the internet will be locked out from these gains [33]. Accessibility of mobile health solutions to the less privileged population continues to be an issue.

Enhanced Patient Engagement and Empowerment

The use of mobile technology greatly improves the patients' participation and freedom, which are crucial in managing their health. On the same note, mobile technology empowers the patient to take charge of his or her care through the provision of tools that facilitate patient-centered care.

Health Tracking and Self-Management: Mobile health apps and wearable devices give users a way to monitor several indices, including physical activity, diet, and vital statistics. This self–management capability enhances patients' autonomy so that they can take an active part in the process of managing their condition through applying, in return, real-time data [34]. For instance, fitness trackers help in the creation of fitness goals and tracking them, while apps for chronic diseases help patients track symptoms and compliance with the drugs.

Educational Resources: The use of Mobile technology ensures that they have a wider list of educational material that the patients can go through to enable them understand the various health conditions and the treatment plans. Mobile applications and websites contain details on health and disease, healthy living, and timely essentials. It enables patients to be knowledgeable about their illness and engage better with the medical practitioners [22].

Communication with Healthcare Providers: Even though mobile technology involves electronic communication of patients' information and information exchange between patients and healthcare providers through secure messaging, and telemedicine consultations and virtual care platforms [23]. Such enhancements facilitate patients' ability to question, rationalize, and deliberate on their conditions with their providers, hence making the patient an active participant in his or her disease process.

Benefits: Informed patient self-management and patient-centered care result in improved clients' compliance with treatment regimens, enhanced health, and greater satisfaction. Patients implement self-care in a better way if they are actively participating in their care, and such participation would make them adhere to various treatments and observe changes in lifestyle that would enhance their health.

Challenges: Nevertheless, the difficulties of such types include digital literacy and user engagement that need to be solved. The use of mHealth technology may also be challenging for some of the users; this means that some patients cannot optimally participate in their care plans [24]. The last consideration is the application of mobile Health solutions, where the concept has to work for all the patients without any form of discrimination.

Real-time Data Collection and Analysis

The use of mobile technology also has the benefit of getting real-time information, accumulating and analyzing, which assists in checking and controlling health conditions. It helps in developing better, timely, and proper decisions in the overall health management.

Continuous Monitoring: Smart watches and mobile health applications offer constant tracking of the different aspects of a person's health, including heart rate, physical activity, and even glucose level. Ongoing surveillance allows the identification of possible cases of ill health, and thus, early intervention is easily made. For instance, the continuous glucose monitors give real-time data regarding the blood sugar level with the opportunity of timely alteration of the insulin management and the food intake [25].

Data Integration and Analysis: Through M2M connectivity and data sharing capabilities, mobile health solutions draw data from wearables, health applications, and EHRs. This integration makes it possible to get a holistic view and understanding of health data, which is important for the assessment of health conditions and the outcomes of the patients [26]. Modern analysis of large sets of numbers allows for the treatment of diseases before they appear and can assess specific needs for the patient.

Benefits: The real-time data collection and analysis improve the opportunity to address health conditions in a better way. It enables changes in the course of the management plan, as well as identifies and manages complications and comorbidities, or monitors chronic diseases. This capability helps in the enhancement of health status and the provision of more proper care.

Challenges: Some of the issues that come with real-time data collection and analysis include issues with data accuracy, integration of data, and issues with data privacy. Preserving the accuracy of the data gathered by wearable devices and handling doubts concerning data safety are important for the usage of real-time health data [27]. Moreover, such information, when combined into a complete and usable format, could be rather challenging and demands effective technology platforms.

Cost-Effectiveness and Efficiency

Mobile technology has shown a high potential in the improvement of cost effectiveness and efficiency when it comes to health management, meaning that it has the potential of improving on the already existing health systems to be more efficient and at the same time cut down on the costs that are incurred by both the patients and the health care facilities.

Reduced Healthcare Costs: They can cut healthcare costs to the extent that they do not need to meet their healthcare provider physically, they would be less likely to be readmitted to the hospital, and they would remove the need for a lot of paperwork. Telemedicine, for instance, minimizes service costs arising from travel and center-based care, mobile health applications, and wearable devices, and averts costly consequences by promoting early therapy of diseases [27].

Improved Resource Utilization: Mobile technology develops resource management by efficiently employing the available resources in healthcare. For example, through the application of telemedicine, depending on healthcare services, possibilities of putting a strain on physical centres may be eliminated, and more patients could be administered by the providers. Wearable devices and health apps also contribute to better control of chronic illnesses, with no need for many follow-up visits and hospitalizations.

Benefits: The characteristics of the mobile technology advocate for reductions in healthcare costs as well as increases in resource utilization and access to the services. This benefit, in one way or another, increases the sustainability and efficiency of the healthcare systems in terms of resource management towards improvement in patients' health status.

Challenges: However, there is a cost advantage; certain issues like initial investments, technology concerns, and maintenance cannot be escaped. Mobile technology adoption in delivering health care is, however, limited by capital investment and technological support that is needed in enhancing roll-out constraints that may exist in some health care systems/organizations, according to [28]. This means that to popularize mobile technological solutions, the solutions have to be affordable in the long run and should offer a good gross return on investment.

CHALLENGES AND LIMITATIONS

The study, however, revealed that, inasmuch as mobile technology has brought about so many positive changes in health management, it also has some challenges and limitations that need to be worked out for it to be of equivalent benefit to all sections of society. This section provides insights with regard to some of the substantive problems related to the use of mobile technology in health management, which comprise privacy and security, digital divide and accessibility issues, regulatory and compliance issues, and data quality and credibility.

Privacy and Security Concerns

Privacy and security are two of the most important issues associated with mobile technology in health management. From the analysis of the risks of the collection, storage, and transmission of sensitive health data *via* mobile devices and applications, various concerns that patients have require some form of protection to enhance patients' trust.

Data Breaches and Cybersecurity Threats: Mobile health applications and devices hold PHI, and thus, they can be a good target for malicious activities. Whenever data breaches occur, or rather whenever there are cases of unauthorized access to health details, it can have severe ramifications for the affected persons since their health information is at the center of such breaches; besides, details such as identity theft and sharing of personal health information can result in fraudulent exercise of a person's identity [31]. To avoid such threats, strong cybersecurity compliance, including the use of encryption, mfa, and security procedures checks, is mandatory.

Privacy Regulations: The privacy operations of health data are covered by different privacy acts that include the HIPAA Act in the United States and the GDPR in the E.U. These regulations put forward specific guidelines to fulfill in the data collection, data storage, and data sharing processes related to health information [34]. Here, it becomes crucial for the mobile health applications to follow the following regulations to avert legal consequences negatively affecting the patients' trust.

Patient Consent and Data Use: The other major element of privacy is the use of valid consent in the management of patients' information. For the data to be collected from patients, they need to be clearly informed on how the data is going to be used, who will be allowed to use the information collected, and the risks that are likely to be involved. Transparency of data usage and giving the control of the data in their hands to the patients makes patients trust the data that is being used and helps in following the privacy regulation [31].

Benefits: To summarize, measures that enhance the privacy and security of information in connection with the use of m-Health technologies are crucial in the establishment of confidence among patients. Through measures used as security steps and by adherence to state and federal laws regarding privacy of health information, the healthcare organizations and IT professionals can prevent and minimize the incidences of loss of data in the health sector.

Challenges: Nevertheless, it is always necessary to maintain the user's confidentiality and security, but the implementation of these measures may be very difficult and costly. Mobile health applications need constant investments in cybersecurity to boost the basic framework and hire cybersecurity experts. Also, the management of the demand for data privacy and the drive for change and data usage in healthcare can be challenging [34].

Digital Divide and Accessibility Issues

A key challenge of mobile health technology is the lack of technology access and 'digital divide' that affects its usage across populations and for people with disabilities. The digital divide is the gap that exists as a result of the difference in the ability of people to use telecommunication and computing technologies, particularly smartphones and the internet. This gap may reduce the probability of involving targeted populations in mobile health solutions, implying that health end-users represent a wide group of people.

Socioeconomic Factors: POS stands out as one of the most powerful variables used to measure the social influences that affect the accessibility of mobile technology. Patients who can be categorized as having low health literacy, low income, or limited access to smartphones or reliable internet, or who may be living in rural or remote areas, may not be able to optimally utilize the mobile health applications [33]. It also results in a digital or technology divide that will clearly widen the health divide, as those who are unlikely to afford the gadgets that support Mobile Health technology will further be locked out of the concept.

Elderly and Technologically Challenged Populations: However, at present, to use the mobile health technology, several challenges are likely to be observed, such as elderly people and those having low health literacy concerning IT. It is easy for the elderly to have impaired faculties, which make it very hard for them to maneuver mobile applications; they may also have physical challenges that see them struggle in touching and working with small screens [29]. Other risks inherent in mHealth solutions include: There is a need to incorporate measures that make them easy to use, including textual size and voice commands.

Language and Cultural Barriers: Linguistic variations and other issues in culture can also form problems in the arrangement of the mobile health technology. Applications that are not developed for more than one language or that do not incorporate differences in beliefs and practices to control or improve health may be less relevant to these groups [30]. Mobile health solutions should also be culturally sensitive as well as linguistically sensitive because health solutions should be made available to an equal proportion.

Benefits: Several researchers have underscored the prospect that digital divide and accessibility concerns can be useful in expanding the uptake of MHT among a diversified populace. Through raising the availability of these applications to healthcare workers, the healthcare of the minority sections, along with the suppressed groups, is enhanced, thus decreasing health inequality.

Challenges: To tip the scale and give people from all backgrounds a fair fighting chance when it comes to going digital, more needs to be done to bridge the gap when it comes to people's access to technology and their abilities to effectively use it. This may include policy measures like subsidies for internet or the most basic means of getting online, like the provision of affordable handsets to the needy ones [33]. Also, time and again, the designers of the mobile health applications have the social responsibility to ensure that the applications are accessible to all people, irrespective of their level of technical expertise or their physical disability.

Regulatory and Compliance Challenges

What makes mobile health technology exciting is the fact that the field is developing at a very fast pace; however, this causes problems of regulation and compliance. These are conceived as emerging from the conflicts between the push towards rigorous safety, effectiveness, and data security of mHealth apps and devices on one hand, and the development and innovation on the other.

Regulatory Frameworks: Generally, the specific laws and policies of M-health technology differ from one country to another, and therefore, there are conflicting policies that are confusing for the developers who are in healthcare practices. The FDA approves some mHealth apps and devices applicable in the United States as medical devices and thus needs to undergo a strict approval process and testing. However, whether an application comes under the jurisdiction of the FDA can often be ambiguous and depends on many factors, and the field remains dynamic.

Compliance with Standards: There are several regulations that have to be met by mobile health applications because they have to be proven to be safe, effective, and able to integrate with other health systems. For example, an HL7 application that gathers and processes health data needs to meet certain standards regarding data protectionism, including the HIPAA and GDPR, whenever retrieving data from different jurisdictions [34]. Further, if an app offers CDS or diagnostic services, then its clinical accuracy and reliability are also expected benchmarks, which makes it hard for developers to manage.

Innovation *vs.* Regulation: The regulation of mobile health technology is always a concern due to the increased time that is taken in the formulation of rules and regulations to address the mobile health technology issues, while at the same time considering safety and compliance levels. High regulation levels may limit innovation by putting a ready blockage to the entry of new technologies for their implementation, while low regulation levels may make the patients vulnerable to the imagined or fake applications. The regulatory agencies often face the challenge of having to constantly reposition themselves as mobile health technology evolves, while, at the same time, ensuring that they are protecting the interests of the consumers.

Benefits: There is a need to regulate such technologies so that they are safe and efficacious when delivering health care to patients out in the field. In mobile health app development, guidelines help the developers to gain the confidence of the users and the healthcare providers to embrace the mHealth solutions in practice.

Challenges: Experiences regarding the regulatory environment structure may be a major concern for developers and healthcare providers. The measures involved in gaining regulatory approval or meeting the standards can take time and resources, hence may hinder the development and implementation of new innovative mHealth technologies. Further, due to the fact that mobile health technology can be implemented on a global level, one discovers that the developers are likely to operate in at least two jurisdictions, each of which will offer different regulated and regulating environments.

Data Accuracy and Reliability

Mobile health technology has to rely on data accuracy and reliability in order to be effective. This will compromise the reliability and acceptability of mobile health solutions, resulting in wrong diagnoses, wrong treatment, and poor health.

Accuracy of Wearable Devices: Smart accessories like wearable devices that include the application of fitness trackers and continuous glucose monitors in health management are commonly used to track different physiological values. Nevertheless, these devices are not always accurate, and their accuracy depends on the quality of sensors used, the device's design, as well as the conditions of usage [27]. Data from wearable devices can therefore be distorted, and this can lead to the dissemination of wrong health information, thus wrong medical decisions, or even bad behavior on the part of the patient.

Reliability of Mobile Health Applications: Any m-Health applications that incorporate a diagnosing, symptom checking, or clinical decision support tool need to ensure that the algorithms used are accurate and evidence-based. Mistakes in these fields are not trivial and may lead to missed diagnoses and wrong treatment advice [28]. For such applications to be reliable, the testing methodologies must be stringent, coupled with a validation procedure to identify and fix the problem.

Integration with Electronic Health Records (EHRs): Personal beacon can become an integration point between data generated by mHealth apps and wearables and an EHR. Nevertheless, it is often difficult to ascertain and synchronize the exactness of this integrated data. Differences in information gathered through mobile devices and the information captured in the patient's EHR can cause confusion and mistakes in the process of patient care [32]. Data sharing underutilization requires other procedures, such as data feed complexities and information interchangeability, to be developed, hence converting mobile health data into EHRs.

Benefits: The quality of data gathered and used in mobile health technology increases the reliability and credibility of the technology. High-quality data will help health care providers and patients make the right decisions, therefore improving health care.

Challenges: As is the case with any data, it is difficult to maintain data's accuracy and reliability, and as such, it is a constant process that has to be monitored, validated, and improved within mobile health technologies. It is up to the developers to spend on quality sensors, strong algorithms, and efficient testing techniques so as to ensure that the data resulting from the developed products is accurate and reliable. Thirdly, there is a need to monitor the kind of data produced by mobile health applications and devices from a healthcare delivery perspective, and how to correctly incorporate them into clinical environments.

CASE STUDIES AND REAL-WORLD EXAMPLES

This chapter utilizes empirical case studies to illustrate how mobile technology is applied in healthcare management. It provides a brief demonstration of successful implementations while addressing the practical challenges encountered during deployment. It also provides the guidelines and findings, and presents the future of the mobile health solutions.

Successful Implementation of Mobile Health Solutions

This section focuses on some of the mobile health solutions that have been deployed to advance patient care and health care services. The following are some of the ways in which mobile technology is able to alter the techniques in health facilities, as shown in Table **1**.

Table 1. Real-life examples of successful mobile health solutions.

Case Study	Description	Outcome
Diabetes Management App	A mobile app that allows patients to monitor blood glucose levels and share data with healthcare providers.	Improved glucose control and patient adherence to treatment plans.
Telemedicine in Rural Areas	Implementation of telemedicine platforms to provide remote consultations in underserved areas.	Increased access to healthcare services for rural populations.
Wearable Cardiac Monitors	Use of wearable devices to continuously monitor heart activity and detect irregularities early.	Early detection of cardiac events, leading to timely interventions.

Explanation: Any constructive mHealth utilization implies that patients are often more engaged, and their cases are followed up more closely and individually. For instance, in the apprehension of chronic diseases like Diabetes, improved levels of self-management and compliance with the recommended regimes are depicted in the use of mobile applications.

Lessons Learned from Mobile Health Initiatives

This talks about the stories and the challenges that organizations and individuals encountered while implementing mHealth projects, providing valuable information on what has been done right and what one could have done otherwise.

Explanation: The mobile health activities shown in Table **2** indicate how the applications were designed, engaging the stakeholders, and how private matters were dealt with. For example, some of the related efforts are not popular, and some do experience a problem in terms of a very small usage rate; in such cases, there is a lot of user orientation and training needed.

Future Prospects of Mobile Technology in Healthcare

The section features an outlook of future prospects of further utilization of mobile technology in the delivery of health care services, extension of the new trends in medication, ideas related to new innovations, as well as a prognosis of long-term medication.

Table 2. Lessons learned from mobile health initiatives.

Case Study	Challenge Encountered	Lesson Learned
Chronic Disease Management App	Low user adoption due to the complexity of the app interface.	Importance of simple, intuitive design and user training.
Mobile Mental Health Support	Privacy concerns among users regarding data security.	Necessity of strong data encryption and transparent privacy policies.
Remote Patient Monitoring in Hospitals	Integration issues with existing Electronic Health Records (EHR) systems.	Need for interoperability standards and seamless integration with EHRs.

Explanation: Some of the future developments in mobile healthcare, as shown in Table **3**, are: usage of artificial intelligence and machine learning for diagnosis, more use of wearables, and a complex client-involved model of treatment. Consequently, such novelties should contribute to the further development of the healthcare sector.

Table 3. Future prospects of mobile technology in healthcare.

Emerging Trend	Description	Potential Impact
AI and Predictive Analytics in Mobile Health	Use of AI to analyze health data and predict potential health issues before they occur.	Improved preventive care and early intervention.
Expansion of Wearable Health Devices	Development of advanced wearables for continuous monitoring of various health metrics.	More comprehensive and real-time health monitoring.
Personalized Health Apps	Mobile apps that tailor healthcare recommendations based on individual health data.	Enhanced personalization of healthcare, leading to better patient outcomes.

FUTURE DIRECTIONS AND INNOVATIONS

Regarding the mobile technology for health management, there is a lot of promise as the future of mobile technology for health inventions is expected to radically change the course of the healthcare system. The various emerging technologies in the multifacets of healthcare, as shown in Table **4**, include the application of Augmented reality, Virtual reality, and blockchain technologies. Furthermore, the use of Artificial Intelligence (AI) and Machine Learning (ML) added to the MH applications shifts the practices in healthcare by enabling biomarker-based diagnostics and prognostics, personalized therapeutic interventions, as well as the efficient organizational management of the care processes. One thing that the current predictive analytics, AI, and modern ML are helping the healthcare industry to do today is to predict the probable future health problems and plan the treatment of every individual person in a comprehensive manner. Lastly, because of these developments, telemedicine and remote care are getting closer to being feasible and increasing the expansion of health care, particularly to the minority. Together, these advances are to improve the support of clients and to determine the organization of health care with the current and future demand for medical services.

Table 4. Real-life examples of future innovations in mobile health management.

Innovation Area	Technology/Innovation	Example	Description	Impact
Emerging Technologies in Mobile Health	Augmented Reality	AR-based patient education platforms.	AR provides interactive, visual explanations of medical procedures and conditions.	Improved patient understanding and engagement in their care.
	Blockchain	Blockchain-based Electronic Health Records (EHR) systems.	Secure, decentralized management of health data, ensuring privacy and data integrity.	Enhanced patient control and security of personal health data.
AI and Machine Learning	AI-powered diagnostics	AI tools for analyzing medical images, such as X-rays or MRIs.	AI algorithms provide rapid and accurate diagnoses by evaluating medical images.	Improved diagnostic speed and accuracy, leading to better outcomes.
	ML-driven wearable health devices	Wearable devices that use ML to predict heart attacks based on continuous monitoring.	Continuous health monitoring with real-time data analysis and predictive alerts.	Prevention of critical health events through early intervention.
Predictive Analytics and Personalized Health	Predictive analytics for chronic disease management	Mobile apps that predict diabetes-related complications based on user data.	Continuous monitoring and analysis of health metrics to prevent disease flare-ups.	Reduced hospitalizations and better chronic disease management.
	Personalized health plans	AI-driven apps that create custom fitness or nutrition plans.	Apps analyze user data to offer personalized recommendations that adapt over time.	Enhanced health outcomes through tailored interventions.

(Table 4) cont.....

Innovation Area	Technology/Innovation	Example	Description	Impact
The Future of Telemedicine and Remote Care	Virtual care platforms	Telemedicine services provide remote consultations.	Patients receive healthcare services *via* video calls, reducing the need for physical visits.	Increased access to healthcare, especially in remote or underserved areas.
	Remote monitoring tools	Systems that allow continuous monitoring of patients with chronic conditions at home.	Vital signs and health data are transmitted to healthcare providers in real-time.	Early detection and management of health issues reduces the need for hospital visits.

CONCLUSION

Mobile technology has therefore enhanced health in terms of new strategies to deliver health care to patients and reorganizing the health system. This chapter has discussed the future trajectory of mhealth technologies, the traditional and contemporary use of mobile devices, and particular applications in relation to telemedicine, wearable devices, and mental health. The benefits of those technologies are: enhanced access, engagement, real-time data capture, and cost-saving. Nevertheless, issues like privacy, the issue of the divide between the information 'haves' and 'have nots', and that of regulation are still barriers that have not been eradicated to date. As to the future, mobile health is the prospect with serious development intentions connected with the use of such technologies as augmented reality, Blockchain, and the new, more effective, AI-based diagnostic systems. Health care experiences should be enhanced by predictive analysis that offers anticipatory treatment as well as telemedicine and distant consultation that will assist patients from all over the globe. Mobile technology in the healthcare sector is already making the role of technology profound, and as there is advancement in the mobile technology sector, the contribution to improvement in healthcare management is projected to grow incredibly. The further advancement of these technologies will be sure to create a future wherein healthcare is more accessible, individualized, and streamlined: a revolutionary advancement as far as the patients' health is concerned in the optimization of the same.

REFERENCES

[1] R.S.H. Istepanian, "Mobile health (m-Health) in retrospect: the known unknowns", *Int. J. Environ. Res. Public Health,* vol. 19, no. 7, p. 3747, 2022. [http://dx.doi.org/10.3390/ijerph19073747] [PMID: 35409431]

[2] C. Free, G. Phillips, L. Watson, L. Galli, L. Felix, P. Edwards, V. Patel, and A. Haines, "The effectiveness of mobile-health technologies to improve health care service delivery processes: a

systematic review and meta-analysis", *PLoS Med.,* vol. 10, no. 1, p. e1001363, 2013. [http://dx.doi.org/10.1371/journal.pmed.1001363] [PMID: 23458994]

[3] C.S. Kruse, N. Krowski, B. Rodriguez, L. Tran, J. Vela, and M. Brooks, "Telehealth and patient satisfaction: a systematic review and narrative analysis", *BMJ Open,* vol. 7, no. 8, p. e016242, 2017. [http://dx.doi.org/10.1136/bmjopen-2017-016242] [PMID: 28775188]

[4] M. Wu, and J. Luo, "Wearable technology applications in healthcare: a literature review", *Online J. Nurs. Inform.,* vol. 23, no. 3, 2019.

[5] M. Gallichan, "Self monitoring of glucose by people with diabetes: evidence based practice: Fig 1", *BMJ,* vol. 314, no. 7085, pp. 964-967, 1997. [http://dx.doi.org/10.1136/bmj.314.7085.964] [PMID: 9099125]

[6] T. Loncar-Turukalo, E. Zdravevski, J. Machado da Silva, I. Chouvarda, and V. Trajkovik, "Literature on wearable technology for connected health: scoping review of research trends, advances, and barriers", *J. Med. Internet Res.,* vol. 21, no. 9, p. e14017, 2019. [http://dx.doi.org/10.2196/14017] [PMID: 31489843]

[7] P. Agarwal, D. Gordon, J. Griffith, N. Kithulegoda, H.O. Witteman, R. Sacha Bhatia, A.W. Kushniruk, E.M. Borycki, L. Lamothe, E. Springall, and J. Shaw, "Assessing the quality of mobile applications in chronic disease management: a scoping review", *NPJ Digit. Med.,* vol. 4, no. 1, p. 46, 2021. [http://dx.doi.org/10.1038/s41746-021-00410-x] [PMID: 33692488]

[8] Y. El-Miedany, "Telehealth and telemedicine: how the digital era is changing standard health care", *Smart Homecare Technol. Telehealth,* vol. 4, pp. 43-51, 2017. [http://dx.doi.org/10.2147/SHTT.S116009]

[9] A. Meiliana, N.M. Dewi, and A. Wijaya, "Personalized medicine: The future of health care", *Indones. Biomed. J.,* vol. 8, no. 3, pp. 127-146, 2016. [http://dx.doi.org/10.18585/inabj.v8i3.271]

[10] B. Martínez-Pérez, I. de la Torre-Díez, and M. López-Coronado, "Privacy and security in mobile health apps: a review and recommendations", *J. Med. Syst.,* vol. 39, no. 1, p. 181, 2015. [http://dx.doi.org/10.1007/s10916-014-0181-3] [PMID: 25486895]

[11] S.P. Bhavnani, J. Narula, and P.P. Sengupta, "Mobile technology and the digitization of healthcare", *Eur. Heart J.,* vol. 37, no. 18, pp. 1428-1438, 2016. [http://dx.doi.org/10.1093/eurheartj/ehv770] [PMID: 26873093]

[12] S. Kumar, W.J. Nilsen, A. Abernethy, A. Atienza, K. Patrick, M. Pavel, W.T. Riley, A. Shar, B. Spring, D. Spruijt-Metz, D. Hedeker, V. Honavar, R. Kravitz, R. Craig Lefebvre, D.C. Mohr, S.A. Murphy, C. Quinn, V. Shusterman, and D. Swendeman, "Mobile health technology evaluation: the mHealth evidence workshop", *Am. J. Prev. Med.,* vol. 45, no. 2, pp. 228-236, 2013. [http://dx.doi.org/10.1016/j.amepre.2013.03.017] [PMID: 23867031]

[13] N.F. BinDhim, A. Hawkey, and L. Trevena, "A systematic review of quality assessment methods for smartphone health apps", *Telemed. J. E Health,* vol. 21, no. 2, pp. 97-104, 2015. [http://dx.doi.org/10.1089/tmj.2014.0088] [PMID: 25469795]

[14] R. Ganapathy, A. Grewal, and J.S. Castleman, "Remote monitoring of blood pressure to reduce the risk of preeclampsia related complications with an innovative use of mobile technology", *Pregnancy Hypertens.,* vol. 6, no. 4, pp. 263-265, 2016. [http://dx.doi.org/10.1016/j.preghy.2016.04.005] [PMID: 27939464]

[15] M. Martínez-García, and E. Hernández-Lemus, "Data integration challenges for machine learning in precision medicine", *Front. Med. (Lausanne),* vol. 8, p. 784455, 2022. [http://dx.doi.org/10.3389/fmed.2021.784455] [PMID: 35145977]

[16] K.F. Foreman, K.M. Stockl, L.B. Le, E. Fisk, S.M. Shah, H.C. Lew, B.K. Solow, and B.S. Curtis, "Impact of a text messaging pilot program on patient medication adherence", *Clin. Ther.,* vol. 34, no.

5, pp. 1084-1091, 2012.
[http://dx.doi.org/10.1016/j.clinthera.2012.04.007] [PMID: 22554973]

[17] E. Mehraeen, S. SeyedAlinaghi, M. Heydari, A. Karimi, A. Mahdavi, M. Mashoufi, A. Sarmad, P. Mirghaderi, A. Shamsabadi, K. Qaderi, P. Mirzapour, A. Fakhfouri, H.A. Cheshmekabodi, K. Azad, S. Bagheri Zargande, S. Oliaei, P. Yousefi Konjdar, F. Vahedi, and T. Noori, "Telemedicine technologies and applications in the era of COVID-19 pandemic: A systematic review", *Health Informatics J.*, vol. 29, no. 2, p. 14604582231167431, 2023.
[http://dx.doi.org/10.1177/14604582231167431] [PMID: 37076954]

[18] A. Barak, L. Hen, M. Boniel-Nissim, and N. Shapira, "A comprehensive review and a meta-analysis of the effectiveness of internet-based psychotherapeutic interventions", *J. Technol. Hum. Serv.*, vol. 26, no. 2-4, pp. 109-160, 2008.
[http://dx.doi.org/10.1080/15228830802094429]

[19] Y. Moussa, A.A. Mahdanian, C. Yu, M. Segal, K.J. Looper, I.V. Vahia, and S. Rej, "Mobile health technology in late-life mental illness: a focused literature review", *Am. J. Geriatr. Psychiatry*, vol. 25, no. 8, pp. 865-872, 2017.
[http://dx.doi.org/10.1016/j.jagp.2017.04.003] [PMID: 28495467]

[20] L. Lu, J. Zhang, Y. Xie, F. Gao, S. Xu, X. Wu, and Z. Ye, "Wearable health devices in health care: narrative systematic review", *JMIR Mhealth Uhealth,* vol. 8, no. 11, p. e18907, 2020.
[http://dx.doi.org/10.2196/18907] [PMID: 33164904]

[21] M. Farzandipour, E. Nabovati, R. Sharif, M. Arani, and S. Anvari, "Patient self-management of asthma using mobile health applications: a systematic review of the functionalities and effects", *Appl. Clin. Inform.*, vol. 8, no. 4, pp. 1068-1081, 2017.
[http://dx.doi.org/10.4338/ACI-2017-07-R-0116] [PMID: 29241254]

[22] R. Roine, A. Ohinmaa, and D. Hailey, "Assessing telemedicine: a systematic review of the literature", *CMAJ,* vol. 165, no. 6, pp. 765-771, 2001.
[PMID: 11584564]

[23] J.H.L. Lui, D.K. Marcus, and C.T. Barry, "Evidence-based apps? A review of mental health mobile applications in a psychotherapy context", *Prof. Psychol. Res. Pr.*, vol. 48, no. 3, pp. 199-210, 2017.
[http://dx.doi.org/10.1037/pro0000122]

[24] Y. Wang, J. Min, J. Khuri, H. Xue, B. Xie, L. A Kaminsky, and L. J Cheskin, "Effectiveness of mobile health interventions on diabetes and obesity treatment and management: systematic review of systematic reviews", *JMIR Mhealth Uhealth,* vol. 8, no. 4, p. e15400, 2020.
[http://dx.doi.org/10.2196/15400] [PMID: 32343253]

[25] J. Liang, X. He, Y. Jia, W. Zhu, and J. Lei, "Chinese mobile health apps for hypertension management: a systematic evaluation of usefulness", *J. Healthc. Eng.*, vol. 2018, no. 1, pp. 1-14, 2018.
[http://dx.doi.org/10.1155/2018/7328274] [PMID: 29744027]

[26] R. Melia, K. Francis, E. Hickey, J. Bogue, J. Duggan, M. O'Sullivan, and K. Young, "Mobile health technology interventions for suicide prevention: systematic review", *JMIR Mhealth Uhealth,* vol. 8, no. 1, p. e12516, 2020.
[http://dx.doi.org/10.2196/12516] [PMID: 31939744]

[27] M.H. Iqbal, A. Aydin, O. Brunckhorst, P. Dasgupta, and K. Ahmed, "A review of wearable technology in medicine", *J. R. Soc. Med.*, vol. 109, no. 10, pp. 372-380, 2016.
[http://dx.doi.org/10.1177/0141076816663560] [PMID: 27729595]

[28] C.S. Kruse, S. Bouffard, M. Dougherty, and J.S. Parro, "Telemedicine use in rural Native American communities in the era of the ACA: a systematic literature review", *J. Med. Syst.*, vol. 40, no. 6, p. 145, 2016.
[http://dx.doi.org/10.1007/s10916-016-0503-8] [PMID: 27118011]

[29] A. Chesser, A. Burke, J. Reyes, and T. Rohrberg, "Navigating the digital divide: A systematic review of eHealth literacy in underserved populations in the United States", *Inform. Health Soc. Care,* vol. 41,

no. 1, pp. 1-19, 2016.
[http://dx.doi.org/10.3109/17538157.2014.948171] [PMID: 25710808]

[30] L. Whitehead, J. Talevski, F. Fatehi, and A. Beauchamp, "Barriers to and facilitators of digital health among culturally and linguistically diverse populations: qualitative systematic review", *J. Med. Internet Res.,* vol. 25, p. e42719, 2023.
[http://dx.doi.org/10.2196/42719] [PMID: 36853742]

[31] S. Arora, J. Yttri, and W. Nilse, "Privacy and security in mobile health (mHealth) research", *Alcohol Res.,* vol. 36, no. 1, pp. 143-152, 2014.
[http://dx.doi.org/10.35946/arcr.v36.1.15] [PMID: 26259009]

[32] J. Miró, and P. Llorens-Vernet, "Assessing the quality of mobile health-related apps: interrater reliability study of two guides", *JMIR Mhealth Uhealth,* vol. 9, no. 4, p. e26471, 2021.
[http://dx.doi.org/10.2196/26471] [PMID: 33871376]

[33] C. Kruse, J. Betancourt, S. Ortiz, S.M. Valdes Luna, I.K. Bamrah, and N. Segovia, "Barriers to the use of mobile health in improving health outcomes in developing countries: systematic review", *J. Med. Internet Res.,* vol. 21, no. 10, p. e13263, 2019.
[http://dx.doi.org/10.2196/13263] [PMID: 31593543]

[34] Galvin, H. K., & DeMuro, P. R. (2020). Developments in privacy and data ownership in mobile health technologies, 2016-2019. Yearbook of medical informatics, 29(01), 032-043.

CHAPTER 2

Transforming Healthcare Through AI: Adoption Trends and Challenges in Modern Medicine

Sangeeta Patil[1,*] and **Reshma K.P.**[1]

[1] *Department of Chemistry, Rungta College of Engineering and Technology, Bhilai, Chhattisgarh, India*

Abstract: The chapter probes how Artificial Intelligence (AI) is altering existing medicine. An essential part of treatment is design, empowering precision medicine, and using robotic technologies to enhance medical processes. AI also improves patient care by enabling remote nursing, managing long-term infections, and encouraging psychological wellness *via* virtual aides. Despite these benefits, bias, statistics secrecy, and the requirement for open and transparent monitoring outlines are some of the ethical and permissible concerns that arise when AI is used in medicine. The assistance of AI adoption for patients and the pharmaceutical trade is twofold: first, it has reduced the time and cost related to medication development. In general, a medication used in medical exercise has gone through manifold phases, including safety validation, response, screening, and detection. AI systems could help estimate three-dimensional structures and protein utility, which could support recognizing potential action targets.

Medication delivery, absorption, biotransformation, and excretion are important pharmacokinetic aspects that disturb how they work in the body. Consequently, researchers tried to apply AI measures to the day-to-day actions of medical chemists. The research on AI-based methodologies executed with 84% to 87% accuracy, which shows AI could help in pharmacokinetic technique assessment. AI has the potential to enable effective drug design and its synthesis. AI in medication research is in an early stage, with more significant complementary development, and ethical concerns are required for a well-organized and modified health organization. This chapter provides a comprehensive overview of AI's existing uses and forthcoming prospects in medicine.

Keywords: Activity scoring, AiCure, Alpha fold, Coarse-grained simulation, DeepChem, Deep learning models, Drug Design, DTINet protein-protein interactions, Monte-Carlo Tree Searches, Nanomedicine, Natural Language Processing, NNScore, Pharmacokinetic Parameters, silicasomes, Synthia, toxicity, XenoSite.

* **Corresponding author Sangeeta Patil:** Department of Chemistry, Rungta College of Engineering and Technology, Bhilai, Chhattisgarh, India;
E-mail: dr.sangeeta.patil@rungta.ac.in

Arun Kumar Rana, Mandeep Kaur & Sumit Kumar Rana (Eds.)

INTRODUCTION

AI includes the practice of statistical computational practices using emerging algorithms that mimic human intelligence. AI identified mathematical models suitable for problem-solving, and Algorithms are used to obtain results to the initial question, and these results are further analyzed and then implemented using a programming language [1]. AI has forecasted the progress of therapeutic consequences, boost workflows, and amend patient care, to achieve the patient requirements, and the pursuit of accurate medication [2 - 5]. The technique of emergent new medications includes a sustained investment of time and money. It is essential to improve both the efficacy and effectiveness of this procedure. For the pharmaceutical industry and patients, the implications of AI adoption are twofold: first, it has shortened the time and expense related to medication development. Discovery, Screening, response, validation, and safety are the main steps in drug development applied in clinical practice [6]. Second, AI has proven helpful in finding new applications for already-approved medications by forecasting how they will interact with various protein targets [7].

AI IN PHARMACEUTICAL RESEARCH AND ADVANCEMENT

Artificial intelligence is altering pharmaceutical development and research through the acceleration of medication discovery, enhancement of medical trial accuracy, and optimization of drug development techniques. In Drug discovery, the first step is target identification. Big datasets may be evaluated by AI to find genes or proteins that may be disease-related targets, or other possible biological targets, for novel medications. Algorithms can forecast which targets will react to the remedy the most. Python-assisted AI technique called DeepChem uses a DL algorithm for chemical recognition to anticipate different drug development workflows. Hit Dexter, InnerOuterRNN, JunctionTree VAE, PPB2, QML, and REINVENT are some AI tools used for drug discovery.

PROTEIN STRUCTURE PREDICTION

Amino acids are natural compounds that are safely used in the pharmaceutical industry. Their assembly in protein can be easily predicted by using AI. X-ray Crystalography [8], Cryo-electron microscopy [9], and NMR spectroscopy [10] are some traditional techniques that are costly and cannot easily handle complex proteins. Recently, a significant advancement in protein structural modelling has seen. Firstly, advances in global statistical models and then deep learning for residue-residue contact forecast were the main drivers of advancement. Later, a more extensive implementation of deep learning methodologies was made for protein structure modelling, initially employing Convolutional Neural Networks and subsequently transitioning to Natural Language Processing, incorporating attention models and Geometric Deep Learning. Two AI approaches, deep learning models [11, 12] and AlphaFold [13, 14], are used for computing Protein structure. Several researchers' review of the most recent developments in models utilising deep learning for protein structure prediction, as well as well-established protein modelling [15]. Deep learning computational methods have also been used to extract complex characteristics from protein sequence data. Deep Learning for 3D protein structure prediction follows the following important steps: First, Identification of sequence homologs and generation of multiple sequence alignment, second, residue-residue distance prediction or residue contact prediction, third, ab initio 3D modeling driven by distance/contact, and fourth, the Quality Assessment of the model [16]. Precisely anticipated protein shapes have applications in drug development, comprehension of protein-protein interactions, and molecular interactions.

With the application of deep learning algorithms, AlphaFold is able to precisely forecast the three-dimensional assembly of proteins based just on their amino acid sequences. Combining AI forecasts with trial data allows for the refinement of structures and the understanding of protein dynamics. The DeepMind AlphaFold combines scientific and physical understanding of protein structures with deep learning, primarily using multilayer neural networks. Multi-sequence alignments are used by it to improve its predictions. AlphaFold2, a more recent version of the program, is based on the architecture of neural networks called a Transformer. Transformers have powerful tools in the fields of natural language processing, since they can capture intricate associations and designs in entire sequences

by using attention mechanisms. AlphaFold2 capitalizes on this ability. It performed significantly better than other prediction methods in the critical Assessment of Structure Prediction (CASP14) competition. CASP is a biennial communal trial utilized to identify the state-of-the-art approaches in protein assembly modeling.

AI IN DRUG DESIGN

For the design of the desired amino acid sequence, generative adversarial and variation autoencoders are used. Machine learning algorithms help in examining the 3D structure of target proteins by developing improved small molecules that bind selectively to certain targets [17, 18]. These forecasts are supported by analysis of protein and earlier screening data. AI also expedites the enhancement of novel treatment by modeling interactions between protein-ligand and forecasting their binding affinities [19]. AI tool NNScore used a neural network-aided scoring function to predict protein-ligand binding affinity, whereas the Potential Net AI tool predicts ligand-binding affinity by engaging a graph CNN.

Nowadays, the traditional technique for the creation of novel medications and the prediction of certain therapeutic pathways is replaced by the AI-based skill "Synthia". It can offer workable synthesis paths for eight medically unnecessary targets and decipher a set of axioms into the machine. Synthia has demonstrated effectiveness in terms of improving the crop and curtailing the budget. The application is ideal for supporting alternative synthesizing designs for patentable products and is thought to be useful in the synthesis of molecules that have not yet been discovered. In the same vein, DNN highlights based on rules of organic chemistry and retrosynthesis, which, in conjunction with the assistance of AI and "Monte-Carlo Tree Searches (MCTS) [20]," help in response predictions and the drug's design and unravelling mechanism, which is far more agile than traditional methods.

The neural network-based platforms "The Reinforced Adversarial Neural Computer (RANC)" and "The Reinforcement-Learning for Structural Evolution program (RLSE)" are used for the production of chemical compounds that may have response rates [21, 22]. This system was trained using substances known as SMILES strings. After that, molecules with predetermined chemical descriptors for logP, MW, and Topological Polar Surface Area were produced. RANC was tested on one distinct platform, ORGANIC, where it was successful and more adept at creating original structures without noticeably shortening the duration of their arrangement. It has been recognized that the Reinforcement Learning for Structural Evolution (RLSE) software handles de novo drug synthesis by using both predictive and generative DNNs to develop new compounds. The generative paradigm provides more exclusive results for these molecules concerning SMILE strings based on a stack memory, although the predictive practices are applied to anticipate the features of the original molecule.

AI IN DRUG SCREENING, ACTIVITY SCORING, PHARMACOKINETIC PARAMETERS, TOXICITY (ADME/T) ATTRIBUTES, AND TOXICITY ASSESSMENT

To identify bioactive molecules (hits) from commercial chemical libraries or in-house compound assemblies, virtual screening entails using an AI system. AI helps effectively to find new hits and weed out compounds with unfavourable scaffolds in the initial phase of drug development. Virtual screening techniques include similarity searches, pharmacophore-based [23], and molecular docking [24]. SIEVE-score is an upgraded AI technique of structure-aided computer-generated. screening through interaction-energy-based learning. The AI role in activity scoring is to assess disease severity, treatment consequences, and patient prognosis. Natural Language processing algorithms help in finding suitable medical evidence from electronic patient health records. In the BI-RADS

(Reporting and Data System) score, AI increases the consistency and reliability of radiological assessments, supporting more precise diagnoses. For the SOFA (Sequential Organ Failure Assessment) score, AI increases the forecast of organ failure in critical care. The APACHE (Acute Physiology And Chronic Health Evaluation) score helps in speedy and precise condition severity assessments. AI tool The DeltaVina combines the random forest and Auto Dock scoring functions to forecast the affinity of small molecules with drugs. Open Drug Discovery Toolkit is utilized for chemoinformatics and molecular modelling employing random forest Score-Score as well as NNScore.

Absorption, distribution, biotransformation, and excretion are important pharmacokinetic factors that affect how a medication works medicinally when consumed. The research on AI-based methods all performed well, with accuracy ranging from 84 to 87%, suggesting that AI might help in pharmacokinetic procedure appraisal [25]. A therapeutic chemist can more easily adjust a compound's absorption properties by anticipating its bioavailability. An investigation team obtained a dataset with 1014 substances and applied the MLR paradigm to chemical features and structural signatures that support potent bioavailability. The ratio of a drug's dose *in vivo* to its steady-state plasma concentration is known as its steady-state distribution (VDss). The VDss represents the degree to which a therapeutic molecule is distributed throughout the tissue. VDss can make it easier for medicinal chemists to predict the use of instructional modifications for improved pharmacokinetic properties. A team of researchers assembled an array of 1096 molecules using Partial Least Squares and Random Forest models to predict VD's chemical characteristics and structural signatures that support potent bioavailability.

Predicting the biotransformation sites with precision helps in enhancing the structure to ensure the metabolite endurance of the moiety. With the 87% gross precision, the neural network method “XenoSite” can determine the site of small molecules biotransformed by cytochrome P450, while some pharmaceuticals can be disposed of directly without biotransformation; most biotransformed metabolites are water-soluble and excreted easily from the body. Lombardo *et al.* [26] utilized Principal Components Analysis to predict the main clearance pathway, and among several methods, the algorithm demonstrated good discrimination results, with a forecast accuracy of 84%. Drug selection can benefit from the prediction of toxicity, which plays a significant role in minimizing the number of lead moieties. It has been demonstrated that DL algorithms that predict toxicity outperform conventional techniques [27]. DeepTox is used for the Toxicity predictions of chemical agents that utilize a DL algorithm. While single-task and multi-task neural networks were compared using Vertex Pharmaceuticals' ADME/T experimental datasets, it was found that multitasking algorithms would produce better output, as expected. In the meantime, multi-task neural networks can improve the capacity for prediction of both pharmacokinetic procedures and toxicity [28 - 30].

CLINICAL TRIAL STRATEGY AND ANALYSIS

Clinical trial strategy plays an important role in drug design due to the high failure rate in effectiveness and safety tests. Hence, the attainment of the clinical trial depends on the right target patient population, the right dosage regimen, the endpoint that measures the therapeutic effect, and trial monitoring. AI tools like predictive analytics and natural language processing accelerate patient recruitment, track trial progress in real time, and increase data accuracy, all of which ultimately result in lower costs and improved outcomes. AI automation assists in emphasizing the critical traits of the clinical trials. It also leads to faster data collection and analysis, expediting the complete trial process. In the process of clinical trials, AI brings up validity and integrity, which improve the patient-physician interaction and build a solid base for the medical statistics management. Clinical data generated and managed by an AI system guarantees the validity and integrity of research. Personalised medication assistance from advanced analytics' ability to forecast patient outcomes and improve clinical decision-making.

AI identifies which patients would benefit the most from the prescribed drugs and helps them follow the exact protocol [31]. AI also makes adaptive clinical trials possible by permitting the new design to be adjusted in response to previous findings, which might result in more fruitful trials."AiCure" has introduced mobile software that supervised schizophrenia patients' regular medication usage in a Phase II experiment. As a result, patients' compliance frequency increased by 25%, ensuring an effective outcome of the study. The 'MedAdhere' app uses the camera on a smartphone to recognize the faces, medications, and medication-taking habits of patients. Patients with schizophrenia may see a substantial enhancement in medication adherence with the use of this easily available tool [32, 33]. Even though AI has numerous applications in clinical trials, disputes like ethical concerns and the requirement for standardization still exist. Resolving these problems is essential to enhancing AI's ability to reduce diagnostic errors and increase healthcare delivery.

DRUG REPURPOSING AND SAFETY

AI plays a crucial role in drug repurposing, as it identifies new therapeutic uses for the medications that have previously received approval. AI generates new indications for medicines that have been certified, speeding up progress and reducing risks. This is achieved by estimating drug-disease interactions through past data analysis. Adverse drug responses monitoring and possible safety issues predictions, an AI system enhances pharmaceutical safety profiles and increases pharmacovigilance. Medication and illness are the two main factors in medication repurposing. Drug repurposing is also linked to auxiliary factors, such as medicine targets and disease-causing genes. Because of how diverse the relations are, network analysis may be used to demonstrate how these elements relate to one another. Nine classes of important networks exist for the purpose of drug design: metabolic, protein-protein, drug-target, drug-drug, drug-disease, target-disease, gene regulatory negative impact, and networks of diseases. The network-dependent scheme's main premise is that similar medications normally have comparable targets. Since the singleton network's data is limited and fractional, it is vital to combine many networks to create the conglomerate network needed to relocate a single medication. In particular, it's imperative to combine medicine repurposing with medicine predicting, as the target may be thought of as a link from the medicine to treat the illness. DTINet is a diverse network that unifies the data of multiple networks using the dimensionality reduction and network diffusion method approach, which was used to predict the new target and treatment niche [34].

AI ADAPTATION IN NANOMEDICINE

Nanomedicines cure, diagnose, and monitor complex diseases such as HIV, malaria, cancer, inflammatory illnesses, and asthma by combining drugs with nanotechnology. Recently, medication delivery by nanoparticle modulation has gained popularity. Nanoparticle-modulated drug delivery improves diagnosis and therapy as they have enhanced therapeutic efficiency [35]. Combining AI and nanotechnology might provide solutions for a number of problems with the evolution of formulation. Nanomedicines reduce adverse effects and increase treatment effectiveness. This is very effective, where drugs that would normally be too toxic to deliver in traditional forms can be. Low solubility of the drugs restricts their efficacy. Nanomedicines help in improving the body's ability to absorb and use. Drug discharge can be sustained over time by designing nanomedicines to release their therapeutic payloads in a controlled way. By lowering the frequency of the dose, this can enhance patient compliance and treatment results. Harmful drug exposure to healthy tissues may be minimised by enclosing drugs in nanocarriers, which helps to reduce the adverse effects. This is mainly beneficial for chemotherapy drugs that may damage healthy cells. It also increases stability, which guards against deterioration and guarantees that they continue to work until they reach their intended site. Proteins, nucleic acids, and small molecules are a few of the therapeutic agents that nanomedicines may be made to transport, making them appropriate for a variety of applications. Greater Surface Area to Volume Ratio: Compared to bulk materials, nanomaterials have a considerably greater surface area to volume ratio. For improving reactivity, this increased surface area can produce special surface phenomena that are not seen in bigger materials, such as higher catalytic activity or changed adsorption qualities. They have the ability to absorb and emit light, which can be altered by quantum phenomena. Size-dependent fluorescence, for instance, is a phenomenon in which the colour of light produced by quantum dots varies according to the particle's size. Imaging and sensing are two of the many applications that take advantage of this capability.

Methotrexate, a nanosuspension, has been algorithmically analyzed by computing the energy released during drug molecule admixture and looking for variables that can encourage formulation clumping [36]. "Coarse-grained simulation" can assist with the interactive assessment of the drug-dendrimer and the assessment of the drug encapsulation inside the dendrimer when used in conjunction with chemical estimation. Additionally, programs like LAMMPS and GROMACS4 are used to investigate the effect of surface chemistry on nanoparticle absorption by cells. The blend of internalising arginine glycine-aspartic acid sequences (iRGD), a peptide that pierces tumours and multifunctional mesoporous silica nanoparticles laden with irinotecan, caused the manufacture of silicasomes, which were made possible by AI. As iRGD stimulates silicasome transcytosis, this internalisation of silicasomes may be augmented three- or four-fold, with improved action results and favourable long-term survival [37].

FUTURE AND CHALLENGES

According to Global Market Insight, the market is expected to increase at a CAGR of 29.6% between 2024 and 2032, from its estimated market size of USD 1.9 billion in 2023, for the utilization of AI for Medicine Discovery. An increase in financing and investment from pharmaceutical corporations, government agencies, and venture capital firms is the reason for the high development of the industry. AI advancement in the field of genomics and predicting specific treatment for the patient will result in improved and targeted therapies. It permits the improved and speedy medical imaging analysis, assisting radiologists and pathologists in diagnosing conditions with greater precision. The AI system also supports remote monitoring and virtual assistance. AI will optimize resource management, predictive analytics, drug development, rehabilitation, and assistive devices. AI uses huge amounts of patient data, which raises concerns about data privacy and security. Concerns about privacy are raised by the use of genetic and protein sequence data, particularly when it is connected to private medical data [38].

An AI system must comply with stringent healthcare guidelines and other regional data protection laws that can be complex and differ by jurisdiction. The functioning mechanics of the operating system used to construct models are difficult for consumers to understand, and it remains opaque. Due to this, many problems arise, such as prejudice, rigidity, accountability, and security holes. More prospective studies are essential to address such issues and guarantee the validity of the findings. The problems and ethical matters that come with using AI in modern medicine must be resolved. The increasing usage of these tools raises vital glitches about algorithmic bias, confidentiality of data, and the necessity for robust control frameworks. Clinical validations, Transparency, and implementation cost are some other future challenges in this area.

CONCLUSION

AI has demonstrated incremental promise and a bright future in medicine. Its use has introduced a revolutionary variation and altered both the conventional approaches to illness diagnosis and treatment used by healthcare consultants. Medical AI is still in its infancy and is beset by difficulties in execution. To verify repeatability, security, and dependability of AI technology, more research is required in this field. The efforts AI uses in modern medicine will prove to be a useful and sophisticated strategy that helps patients and medical professionals alike. AI incorporation has the potential to transform pharmaceutical research and development, improving the efficacy, accessibility, and safety of the medications for patients globally, despite obstacles like data privacy and legal barriers.

ACKNOWLEDGEMENTS

One of the authors is thankful to the Rungta College of Engineering and Technology for providing assistance.

REFERENCES

[1] P.B. Bhattad, and V. Jain, "Artificial Intelligence in Modern Medicine – The Evolving Necessity of the Present and Role in Transforming the Future of Medical Care", *Cureus,* vol. 12, no. 5, p. e8041, 2020.
[http://dx.doi.org/10.7759/cureus.8041] [PMID: 32528777]

[2] K. Manoj, "M, K., Ms., Mahalakshmi. A Review on Artificial Intelligence in Medicine. International Journal of Advanced Research in Science", *Tongxin Jishu,* vol. 4, no. 1, 2024.
[http://dx.doi.org/10.48175/IJARSCT-19338]

[3] A. Isha, K. Bhagat, W. Gajanan, A. Navoday, and D. Kopawar, "Artificial Intelligence in Healthcare : A Review", *Int. J. Sci. Res. Sci. Eng. Technol.,* vol. 11, no. 4, pp. 133-138, 2024.
[http://dx.doi.org/10.32628/IJSRSET24114107]

[4] J. Mansi, "Artificial Intelligence in Healthcare Domain", *Indian Scientific Journal of Research in Engineering and Management,* 2024.
[http://dx.doi.org/10.55041/IJSREM35690]

[5] B. Liudmyla, "I., B., Kɪт., Yury, Havryshchuk., Anatolija, Krasnova., S., V., Vasylyuk. Comprehensive Review of Artificial Intelligence in Medical Diagnostics and Treatment: Challenges and Opportunities", *Futurity Medicine,* vol. 3, no. 3, 2024.

[http://dx.doi.org/10.57125/FEM.2024.09.30.07]

[6] Saurabh, Singhal., Ajeet, Kumar, Sharma., Akhilesh, Kumar, Singh., Abhinav, Pandey., Avinash, Kumar, Sharma. Industry-Specific Applications of AI and ML. Advances in systems analysis, software engineering, and high performance computing book series, 2024. [http://dx.doi.org/10.4018/979-8-3693-3502-4.ch008]

[7] N. Sheliemina, "The Use of Artificial Intelligence in Medical Diagnostics: Opportunities, Prospects and Risks", *Health Economics and Management Review,* vol. 5, no. 2, pp. 104-124, 2024. [http://dx.doi.org/10.61093/hem.2024.2-07]

[8] M.S. Smyth, and J.H.J. Martin, "x Ray crystallography", *Mol. Pathol.,* vol. 53, no. 1, pp. 8-14, 2000. [http://dx.doi.org/10.1136/mp.53.1.8] [PMID: 10884915]

[9] K. Namba, and F. Makino, "Recent progress and future perspective of electron cryomicroscopy for structural life sciences", *Microscopy (Oxf.),* vol. 71, suppl. Suppl. 1, pp. i3-i14, 2022. [http://dx.doi.org/10.1093/jmicro/dfab049] [PMID: 35275178]

[10] J. Koehler Leman, and G. Künze, "Recent Advances in NMR Protein Structure Prediction with ROSETTA", *Int. J. Mol. Sci.,* vol. 24, no. 9, p. 7835, 2023. [http://dx.doi.org/10.3390/ijms24097835] [PMID: 37175539]

[11] L. Chen, Q. Li, K.F.A. Nasif, Y. Xie, B. Deng, S. Niu, S. Pouriyeh, Z. Dai, J. Chen, and C.Y. Xie, "AI-Driven Deep Learning Techniques in Protein Structure Prediction", *Int. J. Mol. Sci.,* vol. 25, no. 15, p. 8426, 2024. [http://dx.doi.org/10.3390/ijms25158426] [PMID: 39125995]

[12] K.H. Nam, "AI-based protein models enhance the accuracy of experimentally determined protein crystal structures", *Front. Mol. Biosci.,* vol. 10, p. 1208810, 2023. [http://dx.doi.org/10.3389/fmolb.2023.1208810] [PMID: 37426417]

[13] L.M.F. Bertoline, A.N. Lima, J.E. Krieger, and S.K. Teixeira, "Before and after AlphaFold2: An overview of protein structure prediction", *Front. Bioinform.,* vol. 3, p. 1120370, 2023. [http://dx.doi.org/10.3389/fbinf.2023.1120370] [PMID: 36926275]

[14] Z. Yang, X. Zeng, Y. Zhao, and R. Chen, "AlphaFold2 and its applications in the fields of biology and medicine", *Signal Transduct. Target. Ther.,* vol. 8, no. 1, p. 115, 2023. [http://dx.doi.org/10.1038/s41392-023-01381-z] [PMID: 36918529]

[15] Lane, T. J. (2023). Protein structure prediction has reached the single-structure frontier. *Nature Methods*, 20 (2), 170-173.

[16] S. Saharkhiz, M. Mostafavi, A. Birashk, S. Karimian, S. Khalilollah, S. Jaferian, Y. Yazdani, I. Alipourfard, Y.S. Huh, M.R. Farani, and R. Akhavan-Sigari, "The State-of-the-Art Overview to Application of Deep Learning in Accurate Protein Design and Structure Prediction", *Top. Curr. Chem. (Cham),* vol. 382, no. 3, p. 23, 2024. [http://dx.doi.org/10.1007/s41061-024-00469-6] [PMID: 38965117]

[17] B. Kuhlman, and P. Bradley, "Advances in protein structure prediction and design", *Nat. Rev. Mol. Cell Biol.,* vol. 20, no. 11, pp. 681-697, 2019. [http://dx.doi.org/10.1038/s41580-019-0163-x] [PMID: 31417196]

[18] D.B. Kitchen, H. Decornez, J.R. Furr, and J. Bajorath, "Docking and scoring in virtual screening for drug discovery: methods and applications", *Nat. Rev. Drug Discov.,* vol. 3, no. 11, pp. 935-949, 2004. [http://dx.doi.org/10.1038/nrd1549] [PMID: 15520816]

[19] M. Ragoza, J. Hochuli, E. Idrobo, J. Sunseri, and D.R. Koes, "Protein–Ligand Scoring with Convolutional Neural Networks", *J. Chem. Inf. Model.,* vol. 57, no. 4, pp. 942-957, 2017. [http://dx.doi.org/10.1021/acs.jcim.6b00740] [PMID: 28368587]

[20] X. Zhao, D. Rangaprakash, B. Yuan, T.S. Denney Jr, J.S. Katz, M.N. Dretsch, and G. Deshpande, "Investigating the correspondence of clinical diagnostic grouping with underlying neurobiological and phenotypic clusters using unsupervised machine learning", *Front. Appl. Math. Stat.,* vol. 4, p. 25,

2018.
[http://dx.doi.org/10.3389/fams.2018.00025] [PMID: 30393630]

[21] C. Sarkar, B. Das, V.S. Rawat, J.B. Wahlang, A. Nongpiur, I. Tiewsoh, N.M. Lyngdoh, D. Das, M. Bidarolli, H.T. Sony, and Artificial Intelligence, "Artificial Intelligence and Machine Learning Technology Driven Modern Drug Discovery and Development", *Int. J. Mol. Sci.,* vol. 24, no. 3, p. 2026, 2023.
[http://dx.doi.org/10.3390/ijms24032026] [PMID: 36768346]

[22] A. Lavecchia, and C. Giovanni, "Virtual screening strategies in drug discovery: a critical review", *Curr. Med. Chem.,* vol. 20, no. 23, pp. 2839-2860, 2013.
[http://dx.doi.org/10.2174/09298673113209990001] [PMID: 23651302]

[23] B. Lotfi, O. Mebarka, S.U. Khan, and T.T. Htar, "Pharmacophore-based virtual screening, molecular docking and molecular dynamics studies for the discovery of novel neuraminidase inhibitors", *J. Biomol. Struct. Dyn.,* vol. 42, no. 10, pp. 5308-5320, 2024.
[http://dx.doi.org/10.1080/07391102.2023.2225007] [PMID: 37334701]

[24] P.C. Agu, C.A. Afiukwa, O.U. Orji, E.M. Ezeh, I.H. Ofoke, C.O. Ogbu, E.I. Ugwuja, and P.M. Aja, "Molecular docking as a tool for the discovery of molecular targets of nutraceuticals in diseases management", *Sci. Rep.,* vol. 13, no. 1, p. 13398, 2023.
[http://dx.doi.org/10.1038/s41598-023-40160-2] [PMID: 37592012]

[25] S. Tripathi, A.I. Augustin, A. Dunlop, R. Sukumaran, S. Dheer, A. Zavalny, O. Haslam, T. Austin, J. Donchez, P.K. Tripathi, and E. Kim, "Recent advances and application of generative adversarial networks in drug discovery, development, and targeting", *Artif. Intell. Life Sci.,* vol. 2, p. 100045, 2022.
[http://dx.doi.org/10.1016/j.ailsci.2022.100045]

[26] F. Lombardo, R.S. Obach, M.V. Varma, R. Stringer, and G. Berellini, "Clearance mechanism assignment and total clearance prediction in human based upon in silico models", *J. Med. Chem.,* vol. 57, no. 10, pp. 4397-4405, 2014.
[http://dx.doi.org/10.1021/jm500436v] [PMID: 24773013]

[27] Ashfaq Ur Rehman , Mingyu Li , Binjian Wu , Yasir Ali , Salman Rasheed , Sana Shaheen , Xinyi Liu , Ray Luo , Jian Zhang , Role of Artificial Intelligence in Revolutionizing Drug Discovery, Fundamental Research. 2024.
[http://dx.doi.org/10.1016/j.fmre.2024.04.021]

[28] B. Reber, L. Van Dijk, B. Anderson, A.S.R. Mohamed, C. Fuller, S. Lai, and K. Brock, "Comparison of Machine-Learning and Deep-Learning Methods for the Prediction of Osteoradionecrosis Resulting From Head and Neck Cancer Radiation Therapy", *Adv. Radiat. Oncol.,* vol. 8, no. 4, p. 101163, 2023.
[http://dx.doi.org/10.1016/j.adro.2022.101163] [PMID: 36798732]

[29] C. Romal, *Intelligent systems for healthcare diagnostics and treatment.* World Journal Of Advanced Research and Reviews, 2024.
[http://dx.doi.org/10.30574/wjarr.2024.23.1.2015]

[30] Ejike, Innocent, Nwankwo., Ebube, Victor, Emeihe., Mojeed, Dayo, Ajegbile., Janet, Aderonke, Olaboye., Chukwudi, Cosmos, Maha. AI in personalized medicine: Enhancing drug efficacy and reducing adverse effects. International medical science research journal. 2024; 4 (8).
[http://dx.doi.org/10.51594/imsrj.v4i8.1453]

[31] A. Sahu, J. Mishra, and N. Kushwaha, "Artificial Intelligence (AI) in Drugs and Pharmaceuticals", *Comb. Chem. High Throughput Screen.,* vol. 25, no. 11, pp. 1818-1837, 2022.
[http://dx.doi.org/10.2174/1386207325666211207153943] [PMID: 34875986]

[32] H.H. Chen, H.T. Hsu, P.C. Lin, C.Y. Chen, H.F. Hsieh, and C.H. Ko, "Efficacy of a Smartphone App in Enhancing Medication Adherence and Accuracy in Individuals With Schizophrenia During the COVID-19 Pandemic: Randomized Controlled Trial", *JMIR Ment. Health,* vol. 10, p. e50806, 2023.
[http://dx.doi.org/10.2196/50806] [PMID: 38096017]

[33] Mustafa, Öztatlıcı., Seçil, Eroğlu., Hülya, Birinci., Mehmet, Göl. "6. Artificial Intelligence in Diagnosis and Treatment. Gaziantep Islam Science and Technology University, 2024. [http://dx.doi.org/10.46871/eams.1470170]

[34] K. Elumalai, S. Srinivasan, and A. Shanmugam, "Review of the efficacy of nanoparticle-based drug delivery systems for cancer treatment", *Biomedical Technology,* vol. 5, pp. 109-122, 2024. [http://dx.doi.org/10.1016/j.bmt.2023.09.001]

[35] Y. Luo, X. Zhao, J. Zhou, J. Yang, Y. Zhang, W. Kuang, J. Peng, L. Chen, and J. Zeng, "A network integration approach for drug-target interaction prediction and computational drug repositioning from heterogeneous information", *Nat. Commun.,* vol. 8, no. 1, p. 573, 2017. [http://dx.doi.org/10.1038/s41467-017-00680-8] [PMID: 28924171]

[36] D. Maiti, M. Naseeruddin Inamdar, M. Almuqbil, S. Suresh, S. Mohammed Basheeruddin Asdaq, S. Alshehri, S. Ali Al Arfaj, A. Musharraf Alamri, M. Meshary Aldohyan, M. Theeb Alqahtani, T. Mohammed Alosaimi, S. Haran Alenazi, M.E. Almadani, J. Ahmed S Mulla, and S. Imam Rabbani, "Evaluation of solid-lipid nanoparticles formulation of methotrexate for anti-psoriatic activity", *Saudi Pharm. J.,* vol. 31, no. 6, pp. 834-844, 2023. [http://dx.doi.org/10.1016/j.jsps.2023.04.007] [PMID: 37228325]

[37] D. Ho, P. Wang, and T. Kee, "Artificial intelligence in nanomedicine", *Nanoscale Horiz.,* vol. 4, no. 2, pp. 365-377, 2019. [http://dx.doi.org/10.1039/C8NH00233A] [PMID: 32254089]

[38] Chopra H, Annu, Shin DK, *et al.* Revolutionizing clinical trials: the role of AI in accelerating medical breakthroughs. Int J Surg. 2023;109(12):4211-4220. Published, 2023. [http://dx.doi.org/10.1097/JS9.0000000000000705]

CHAPTER 3

Advancements in Wearable Health Tech: Applications, Challenges, and Future Directions

Muhammad Thesa Ghozali[1,*] and **Anita Agustina Styawan**[2]

[1] *School of Pharmacy, Faculty of Medicine and Health Sciences, Universitas Muhammadiyah Yogyakarta, Yogyakarta, Indonesia*

[2] *Faculty of Health and Technology, Universitas Muhammadiyah Klaten, Central Java, Indonesia*

Abstract: Wearable technologies and smart medical devices are transforming healthcare by enabling users to monitor vital signs continuously and in real time, thus supporting more individualized and data-driven medical care. By examining core components such as biosensors, microcontrollers, and wireless communication systems, this chapter explores wearable technologies within the context of the Internet of Things (IoT) and data analytics. It further investigates the applications of wearables in healthcare, including remote monitoring, rehabilitation, disease prevention, and elderly care. Key challenges such as battery limitations, sensor accuracy, and the ethical and legal concerns surrounding these technologies are also discussed. Additionally, the chapter highlights the integration of Artificial Intelligence (AI) and Machine Learning (ML) in wearable systems, the evolution of next-generation devices, and their implications for public health, especially in epidemic preparedness. Finally, it identifies future research directions that encourage multidisciplinary collaboration and the development of patient-centered healthcare. As wearable technology continues to evolve, it holds significant potential to improve patient outcomes and advance community health.

Keywords: Artificial Intelligence, Public health, Smart medical devices, Wearable technology.

INTRODUCTION

The adoption of smart medical devices and wearable technologies has the potential to revolutionize healthcare by providing unprecedented opportunities for continuous monitoring, diagnosis, and treatment outside traditional clinical settings [1]. Smart medical devices enable real-time monitoring of physiological data [2], typically integrating specialized sensors, microprocessors, and wireless

* **Corresponding author Muhammad Thesa Ghozali:** School of Pharmacy, Faculty of Medicine and Health Sciences, Universitas Muhammadiyah Yogyakarta, Yogyakarta, Indonesia; E-mail: ghozali@umy.ac.id

communication technologies to collect, analyze, and transmit data on an individual's health status. From consumer-grade fitness trackers and smartwatches that monitor general wellness to advanced medical-grade wearables such as continuous glucose monitors [3], wearable electrocardiograms [4], and smart implants [5], the range of applications is extensive.

Wearable technologies play an increasingly vital role in modern healthcare, as they offer personalized, real-time data that can enhance clinical decision-making and promote proactive health management. These technologies support personalized medicine by tailoring treatments to individual patients based on continuous health data [6]. For example, wearable ECGs can detect cardiac abnormalities such as arrhythmias in real time, allowing for early diagnosis and intervention. Furthermore, wearables empower patients to actively manage their health, improving treatment adherence and overall health outcomes [7].

Over the past two decades, wearable medical technology has undergone a dramatic transformation. Early devices were bulky, had limited functionality, and could not process data in real time [8]. However, advancements in sensor miniaturization, battery efficiency, and wireless communication have enabled smaller, more powerful devices with enhanced usability. The convergence of the Internet of Things (IoT), artificial intelligence (AI), and wearable technologies has greatly expanded their potential to revolutionize healthcare [9]. Modern healthcare ecosystems increasingly integrate wearables for remote monitoring, diagnostics, and precision medicine.

Focusing on their uses in healthcare, this chapter aims to explore the present scene of wearable technology and smart medical equipment. The chapter specifically focuses on examining the implementation of these tools for real-time monitoring, diagnostics, rehabilitation, and management of chronic diseases. This chapter will give a thorough picture of how wearables support the developing field of customized medicine by looking at the technological bases of these devices, such as the sensors and communication protocols allowing their operation.

This chapter examines the current landscape of wearable technologies and smart medical devices, emphasizing their applications in real-time monitoring, diagnostics, rehabilitation, and chronic disease management. It discusses the technological foundations of wearables, including their sensors, data communication protocols, and architecture. The chapter also explores opportunities and challenges associated with wearable technologies—particularly issues related to data security, usability, and regulatory compliance—and suggests potential solutions to overcome these barriers. Finally, it highlights the development of next-generation wearables incorporating flexible and biodegradable materials, and the integration of AI and ML for predictive health analytics.

THE TECHNOLOGICAL FOUNDATIONS OF WEARABLE DEVICES

Key Components and Architecture

Wearable technology relies on a sophisticated combination of hardware and software that enables continuous data collection and processing. Sensors such as accelerometers, gyroscopes, and biosensors form the foundation of wearable systems. Medical wearables depend heavily on biosensors that detect physiological signals such as temperature, glucose levels, and heart rate [10]. These sensors convert biological signals into electrical outputs, which are then processed and analyzed to generate actionable health insights [11].

Microcontrollers and processing units manage data collection, signal processing, and communication. Algorithms filter and interpret raw sensor data to identify relevant trends and patterns [12]. Power efficiency is a critical design factor, as wearable devices must remain lightweight and energy-efficient to optimize battery life. Wireless communication technologies—including Bluetooth, Zigbee, and Wi-Fi—transmit collected data to external devices or cloud platforms for further analysis [13, 14]. The choice of protocol depends on factors such as transmission range, data rate, and power consumption.

Types of Wearable Medical Devices

Wearable medical devices vary widely in design and application. Common examples include fitness trackers and smartwatches that monitor heart rate, physical activity, and sleep [15]. Although often used for general wellness, these devices are increasingly being adapted for medical purposes, particularly for the long-term monitoring of chronic conditions. Advanced devices include implantable sensors and clothing-integrated systems. Implantable technologies, such as cardiac pacemakers and continuous glucose monitors, enable real-time, long-term physiological monitoring [16]. Smart textiles, embedded with biosensors, can measure parameters such as respiration and muscle activity, providing valuable data for rehabilitation and sports medicine.

Integration with IoT and Data Analytics

The integration of wearable technology with IoT is essential for seamless connectivity and real-time health data sharing. Within an IoT framework, wearables act as nodes in a broader network of interconnected medical systems

[17]. These devices collect and transmit data continuously, facilitating remote patient management and precision healthcare delivery.

The real power of wearables lies in data analytics. AI and ML algorithms process vast amounts of data to detect anomalies, predict health events, and optimize treatment plans [18]. For instance, AI-driven wearables that analyze heart rate variability can predict cardiovascular risks, enabling early intervention. Predictive healthcare—powered by data analytics—is particularly valuable in chronic disease management, where timely insights can significantly improve patient outcomes. For instance, AI-driven wearables that analyze heart rate variability can predict cardiovascular risks, enabling early intervention. Predictive healthcare—powered by data analytics—is particularly valuable in chronic disease management, where timely insights can significantly improve patient outcomes.

Applications in Healthcare

Remote Monitoring and Diagnostics

Wearable devices, shown in Fig. (**1**), have revolutionized remote monitoring by allowing continuous data collection in real time. Devices such as smartwatches, biosensor patches, and implantable monitors track vital signs, including heart rate, glucose levels, and blood pressure [19]. Continuous glucose monitors (CGMs) enable diabetic patients to measure glucose fluctuations throughout the day without traditional finger-prick testing, while wearable blood pressure monitors transmit readings directly to healthcare providers for immediate intervention.

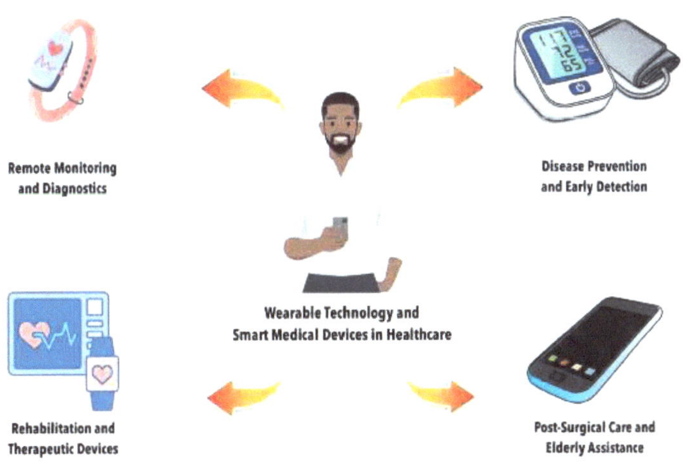

Fig. (1). Applications of wearable technology and smart medical devices in healthcare, including remote monitoring, rehabilitation, disease prevention, and post-surgical or elderly care support.

Advanced wearable ECG and EEG systems are particularly useful for patients with neurological or cardiovascular conditions [20]. These devices detect abnormal heart or brain activity, enabling early diagnosis of disorders such as arrhythmia or epilepsy. Pulse oximeters, commonly used in respiratory conditions, measure oxygen saturation and help detect hypoxemia in patients with COPD or COVID-19. Remote monitoring reduces hospital visits and supports efficient long-term care management.

Therapeutic Devices for Rehabilitation

Wearables play a crucial role in rehabilitation by providing continuous assessment of posture and movement. Devices equipped with gait sensors track parameters such as stride length and walking speed, offering real-time feedback to support recovery after injury or surgery [21]. Smart clothing and posture correction wearables deliver continuous monitoring and corrective feedback, benefiting individuals with musculoskeletal disorders or post-surgical conditions.

Therapeutic wearables, such as insulin delivery systems, have become integral to diabetes management. Unlike traditional injection schedules, these systems adjust insulin delivery dynamically based on glucose data. Wearable pain management devices, such as those employing Transcutaneous Electrical Nerve Stimulation (TENS), offer non-invasive relief for chronic pain conditions like arthritis and neuropathy [22]. These technologies improve quality of life while reducing dependence on medication.

Disease Prevention and Early Detection

AI-enhanced wearables are increasingly used for early disease detection and prevention. By identifying subtle anomalies in continuous physiological data, wearables can detect the onset of diseases such as diabetes and cardiovascular disorders before symptoms manifest [23]. For example, variations in heart rate variability can signal cardiovascular stress, allowing early intervention. Emerging research explores biosensors capable of detecting biomarkers linked to cancer and metabolic diseases [24]. Such preventive monitoring represents a paradigm shift from reactive to proactive healthcare, reducing both disease burden and healthcare costs.

Post-Surgical Care and Elderly Assistance

In post-surgical care, wearables track vital signs, mobility, and wound healing indicators. Smart dressings, capable of monitoring temperature and moisture levels, alert clinicians to potential infections [25]. Rehabilitation wearables ensure patients adhere to recovery protocols, reducing complications such as deep vein thrombosis. For elderly care, smart devices enhance safety and independence. Fall detection systems integrated into wearable pendants or watches automatically alert caregivers in emergencies [26]. Devices that monitor hydration, activity levels, and medication adherence help maintain health and autonomy among older adults, improving their quality of life and reducing caregiver strain.

CHALLENGES AND LIMITATIONS

Technical Challenges

Despite their promise, wearable medical devices face technical constraints. Battery life remains a primary challenge, as continuous monitoring consumes substantial power [27]. Developers must balance functionality with form factor to maintain user comfort and device efficiency. Sensor accuracy is another concern; factors such as placement, temperature, and movement can affect data reliability [28]. Data security and privacy pose significant risks, as wearables handle sensitive health information [29]. Breaches could compromise personal data, emphasizing the need for robust cybersecurity protocols and encrypted communication systems.

Regulatory and Ethical Issues

A comprehensive understanding of regulatory frameworks is essential for successfully translating wearable medical technologies from prototype to clinical practice. In the United States, the Food and Drug Administration (FDA) oversees digital health products through the Digital Health Center of Excellence (DHCoE), which provides guidance on the development, assessment, and regulation of wearable medical devices. The FDA classifies devices according to their intended use and associated level of risk under the Medical Device Classification System (Class I, II, or III). Devices with diagnostic or therapeutic functions typically fall into higher classes and are subject to more rigorous review processes, such as the 510(k) Premarket Notification, De Novo Classification, or Premarket Approval (PMA) pathways. For instance, wearable ECG monitors and continuous glucose sensors that provide real-time clinical data for treatment decisions must demonstrate substantial equivalence to an approved predicate device or undergo extensive clinical validation to ensure safety and efficacy. The DHCoE also promotes innovation through initiatives such as the Software as a Medical Device (SaMD) framework, which addresses emerging regulatory considerations for AI- and ML-enabled wearable technologies.

At the international level, regulatory bodies such as the European Medicines Agency (EMA) and the European Commission's Conformité Européenne (CE) marking system oversee compliance under the EU Medical Device Regulation

(MDR 2017/745). This framework requires manufacturers to provide comprehensive technical documentation, conduct risk assessments, and maintain post-market surveillance to ensure device safety and performance. Furthermore, global initiatives led by organizations such as the International Medical Device Regulators Forum (IMDRF) and ISO/IEC are working toward harmonizing international standards to facilitate cross-border approval of digital health technologies. As wearable devices increasingly integrate artificial intelligence, adaptive algorithms, and continuous software updates, regulators are evolving their frameworks to address key issues such as algorithm transparency, cybersecurity resilience, and real-world performance validation. These evolving regulatory efforts are crucial to ensuring that wearable medical devices achieve a balance between technological innovation, patient safety, and public trust in the rapidly advancing digital healthcare ecosystem.

Ethically, continuous health data collection raises questions about privacy, consent, and data ownership [30]. Patients must clearly understand how their data is stored, accessed, and used. Transparent data governance frameworks are essential to protect autonomy and trust in digital healthcare systems.

User Acceptance and Usability

User acceptance is another critical challenge. Devices must be comfortable, intuitive, and accessible to diverse populations [31]. Older users—who stand to benefit most—often face barriers related to usability and technological literacy. Cost also remains a limiting factor, as advanced wearables may be inaccessible to lower-income populations [32]. Ensuring equitable access requires user-centered design, affordability strategies, and public education on digital health literacy.

NEW DEVELOPMENTS AND EMERGING TRENDS

Integration of AI and ML

AI and ML are transforming wearable technologies into intelligent diagnostic and predictive tools. AI-driven wearables can analyze vast sensor datasets to detect subtle physiological changes, improving diagnostic accuracy [33]. For example, AI-enabled ECG devices identify arrhythmias such as atrial fibrillation with greater precision than manual interpretation [34].

In mental health, AI-integrated wearables track stress, anxiety, and depression indicators such as heart rate variability and skin conductance [35]. These devices provide real-time feedback and adaptive interventions, supporting mental and cognitive well-being.

Future Wearables

Next-generation wearables aim for greater autonomy, flexibility, and sustainability. Flexible and biodegradable materials improve comfort while reducing electronic waste [36]. Self-powered systems that harvest energy from body motion or heat could eliminate the need for frequent charging [37]. Nanotechnology is also revolutionizing wearable sensors—materials like graphene enhance sensitivity, durability, and biocompatibility.

Wearable Sensors for COVID-19 and Future Pandemics

The COVID-19 pandemic highlighted the importance of wearable sensors in public health surveillance [38]. Devices capable of monitoring temperature, respiratory rate, and oxygen saturation provided early warning signals of infection. Contact-tracing wearables also contributed to exposure monitoring in healthcare settings. Beyond COVID-19, wearable technologies will play a pivotal role in future pandemic preparedness by enabling large-scale, real-time health monitoring and decentralized care [39]. Such applications reduce hospital burden and facilitate early outbreak detection.

FUTURE DIRECTIONS AND RESEARCH PROSPECTS

Multidisciplinary Research Projects

Future progress in wearable medical devices depends on collaboration between engineers, clinicians, and data scientists [40]. Engineers develop advanced hardware, data scientists build predictive algorithms, and clinicians ensure clinical relevance [41]. Partnerships with industry stakeholders—such as telecommunications and software firms—are vital for scaling innovation and infrastructure [42].

Models of Patient-Centered Healthcare

Wearables are driving a transition toward patient-centered healthcare models that prioritize personalization and engagement [43]. Continuous monitoring enables physicians to tailor treatments in real time, while patients gain autonomy over their health data [44]. This proactive approach can prevent disease progression, reduce hospitalizations, and improve overall healthcare efficiency.

Wearables in Public Health

Wearable data has immense potential for public health analytics. Aggregated data from millions of users can reveal population-level trends, informing health policies and preventive strategies [45]. During pandemics, wearable data support symptom tracking and early detection of disease outbreaks [46]. As adoption increases, wearables will become vital tools for reducing health disparities and strengthening global health resilience.

CONCLUDING REMARKS

Wearable technology has rapidly evolved into a cornerstone of modern healthcare, enabling real-time insights that enhance diagnosis, prevention, and chronic disease management. Continued innovation in sensor accuracy, AI integration, and power efficiency will further expand their potential. Healthcare professionals should embrace wearable data to deliver personalized treatment, while policymakers must ensure regulatory clarity, data security, and equitable access. With advancements in flexible, self-powered, and AI-enhanced wearables, the coming decade promises a new era of proactive, patient-centered, and globally connected healthcare.

REFERENCES

[1] C. Li, and J. Wang, "Wang S, Zhang Y. A review of IoT applications in healthcare", *Neurocomputing,* vol. 565, p. 127017, 2024.
[http://dx.doi.org/10.1016/j.neucom.2023.127017]

[2] S. Dockray, E. Whelan, and J. Cooney-Quane, "Psychobiological assessments", In: *Encyclopedia of Adolescence.,* W. Troop-Gordon, E.W. Neblett, Eds., 2nd ed. Academic Press: Oxford, 2024, pp. 356-376.
[http://dx.doi.org/10.1016/B978-0-323-96023-6.00028-2]

[3] A.K. Yetisen, J.L. Martinez-Hurtado, B. Ünal, A. Khademhosseini, and H. Butt, "Wearables in Medicine", *Adv. Mater.,* vol. 30, no. 33, p. 1706910, 2018.
[http://dx.doi.org/10.1002/adma.201706910] [PMID: 29893068]

[4] E. Escobar-Linero, L. Muñoz-Saavedra, F. Luna-Perejón, J.L. Sevillano, and M. Domínguez-Morales, "Wearable Health Devices for Diagnosis Support: Evolution and Future Tendencies", *Sensors (Basel),* vol. 23, no. 3, p. 1678, 2023.
[http://dx.doi.org/10.3390/s23031678] [PMID: 36772718]

[5] Verma D, Singh KR, Yadav AK, Nayak V, Singh J, Solanki PR, *et al.* Internet of things (IoT) in nano-integrated wearable biosensor devices for healthcare applications. Biosensors and Bioelectronics: X 2022; 11: 100153.
[http://dx.doi.org/10.1016/j.biosx.2022.100153]

[6] L. Izu, B. Scholtz, and I. Fashoro, "Wearables and Their Potential to Transform Health Management: A Step towards Sustainable Development Goal 3", *Sustainability (Basel),* vol. 16, no. 5, p. 1850, 2024.
[http://dx.doi.org/10.3390/su16051850]

[7] H.H.V. Tran, N.A. Urgessa, P. Geethakumari, P. Kampa, R. Parchuri, R. Bhandari, A.R. Alnasser, A. Akram, S. Kar, F. Osman, G.D. Mashat, and L. Mohammed, "Detection and Diagnostic Accuracy of Cardiac Arrhythmias Using Wearable Health Devices: A Systematic Review", *Cureus,* vol. 15, no. 12, p. e50952, 2023.
[http://dx.doi.org/10.7759/cureus.50952] [PMID: 38249280]

[8] Y.M. de-la-Fuente-Robles, A.J. Ricoy-Cano, A.P. Albín-Rodríguez, J.L. López-Ruiz, and M. Espinilla-Estévez, "Past, Present and Future of Research on Wearable Technologies for Healthcare: A Bibliometric Analysis Using Scopus", *Sensors (Basel),* vol. 22, no. 22, p. 8599, 2022.
[http://dx.doi.org/10.3390/s22228599] [PMID: 36433195]

[9] J. Bajwa, U. Munir, A. Nori, and B. Williams, "Artificial intelligence in healthcare: transforming the practice of medicine", *Future Healthc. J.,* vol. 8, no. 2, pp. e188-e194, 2021. [http://dx.doi.org/10.7861/fhj.2021-0095] [PMID: 34286183]

[10] R. De Fazio, V.M. Mastronardi, M. De Vittorio, and P. Visconti, "Wearable Sensors and Smart Devices to Monitor Rehabilitation Parameters and Sports Performance: An Overview", *Sensors (Basel),* vol. 23, no. 4, p. 1856, 2023. [http://dx.doi.org/10.3390/s23041856] [PMID: 36850453]

[11] V. Vijayan, J.P. Connolly, J. Condell, N. McKelvey, and P. Gardiner, "Review of Wearable Devices and Data Collection Considerations for Connected Health", *Sensors (Basel),* vol. 21, no. 16, p. 5589, 2021. [http://dx.doi.org/10.3390/s21165589] [PMID: 34451032]

[12] R.L. Bulathsinghala, W. Ding, and R.D.I.G. Dharmasena, "Triboelectric nanogenerators for wearable sensing applications: A system level analysis", *Nano Energy,* vol. 116, p. 108792, 2023. [http://dx.doi.org/10.1016/j.nanoen.2023.108792]

[13] A.S. AlShuhail, S. Bhatia, A. Kumar, and B. Bhushan, "Zigbee-Based Low Power Consumption Wearables Device for Voice Data Transmission", *Sustainability (Basel),* vol. 14, no. 17, p. 10847, 2022. [http://dx.doi.org/10.3390/su141710847]

[14] H.N.S. Aldin, M.R. Ghods, F. Nayebipour, and M.N. Torshiz, "A comprehensive review of energy harvesting and routing strategies for IoT sensors sustainability and communication technology", *Sensors International,* vol. 5, p. 100258, 2024. [http://dx.doi.org/10.1016/j.sintl.2023.100258]

[15] R.J. Shei, I.G. Holder, A.S. Oumsang, B.A. Paris, and H.L. Paris, "Wearable activity trackers–advanced technology or advanced marketing?", *Eur. J. Appl. Physiol.,* vol. 122, no. 9, pp. 1975-1990, 2022. [http://dx.doi.org/10.1007/s00421-022-04951-1] [PMID: 35445837]

[16] M.M.H. Shandhi, K. Singh, N. Janson, P. Ashar, G. Singh, B. Lu, D.S. Hillygus, J.M. Maddocks, and J.P. Dunn, "Assessment of ownership of smart devices and the acceptability of digital health data sharing", *NPJ Digit. Med.,* vol. 7, no. 1, p. 44, 2024. [http://dx.doi.org/10.1038/s41746-024-01030-x] [PMID: 38388660]

[17] C. Huang, J. Wang, S. Wang, and Y. Zhang, "Internet of medical things: A systematic review", *Neurocomputing,* vol. 557, p. 126719, 2023. [http://dx.doi.org/10.1016/j.neucom.2023.126719]

[18] Khan I, Rashid D. Internet of Things (IoT) Its Applications and Enabling Technologies in Healthcare: A Review. Educational Administration Theory and Practices 2024; 30. [http://dx.doi.org/10.53555/kuey.v30i4.5031]

[19] K. Guk, G. Han, J. Lim, K. Jeong, T. Kang, E.K. Lim, and J. Jung, "Evolution of Wearable Devices with Real-Time Disease Monitoring for Personalized Healthcare", *Nanomaterials (Basel),* vol. 9, no. 6, p. 813, 2019. [http://dx.doi.org/10.3390/nano9060813] [PMID: 31146479]

[20] Z. Alimbayeva, C. Alimbayev, K. Ozhikenov, N. Bayanbay, and A. Ozhikenova, "Wearable ECG Device and Machine Learning for Heart Monitoring", *Sensors (Basel),* vol. 24, no. 13, p. 4201, 2024. [http://dx.doi.org/10.3390/s24134201] [PMID: 39000979]

[21] S. Díaz, J.B. Stephenson, and M.A. Labrador, "Use of Wearable Sensor Technology in Gait, Balance, and Range of Motion Analysis", *Appl. Sci. (Basel),* vol. 10, no. 1, p. 234, 2019. [http://dx.doi.org/10.3390/app10010234]

[22] V. Elian, V. Popovici, E.A. Ozon, A. Musuc, A. Fița, E. Rusu, G. Radulian, and D. Lupuliasa, "Current Technologies for Managing Type 1 Diabetes Mellitus and Their Impact on Quality of

Life—A Narrative Review", *Life (Basel),* vol. 13, no. 8, p. 1663, 2023. [http://dx.doi.org/10.3390/life13081663] [PMID: 37629520]

[23] A. Hughes, M.M.H. Shandhi, H. Master, J. Dunn, and E. Brittain, "Wearable Devices in Cardiovascular Medicine", *Circ. Res.,* vol. 132, no. 5, pp. 652-670, 2023. [http://dx.doi.org/10.1161/CIRCRESAHA.122.322389] [PMID: 36862812]

[24] Z. Song, S. Zhou, Y. Qin, X. Xia, Y. Sun, G. Han, T. Shu, L. Hu, and Q. Zhang, "Flexible and Wearable Biosensors for Monitoring Health Conditions", *Biosensors (Basel),* vol. 13, no. 6, p. 630, 2023. [http://dx.doi.org/10.3390/bios13060630] [PMID: 37366995]

[25] M.I. Hossain, M.S. Zahid, M.A. Chowdhury, M.M.M. Hossain, N. Hossain, M.A. Islam, and M.H. Mobarak, "Smart bandage: A device for wound monitoring and targeted treatment", *Results in Chemistry,* vol. 7, p. 101292, 2024. [http://dx.doi.org/10.1016/j.rechem.2023.101292]

[26] M. Pech, H. Sauzeon, T. Yebda, J. Benois-Pineau, and H. Amieva, "Falls Detection and Prevention Systems in Home Care for Older Adults: Myth or Reality?", *JMIR Aging,* vol. 4, no. 4, p. e29744, 2021. [http://dx.doi.org/10.2196/29744] [PMID: 34889755]

[27] A.A. Smith, R. Li, and Z.T.H. Tse, "Reshaping healthcare with wearable biosensors", *Sci. Rep.,* vol. 13, no. 1, p. 4998, 2023. [http://dx.doi.org/10.1038/s41598-022-26951-z] [PMID: 36973262]

[28] S. Shajari, K. Kuruvinashetti, A. Komeili, and U. Sundararaj, "The Emergence of AI-Based Wearable Sensors for Digital Health Technology: A Review", *Sensors (Basel),* vol. 23, no. 23, p. 9498, 2023. [http://dx.doi.org/10.3390/s23239498] [PMID: 38067871]

[29] A.G. Silva-Trujillo, M.J. González González, L.P. Rocha Pérez, and L.J. García Villalba, "Cybersecurity Analysis of Wearable Devices: Smartwatches Passive Attack", *Sensors (Basel),* vol. 23, no. 12, p. 5438, 2023. [http://dx.doi.org/10.3390/s23125438] [PMID: 37420605]

[30] C. Erdmier, J. Hatcher, and M. Lee, "Wearable device implications in the healthcare industry", *J. Med. Eng. Technol.,* vol. 40, no. 4, pp. 141-148, 2016. [http://dx.doi.org/10.3109/03091902.2016.1153738] [PMID: 27010250]

[31] C. Buenaflor, and H-C. Kim, "Six human factors to acceptability of wearable computers", *International Journal of Multimedia and Ubiquitous Engineering,* vol. 8, pp. 103-114, 2013.

[32] L.P. Calegari, D.C. Fettermann, L.P. Calegari, and D.C. Fettermann, "Analysis of barriers and benefits associated with e-health technology applications", *J. Technol. Manag. Innov.,* vol. 17, no. 4, pp. 106-116, 2022. [http://dx.doi.org/10.4067/S0718-27242022000400106]

[33] M.A. Muzammil, S. Javid, A.K. Afridi, R. Siddineni, M. Shahabi, M. Haseeb, F.N.U. Fariha, S. Kumar, S. Zaveri, and A.J. Nashwan, "Artificial intelligence-enhanced electrocardiography for accurate diagnosis and management of cardiovascular diseases", *J. Electrocardiol.,* vol. 83, pp. 30-40, 2024. [http://dx.doi.org/10.1016/j.jelectrocard.2024.01.006] [PMID: 38301492]

[34] D.B. Olawade, N. Aderinto, G. Olatunji, E. Kokori, A.C. David-Olawade, and M. Hadi, "Advancements and applications of Artificial Intelligence in cardiology: Current trends and future prospects", *Journal of Medicine, Surgery, and Public Health,* vol. 3, p. 100109, 2024. [http://dx.doi.org/10.1016/j.glmedi.2024.100109]

[35] M.L. González Ramírez, J.P. García Vázquez, M.D. Rodríguez, L.A. Padilla-López, G.M. Galindo-Aldana, and D. Cuevas-González, "Wearables for Stress Management: A Scoping Review", *Healthcare (Basel),* vol. 11, no. 17, p. 2369, 2023. [http://dx.doi.org/10.3390/healthcare11172369] [PMID: 37685403]

[36] G. Shen, "Recent advances of flexible sensors for biomedical applications", *Prog. Nat. Sci.,* vol. 31, no. 6, pp. 872-882, 2021.
[http://dx.doi.org/10.1016/j.pnsc.2021.10.005]

[37] M.T. Ghozali, "Implementation of the IoT-Based Technology on Patient Medication Adherence: A Comprehensive Bibliometric and Systematic Review", *Journal of Information and Communication Technology,* vol. 22, pp. 503-544, 2023.
[http://dx.doi.org/10.32890/jict2023.22.4.1]

[38] W. Jiang, S. Majumder, S. Kumar, S. Subramaniam, X. Li, R. Khedri, T. Mondal, M. Abolghasemian, I. Satia, and M.J. Deen, "A Wearable Tele-Health System towards Monitoring COVID-19 and Chronic Diseases", *IEEE Rev. Biomed. Eng.,* vol. 15, pp. 61-84, 2022.
[http://dx.doi.org/10.1109/RBME.2021.3069815] [PMID: 33784625]

[39] M. Umair, M.A. Cheema, O. Cheema, H. Li, and H. Lu, "Impact of COVID-19 on IoT Adoption in Healthcare, Smart Homes, Smart Buildings, Smart Cities, Transportation and Industrial IoT", *Sensors (Basel),* vol. 21, no. 11, p. 3838, 2021.
[http://dx.doi.org/10.3390/s21113838] [PMID: 34206120]

[40] Z. Johnson, and M.J. Saikia, "Digital Twins for Healthcare Using Wearables", *Bioengineering (Basel),* vol. 11, no. 6, p. 606, 2024.
[http://dx.doi.org/10.3390/bioengineering11060606] [PMID: 38927842]

[41] E. Nasarian, R. Alizadehsani, U.R. Acharya, and K.L. Tsui, "Designing interpretable ML system to enhance trust in healthcare: A systematic review to proposed responsible clinician-AI-collaboration framework", *Inf. Fusion,* vol. 108, p. 102412, 2024.
[http://dx.doi.org/10.1016/j.inffus.2024.102412]

[42] M. Javaid, A. Haleem, and R.P. Singh, "Health informatics to enhance the healthcare industry's culture: An extensive analysis of its features, contributions, applications and limitations", *Informatics and Health,* vol. 1, no. 2, pp. 123-148, 2024.
[http://dx.doi.org/10.1016/j.infoh.2024.05.001]

[43] E. Mbunge, and J. Batani, "Application of deep learning and machine learning models to improve healthcare in sub-Saharan Africa: Emerging opportunities, trends and implications", *Telematics and Informatics Reports,* vol. 11, p. 100097, 2023.
[http://dx.doi.org/10.1016/j.teler.2023.100097]

[44] P. Khatiwada, B. Yang, J.C. Lin, and B. Blobel, "Patient-Generated Health Data (PGHD): Understanding, Requirements, Challenges, and Existing Techniques for Data Security and Privacy", *J. Pers. Med.,* vol. 14, no. 3, p. 282, 2024.
[http://dx.doi.org/10.3390/jpm14030282] [PMID: 38541024]

[45] H.S. Kang, and M. Exworthy, "Wearing the Future—Wearables to Empower Users to Take Greater Responsibility for Their Health and Care: Scoping Review", *JMIR Mhealth Uhealth,* vol. 10, no. 7, p. e35684, 2022.
[http://dx.doi.org/10.2196/35684] [PMID: 35830222]

[46] S. Takahashi, E. Nakazawa, S. Ichinohe, A. Akabayashi, and A. Akabayashi, "Wearable Technology for Monitoring Respiratory Rate and SpO2 of COVID-19 Patients: A Systematic Review", *Diagnostics (Basel),* vol. 12, no. 10, p. 2563, 2022.
[http://dx.doi.org/10.3390/diagnostics12102563] [PMID: 36292252]

CHAPTER 4

Blockchain Technology in Healthcare

Kajal Jain[1,*] and **Sanjeev Rana**[1]

[1] *CSE Department, Maharishi Markandeshwar (Deemed to be University), Mullana, Haryana, India*

Abstract: Blockchain adoption in healthcare is changing the way in which medical information is managed, shared, and secured. As a distributed digital ledger, it helps solve big problems in healthcare, such as scattered data, privacy risks, and slow or inefficient exchange of records. With the help of cryptography and consensus mechanisms, blockchain ensures that records are permanent, transparent, and easy to track. Its applications are wide-ranging, covering Electronic Health Records (EHRs), drug supply chain tracking, insurance claims management, and protecting the accuracy of clinical trial data. Smart contracts can also automate routine tasks, reduce fraud, and cut down operating costs. A key advantage of blockchain is its decentralized design, which gives patients more control and access to their health information, supporting a patient-centered approach to care. However, there are still challenges, such as limited scalability. This chapter reviews current blockchain applications in healthcare, explains its transformative role in improving healthcare delivery, and discusses the technical, ethical, and legal barriers that must be addressed for wider adoption.

Keywords: Blockchain, Cryptography, Distributed ledger, Healthcare ecosystem, Smart contract.

INTRODUCTION

Definition of Blockchain Technology

The core concept of the blockchain is based on security, transparency, and decentralization. It was conceived by Satoshi Nakamoto in 2008, hyped as the backbone of the cryptocurrency Bitcoin, but its utility went far beyond digital currencies. Essentially, the blockchain is a distributed ledger, a continuously growing list of records, called blocks, which are linked and secured using cryptography. Each block normally includes a cryptographic hash of the prior block, a timestamp, and transaction data [1]. It is this structure that makes a blockchain inherently tamper-resistant. The "distributed" aspect is what underlies

* **Corresponding author Kajal Jain:** CSE Department, Maharishi Markandeshwar (Deemed to be University), Mullana, Haryana, India; +91-9253746103; E-mail: Kajal.mittal@mmumullana.org

Arun Kumar Rana, Mandeep Kaur & Sumit Kumar Rana (Eds.)

all the transformative potential of blockchain. While traditional, centrally stored databases rely on a single location to store information, blockchains are maintained by a network of computers, often referred to as nodes. Each node on the network has a complete copy of the blockchain, and the nodes update one another through a consensus mechanism. As such, there is no need for any central intermediary (a central authority) to ensure the data is valid and stored; this reduces vulnerability points and makes the system much more resilient. In many of its implementations, notably in cryptocurrencies, the verification and recording of transactions on a blockchain are done via a procedure called mining. Miners solve mathematical puzzles; this is normally how they are granted the right to add a new block to the chain. This process of Proof of Work ensures the integrity and chronological order of the blockchain. However, there are other consensus mechanisms like Proof of Stake, also widely used in numerous blockchain implementations, with their pros and cons [2]. Perhaps among the biggest features of blockchain technology is its own immutability. It is extremely hard for data to be changed retroactively once it has been recorded on a blockchain. This is because any change in a single block would involve changing all subsequent blocks after it and convincing the majority in the network to accept this changed version of the chain, something that gets more improbable as the chain goes on and gets longer. Such immutability, in addition to the intrinsic transparency and decentralization of the technology, makes blockchain particularly appealing in those applications that require highly trustworthy, secure, and integrity-assured data-management levels, especially in the healthcare sector [3]. Fig. (**1**) shows the structure of blockchain technology implemented with the help of the Merkle root tree.

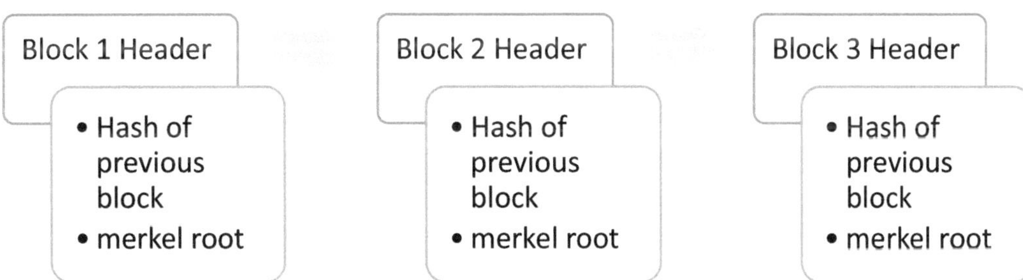

Fig. (1). Blockchain structure with Merkle root.

Brief Overview of Healthcare Industry Challenges

Healthcare is an important pillar of society, which faces everyday challenges that hinder true efficiency and optimization despite the innovation that continues. Major obstacles are data management and interoperability. Across the globe, healthcare systems struggle with fragmented and disconnected information. Data is dispersed among various hospitals, clinics, service providers, and Electronic

Health Record (EHR) platforms. This fragmented nature of data hampers the increase in the chances of medical errors, duplicate testing, coordinated care, and unnecessary expenditure [4]. The main contributing factors include the lack of standardized data formats and the unwillingness of stakeholders to share information. These issues make it difficult to achieve a comprehensive and unified view of a patient's medical history.

Closely linked to this problem are the concerns surrounding data privacy and security. With the steady digital transformation of healthcare, the volume of electronically stored patient data has grown tremendously. Although digitalization offers numerous benefits, it has also made healthcare systems prime targets for cyberattacks. High-profile data breaches have not only compromised patient confidentiality but have also created deep distrust regarding the ability of healthcare institutions to protect sensitive personal information [5 - 7]. Striking the right balance between enabling data sharing for improved care coordination and safeguarding it against unauthorized access remains a major challenge. Fig. (**2**) shows the centralized system of healthcare, which faces multiple challenges.

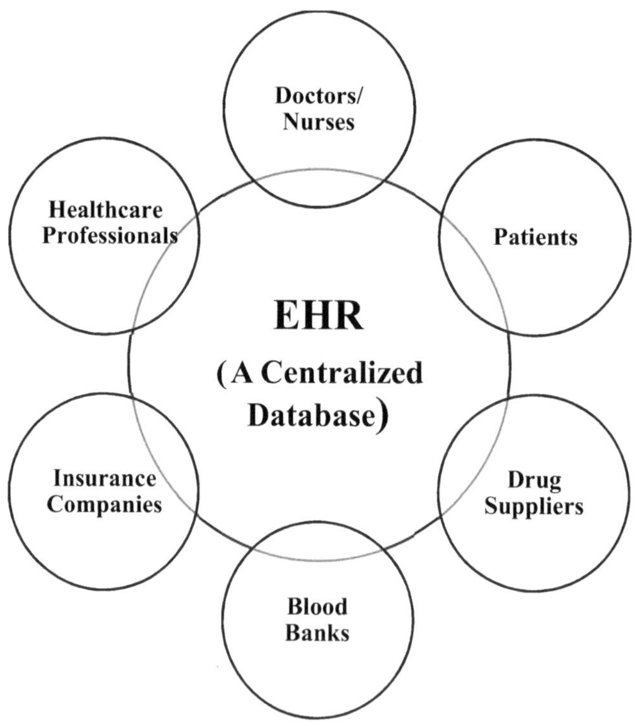

Fig. (2). Centralised healthcare system.

The problem is that global supply chains for medications, even in more regulated markets, are so complex that the full assurance of authenticity and quality throughout the entire process, from manufacturing and distribution to the end consumer, is a very difficult task [8]. Finally, the healthcare industry must address the challenge of knowledge management and utilization in the face of enormous amounts of information generated in research, clinical trials, and patient care. This could lead to medical breakthroughs and vastly improve patient outcomes [9]. However, data ownership, consent management, and the ability to securely share information across institutions and borders make the full realization of this potential difficult to achieve. A lack of incentives to share data and intellectual property concerns makes efforts to promote collaboration in medical research and development even more complicated. While daunting, these challenges also create opportunities for innovation. The following sections discuss how many of these matters can be potentially resolved using blockchain technology to really transform the handling, sharing, and security of healthcare data in the modern-day digital era [10].

CURRENT CHALLENGES IN HEALTHCARE THAT BLOCKCHAIN COULD ADDRESS

Even though it is a very critical and rapidly developing industry, the healthcare sector still faces many challenges, such as efficiency, effectiveness, and optimal patient care. Some of these challenges have certain solution proposals offered by blockchain technology because of its distinctive features. Let us take a closer look at some of the key ones:

Data Security and Privacy Issues

The healthcare sector has become a prime target for cyberattacks in this increasingly digitized world due to the nature of data handled within the industry. Health records of patients carry huge volumes of personal information, hence making them an attractive commodity for malicious actors [6]. Frequent data breaches of sensitive patient information, unauthorized access to EHRs, a balancing act in maintaining the confidentiality of patient data while providing necessary access for care providers, and compliance with stringent data protection regulations such as HIPAA in the United States and GDPR in Europe are major concerns [11]. Therefore, blockchain does have some characteristics that can help in data security: being highly decentralized and cryptographic. With its immutable ledger and advanced techniques of encryption, the data of any patient may become extremely hard to compromise by a hacker. In addition, it could empower patients with fine-grained access control over who has accessed their health information, thereby revolutionizing data privacy in healthcare [12].

Issues of Interoperability between Healthcare Systems

Different stakeholders in the ecosystem include hospitals, clinics, pharmacies, insurance providers, and others, using different systems for storing and managing data [7, 13]. These fragmentations result in huge interoperability issues. Current challenges include that siloed data systems inhibit efficient information sharing among healthcare providers, a lack of standardization in data formats and communication protocols, difficulty in creating a comprehensive patient health record across multiple providers, and inefficient and error-prone manual data reconciliation processes. Blockchain can act as an interoperability layer that provides a single, shared, distributed ledger for patient health information. This may allow frictionless, secure, and timely sharing of patient information across various healthcare providers, thus promoting care coordination and reducing errors due to a lack of information [14].

Drug Supply Chain Integrity

Supply chains for pharmaceutical products are long, with many players across the globe in various geographical regions. Supply chain integrity ensures the safety of patients and is crucial to public health [15]. Prevalence of counterfeit drugs in the global market, difficulties in tracing the origin and journey of pharmaceutical products, inefficient recall processes when issues are identified, and a lack of transparency into the supply chain result in fraud and errors. Blockchain can create an indelible mark on each and every instance of that particular movement of a drug throughout its supply chain. Every transaction in its life cycle, from manufacturing to distribution to dispensing, is recorded on the blockchain in a transparent, tamper-proof audit trail that reduces the infiltration of counterfeit drugs [16]. This would go a long way in reducing massive infiltration of counterfeit drugs and enabling fast, targeted recalls when necessary.

Claims and Billing Inefficiencies

Generally, health care billing and the claims process are very complex and inefficient, generating extraordinarily high administrative burdens or costs and delaying payment [17]. Current challenges facing the healthcare industry include a high rate of billing errors and claim denials, long times to process insurance claims, a lack of transparency in the billing process for patients, and vulnerability to fraud and abuse in the claims process. Smart contracts on a blockchain network could automate much of the claims process. They could check, in real time, insurance coverages, patient eligibility, and the procedure code. This may reduce processing time and minimize errors. The nature of blockchain systems can then help trace potential fraud attempts and prevent fraudulent claims because all transactions would be visible and trackable within the network [18].

In this context, a blockchain brings in the opportunity to enable new ways of health delivery with better patient outcomes by reducing cost and inefficiency. In the following sections, we shall try to delve into the details as to how each of these challenges can be met with blockchain technology, along with opportunities and hurdles in the way. Fig. (**3**) explains the working of the healthcare system using a smart contract through blockchain technology.

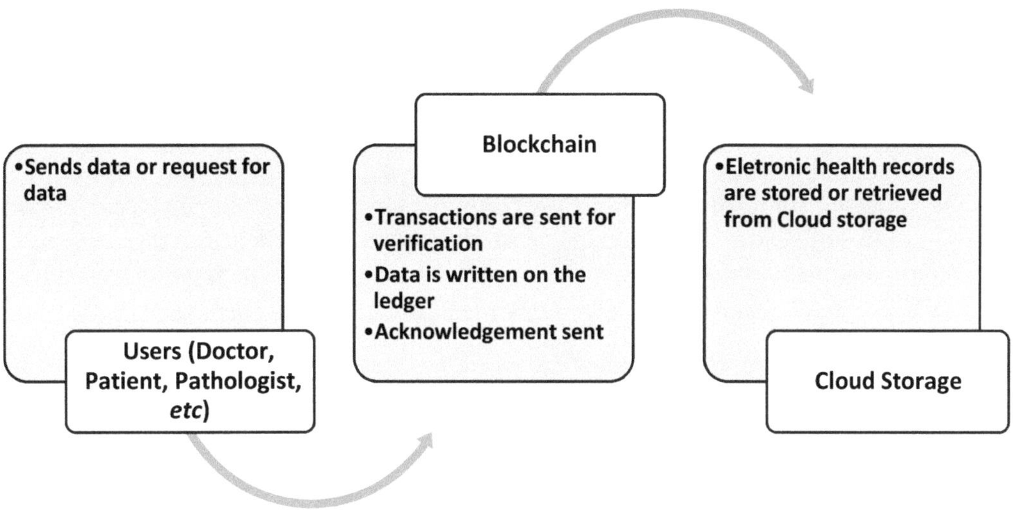

Fig. (3). Working of a decentralised Blockchain-based healthcare system.

POTENTIAL OF BLOCKCHAIN TO ADDRESS HEALTHCARE CHALLENGES

Blockchain is, therefore, emerging as the effective answer to the deep-seated challenges in healthcare. This technology is novel for healthcare in all respects: decentralized, immutable, transparent, and secure. First and foremost, blockchain is a robust answer to data fragmentation and interoperability. It can serve as an interoperability layer between the various healthcare systems by developing a shared, decentralized ledger of patient information [19]. In a blockchain-based healthcare ecosystem, every interaction involving a patient, diagnosis, or treatment could be etched on the chain as a kind of transaction to create a comprehensive chronological health record. This guarantees consistency of data across providers and allows real-time updating and viewing of patient information, thus enabling more coordinated and better-informed delivery of care. Further, the application of smart contracts--self-executing contracts with the terms of the agreement written directly into lines of code--can ensure that specified datasets are automatically shared in a secure fashion based on predetermined and pre-programmed rules [20]. This can further facilitate interoperability while ensuring strict access controls. And in tackling important issues such as data privacy and security, the cryptographic origins of blockchain come with a host of advantages. Every transaction within a blockchain is thus encrypted and linked to the previous transaction in such a way that the audit trail that is automatically generated becomes very difficult to alter retroactively [21]. This aspect of immutability will go a long way in reducing the risk of medical record tampering and unauthorized changes. Moreover, blockchain provides much finer-grained access to who has the key to the data through its use of public-private keys. Patients would be given control over who can access their medical data if they utilize that capability to grant and rescind access to their information, placing the patients in charge of their health information and dampening ongoing debates about ownership and management of consent regarding patient data. The inefficiencies that characterize general healthcare administration could be greatly reduced with the implementation of blockchain. On a blockchain network, smart contracts can automate a good portion of the claims adjudication process, real-time verification of insurance coverage, patient eligibility, and procedure codes [22]. This could well reduce processing times considerably, minimize errors, and reduce administrative costs to a large extent. Besides, transparency built into blockchain systems should deter and detect fraudulent claims since all transactions would become virtually visible and traceable in the network. Indeed, blockchain technology appears as a very viable answer to some insurmountable problems of pharmaceutical supply chain management. It could create an immutable, transparent record of the entire supply chain by recording each step of a drug's journey, right from its manufacturing to its distribution and dispensing, on the blockchain. Transparency to this level would make it exponentially more difficult to allow counterfeit drugs into the supply chain since any attempt to introduce fake products would immediately be detectable [23]. Also, in the case of recalls, blockchain would enable rapid tracking with full accuracy of the batches involved and could save lives while retaining the effort of recall to the minimum scope and cost. Finally, blockchain has the potential to disrupt medical research and clinical trials: offering a secure, transparent platform for sharing research data, blockchain enables collaboration among institutions while ensuring the integrity of the data [24]. Clinical trials might have smart contracts automate processes of informed consent by patients, thereby ensuring that personal data could be used only in the ways agreed. Similarly, the immutability of records on the blockchain may further enhance trial result credibility, since the entire research process, from protocol design to data collection and analysis, might be performed in a tamper-resistant way. It is huge, but this potential of blockchain in healthcare must be put into perspective-the benefits will be fully realized after addressing a set of technical, regulatory, and adoption challenges [25]. As we embark on discussing each of the application areas in detail in subsequent chapters, we shall explore not only the transformative potential of blockchain but also the hurdles to be overcome for its successful implementation in the health sector.

BLOCKCHAIN APPLICATIONS IN HEALTHCARE

Electronic Health Record Management

Electronic Health Records are the digital version of the paper chart, containing the patient's medical history from a single doctor's office or an organization that delivers health care. They are intended to be shared immediately and securely with anyone authorized to look at them--eventually enabling access by and sharing between patients, health care providers, and payers. Although EHRs have gone a long way towards improving health delivery, issues relating to their interoperability, security, and control by the patient do pose concerns that may be benefited by blockchain technologies. Blockchain technology is thus touted as one that will revolutionize the management of EHRs [26].

Enhancing Interoperability

The biggest challenge facing healthcare is the inability of EHR systems to interoperate with one another. Now, blockchain can resolve this in several ways: Blockchain can serve as a shared, decentralized ledger on which different providers of healthcare add and view patient data [27], thus offering a single source of truth-a 'single version of the truth'-on the health history of a patient. If the data is to be put on a blockchain in a standardized format, interoperability among such systems can be enabled. Automation of data exchange between different healthcare providers can also be developed using smart contracts, which again can ensure that the right information is available to those entities at the right time. With blockchain, secure data sharing would be enabled across a range of healthcare institutions, hence enhancing coordination of care for patients receiving treatment from multiple providers [28].

Enhancing Data Security and Privacy

The nature of blockchain means that the security and privacy of EHRs can be enhanced immensely. All data on the blockchain is encrypted; this institutes a high level of security against unauthorized access. All access and modifications to a patient's record are logged in a blockchain to create an immutable audit trail and, therefore, increase accountability, aiding in the prevention of unauthorized changes [29]. Blockchain distributes data across a network of nodes that eliminates single-point failures common in centralized systems, hence making it more resistant to hacks and data breaches. It enables blockchain to support fine-grained access control, whereby a patient can define which parts of the health record can be accessed by which entity.

Empower Patient Control

Blockchain can help in the paradigm shift toward a more patient-centric model of management of EHRs. In blockchain-based EHRs, patients would have possession and ownership of their health records along with the right to decide on access and its revocation [30]. Patients may give consent over specific usages of data using digital signatures, which are recorded on the blockchain. Since the blockchain serves as a source of a common record, it would be quite easy for patients to share their complete health history when switching between healthcare providers or even for the purpose of second opinions. Blockchain might allow the integration of data from a personal health device or application into the formal EHR so that the latter would provide the healthcare professional with a comprehensive and integrated view of the patient's health [31].

Data Integrity

Immutability through Blockchain will ensure that the health records are not tampered with. Inherent in the concept of blockchain, as all blocks are connected, implies that any falsification in a record would alter subsequent blocks, a falsification that is thus easily detectable. Blockchain keeps a transparent history of changes that have been made to a health record, documenting the health history of a patient. Blockchain tracks the origin of every single piece of health data to ensure knowledge of where information comes from, hence ensuring information is trusted [32].

Challenges and Considerations

Although blockchain holds tremendous promise for handling EHRs, some challenges persist. The amount of data generated within a health care system is enormous. Ensuring the volume that blockchain systems can manage is an important challenge. For implementing blockchain-based EHR, integration with the existing healthcare IT infrastructure is required. Any blockchain-based EHR platform would have to be HIPAA-compliant. While the blockchain itself can maintain access permissions and audit logs, large medical files such as imaging studies are impractical to store directly on the blockchain. Hybrid systems may thus be required in this respect, which includes off-chain storage [33]. Fig. (**4**) describes the healthcare challenges and blockchain opportunities.

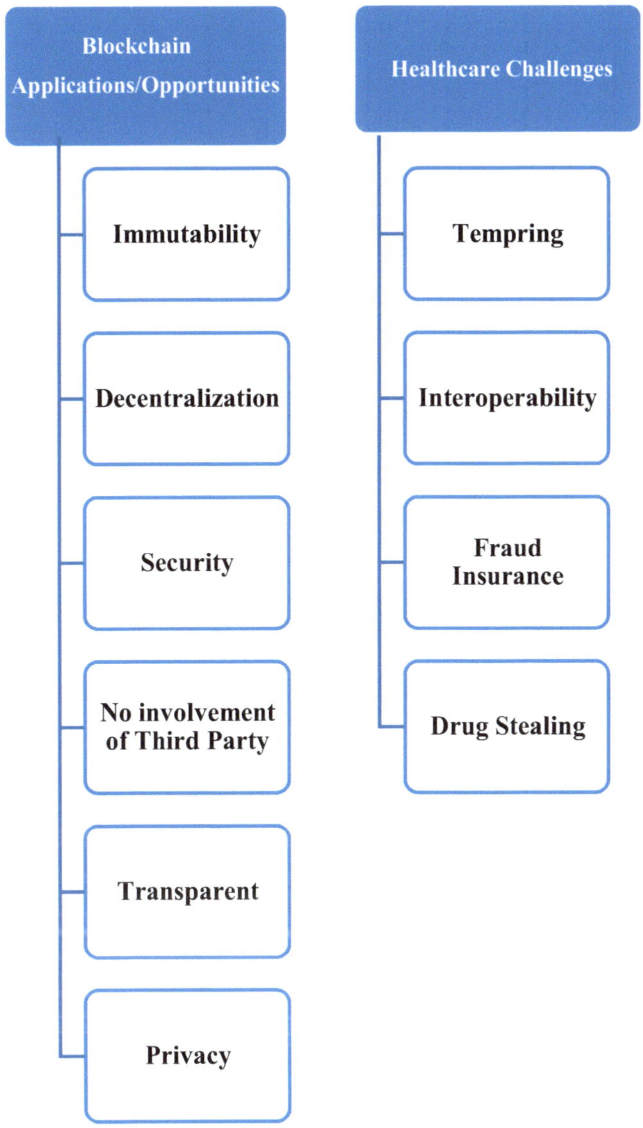

Fig. (4). Healthcare challenges and blockchain opportunities.

However, considering these challenges, the potential of blockchain to generate EHR systems that are, in turn, more interoperable, secure, and patient-centric, thus making it one of the promising technologies for the future of healthcare data management. It would be expected to see more adoptions of blockchain-based EHR solutions within the healthcare industry when the technology matures further and as many of these challenges are sorted out.

Supply Chain Management for Pharmaceuticals

The pharmaceutical supply chain is immensely complex due to the diversified geographical location of its different stakeholders. This implies that it faces a host of problems, including drug counterfeiting, inefficient tracking, and a lack of transparency. Blockchain technology has promising solutions for these issues that may actually revolutionize the management of pharmaceutical supply chains. One of the main uses of blockchain in pharmaceutical supply chain management is enhancing the traceability of drugs and fighting against counterfeit medication [34]. Blockchain can create an immutable record of a drug's journey from the manufacturer to the patient. Every transaction within the supply chain, from production all the way through to distribution and dispensing, can be recorded as a block in the chain. Every package of drugs could be assigned a unique identifier, like a serial number or barcode, that is recorded on the blockchain. The identifier can be scanned at every point in the supply chain to update the status and location of a particular drug. Smart contracts can be used for automatic verification of drugs at every stage of the supply chain. If any discrepancy is found, there can be automated notifications to the relevant parties. This may allow patients or pharmacists to scan the bar code on a drug to verify its authenticity and its entire path in the supply chain for added confidence and safety [35].

Enhanced Efficiency in Recall

Blockchain can significantly contribute to efficiency in the process of a drug recall by being far more accurate in such an event. It could identify with precision exactly which batches were afflicted and where they were within the supply chain. Smart contracts, upon the initiation of a recall, would automatically trigger notifications of the recall to relevant parties-distributors, pharmacies, patients, and so forth. Because the blockchain records all transactions, the progress of recall efforts can be tracked in real time to ensure that every affected product is accounted for. Blockchain could also be used to optimize pharmaceutical inventory management [36]. With a real-time view of inventory levels across the supply chain, blockchain can help prevent stockouts and overstocking. With a complete, accurate record of drug movements, blockchain data could be used to enhance demand forecasting and production planning. Because blockchain monitors the expiration dates of drugs, it helps in the reduction of waste by ensuring that the older stock is used up first.

Maintaining Compliance with Legislation

Blockchain can enable regulatory requirements to be supported. The traceability features of blockchain align quite well with regulations like the Drug Supply Chain Security Act, which ensures prescription drugs are traceable within the

United States. In the case of drugs reliant on specific conditions in storage, IoT sensors could register temperature data directly into the blockchain and ensure that this aspect of storage requirements for such drugs has been fulfilled along the supply chain [37]. Smart contracts can automate the creation and submission of required reports to regulators, thereby reducing administrative burdens and delinquencies.

Supply Chain Efficiency Enhancement

Besides security and compliance, blockchain can make supply chains more effective overall. Smart contracts can automatically execute payment when certain pre-defined conditions or criteria are met, say, an acknowledgement of delivery. While this helps reduce delay in payments and disputes in general, by having the very same information that is current on the status of the supply chain, coordination between manufacturers, distributors, and retailers can be significantly improved. Blockchain can digitize and automate a lot of the paper-based processes in a supply chain and reduce administrative costs and errors [38].

Challenges and Considerations

While it does hold immense promise for the management of pharmaceutical supply chains, a number of challenges persist. First, its implementation involves integrating blockchain into the prevailing systems and processes of supply chain management [39]. Till now, an effective blockchain through the supply chain requires standards for sharing data and protocols for smart contracts. While blockchain does provide enhanced security, careful attention to what data is kept on-chain and off-chain should be done with due diligence to remain in conformance with data privacy regulations. The implementation and adoption must be performed by all stakeholders throughout the supply chain in pharmaceuticals [40].

With these challenges in mind, the potential of blockchain to create more secure, efficient, and transparent pharmaceutical supply chains makes it a promising technology for future healthcare. Once the technology matures and these challenges are overcome, we will see more blockchain-based solutions adopted in the management of pharmaceutical supply chains.

Clinical Trial Data Management

Clinical trials are basic building blocks of medical knowledge and treatment development, while a lot of challenges arise on issues of data integrity, privacy of patients, and efficiency in dealing with data. Blockchain promises much in such areas and may disrupt the way this information from clinical trials is handled.

More Granular Data Integrity and Transparency

Data integrity and transparency form one of the most important aspects of blockchain in clinical trials. Every data entry and modification occurring in a clinical trial can be recorded as a transaction on the blockchain, creating an audit trail that is immutable [39]. It would practically be impossible to retroactively alter any of the data without detection. Blockchain will ensure tamper-proof time-stamping of all data entries, thus guaranteeing chronological integrity of the trial data. Smart contracts could automatically enforce the clinical trial protocol, confirming whether data entry and processes have been executed in accordance with what was agreed upon in advance. Real-time access to trial data by relevant parties would enable increased transparency and allow for early analysis and decision-making.

Strengthening Patient Privacy and Consent Management

With blockchain, there is a significant improvement in maintaining patient privacy and consent management in clinical trials. While it's not advisable to store sensitive patient data on a blockchain chain directly due to privacy concerns, blockchain can be used to manage access to anonymized patient records kept off-chain. It will give the patients fine-grained control over their data. Smart contracts can administer consent by which patients can grant or refuse access to part or all of the data at any moment in time. Events related to patient consent can be tracked on the blockchain; every event of who consented for what and when is clearly attributable. Smart contracts can check that no use of patient data exceeds the consent provided and automatically block unauthorized use of data [41].

Improve Recruitment and Retention

Blockchain can accelerate and streamline patient recruitment, thereby improving retention. Blockchain can maintain a decentralized database of potential participants in trials and hence facilitate screening for appropriate candidates with preservation of patient privacy. Smart contracts can automate the process of screening potential participants against trial criteria and accelerate the recruitment process. Blockchain can manage and track patient incentives, such as the timely issuance of payments for participation, with complete transparency. Blockchain thus allows greater collaboration and sharing of data in multi-centre trials [42]. With blockchain, the sharing of trial data between various research centres will be safely done, thereby fostering collaboration with data integrity. Blockchains that enforce standardized data formats further enhance the interoperability of systems used in multi-center trials. Access rights can be managed by the smart contract, so that each collaborator can see only the data they are supposed to have.

Blockchain can enable regulatory processes in clinical trials to be more efficient. Smart contracts could automate the creation of regulatory reports, ensuring that all required data is present and submitted on time. Regulators can be given permissioned access to the blockchain for such records, thus easily verifying the integrity and completeness of trial data. Auditing processes could highly simplify the immutable audit trails created by blockchain, likely reducing time and costs involved in regulatory audits.

Challenges and Considerations

While blockchain provides a significant opportunity regarding the management of clinical trial data, challenges also exist. Any blockchain solution will have to conform to data privacy regulations such as GDPR and HIPAA. This may involve creative methods of storing and controlling access to the data. Clinical trials generate volumes of data. This, therefore, presents one of the challenges in ensuring that blockchain systems can efficiently manage such a volume [43]. Implementation of blockchain would, therefore, imply the incorporation of existing clinical trial management systems and processes. Standards for data sharing and smart contract protocols would have to be developed for blockchain to be effective across various trials and research centres. Engagement requires educative approaches and buy-in by stakeholders: the researchers, participants, and regulators.

Despite these challenges, the potential of blockchain to create more transparent, secure, and efficient clinical trials is promising for future medical research. As the technology matures through overcoming these challenges, we will be able to realize increased adoption of blockchain-based solutions in clinical trial data management.

KEY BENEFITS OF IMPLEMENTING BLOCKCHAIN TECHNOLOGY IN HEALTHCARE

More Security Regarding Data and Privacy

Cryptography protocols of Blockchain make the platform very secure for maintaining data related to patients. Any transaction or entry of data is encrypted and is interlinked with the previously entered data; thus, it makes it practically impossible to manipulate the records without leaving traces. This could drastically reduce data breaches in healthcare, which, unfortunately, are quite common and often very costly. It might be challenging, though, to implement systems based on blockchain that support the existing privacy regulations in healthcare, like HIPAA in the US or GDPR in Europe. There is also a question regarding how to handle the "right to be forgotten" under GDPR, given the immutable nature of blockchain [44].

Improved Interoperability

Today, most of them have several, usually incompatible EHR systems installed. A blockchain system could offer a single, secure layer for data exchange among these. Care coordination, especially for patients with complex conditions that require seeing multiple specialists, would be particularly improved since each of them uses a different system. The challenge here is to get different healthcare organizations to agree on standards of data sharing and invest in compatible systems. Add to that the technical challenge of scalability: healthcare generates enormous amounts of data, and current blockchain technologies might already struggle with efficient handling.

Drug Traceability

Blockchain can offer an end-to-end tracking system starting from raw materials to manufacturing and, finally, to distribution. It could prevent drug counterfeiting, as noted, which is one of the major health issues nowadays around the world. Any implementation requires collaboration among all actors in the pharmaceutical supply chain: manufacturers, distributors, pharmacies, and regulators. The integration in existing tracking systems and compliance with various national and international regulations are also to be performed [45].

Clinical Trial Management

To that extent, it could provide a tamper-proof record of clinical trial protocols, patient consent, and data collected. It would also make trial results more credible, since they would be more transparent, and perhaps speed up the approval process of new drugs [46]. However, there's a lot of concern about how such a system would protect patient privacy, especially in sensitive trials. Another question is who would control and have access to this blockchain: the pharmaceutical companies, researchers, regulators, or some combination thereof.

Claims and Billing Processing

Smart contracts on a blockchain could automate much of the claims process with potentially fewer errors, fraud, and administrative costs. For example, a smart contract could check whether a treatment is covered under a patient's insurance and automatically forward the claim to the appropriate party. Implementation of such a system would require major changes in existing health-care billing systems and practices. It would also need to be flexible enough to handle the complexities like insurance rules and exceptions [47]. These are just a few areas in which blockchain could potentially revolutionize healthcare. But let's not get carried away: blockchain isn't a panacea. Overall, some of the challenges its implementation faces are: regulatory compliance-healthcare is a highly regulated field, and blockchain systems would need to work within an existing labyrinthine web of regulations; technical challenges-scalability, energy use for proof-of-work blockchains, and integration with legacy systems are concerns that need to be ironed out; while blockchain does greatly enhance security, there are apprehensions regarding patient privacy protection, especially sensitive health data; the cost and length of time it takes to overhaul current systems for blockchain inclusion are holding factors in its adoption; and there is a need for healthcare professionals to adopt new blockchain-based systems, which could be quite a task.

For all these challenges, many believe that blockchain might play a substantial role in improving health care management and delivery. Realization of such great potential would demand prudent planning, substantial investment, and collaboration across the health ecosystem.

CHALLENGES AND LIMITATIONS OF BLOCKCHAIN ADOPTION IN HEALTHCARE

Technical Challenges

Scalability

Health systems generate huge volumes of data. The existing blockchain systems can hardly scale to efficiently store and process this amount of data. Transaction speed is again a problem: most blockchains process transactions much more slowly than traditional databases do. Such conditions can be devastating in urgent healthcare situations. Over time, the size of the blockchain grows, and with it, the increased storage requirement for each node may result in unwanted centralization since fewer entities would be able to run full nodes.

Energy Use

Several blockchain networks apply consensus mechanisms of Proof-of-Work, which are very energy-intensive. While blockchains in health may apply more environmentally friendly consensus mechanisms, such as Proof-of-Stake, even these require resources in the form of computers [47]. On a large scale, the environmental footprint of blockchain adoption across the health sector could be enormous and even run directly against the sustainability goals of our time.

Interoperability

Ensuring that different blockchain systems can communicate with each other, as well as with already existing healthcare IT infrastructure, is a major technical hurdle. Standardization of data formats and protocols among various blockchain platforms in healthcare is very desirable; their actual implementation is very hard to achieve.

Regulatory and Compliance Issues

If applied to regulatory compliances like HIPAA in the USA, GDPR in the EU, or PIPEDA in Canada, blockchain has a very transparent and immutable nature that makes compliance cumbersome. The "right to be forgotten" under GDPR is in conflict with the immutability of the blockchain. A few jurisdictions restrict health information from being taken out of country borders, which can be difficult to implement with decentralized blockchains. In most jurisdictions, it is still unclear whether healthcare-related smart contracts on a blockchain are legally enforceable. In this regard, blockchain-based healthcare solutions may need to invest a lot of time getting through bodies like the FDA, which will, in turn, delay overall adoption [48].

Adoption Barriers and Resistance to Change

Because of the huge investments made in existing systems, health care organizations may be resistant or leery of the wholesale changes required to accommodate blockchain. Due to the critical nature of their service, the healthcare industry is often very conservative in the adoption of new technologies. Transitioning to blockchain-based systems would require substantial financial investment, perhaps limiting it for many health care providers. The return on investment for blockchain in healthcare is not clearly seen; hence, its cost is hard to justify. There is a shortage of blockchain experts in the healthcare industry; hence, there is difficulty in implementation and maintenance. In any case, training health professionals to use blockchain-based systems would be a daunting task. Success in implementation requires the cooperation of key stakeholders-providers, insurers, patients, and regulators-each of whom has a different interest and concern. In itself, this is quite a multi-dimensional challenge: it requires convincing all parties of the benefits while addressing specific misgivings. Second, there is a huge challenge in migrating existing healthcare data into blockchain systems, given the quantity and sensitivity of such data. Maintaining integrity and continuity of this data during migration is paramount yet challenging [49]. The interfaces for blockchain may be less user-friendly compared to existing systems, and this could provide a significant amount of resistance for healthcare professionals. Blockchain is representative of a big change from centralized control that has dominated data in health, and such a shift may face resistance from those who have benefited from such control.

These challenges are, however, not impossible to surmount. In the process of solving them, there will be a need for collaboration between technologists, healthcare professionals, policymakers, and other stakeholders. Most of these barriers will fade away with increased successful use cases as blockchain technology matures. Careful consideration of these challenges is indeed very necessary in the case of any organization thinking about the adoption of blockchain in health care.

FUTURE OUTLOOK FOR BLOCKCHAIN IN HEALTHCARE

The future landscape for blockchain in healthcare is an intoxicating blend of promising prospects and emergent challenges. Let's look at some of the recent trends, innovations, and possible impacts:

Trends and Innovations Coming Up

While EHRs are becoming the norm, DHRs could take it to the next step in making patients the sole guardians of their personal health information. Granular access to data, or the ability to allow and deny permissions in a granular fashion, can be provided to the patient. This will increase privacy and data sharing for patients. Integrating AI with blockchain might enable the secure and decentralized analysis of huge amounts of healthcare data. This could accelerate drug discovery, improve the diagnosis, and allow for more personalized treatment. Blockchain can secure and manage wearable device and home health monitoring equipment data. It will thus facilitate better remote patient monitoring and preventive care. Incentivizing patients to share anonymized health data for research using cryptocurrency tokens would be one way. This could increase the amount of data available in medical research manifold while considering the privacy of patients [50]. Global telemedicine would be possible on secure, blockchain-based platforms. Payment automation and regulatory compliance across borders might be possible with smart contracts.

Potential Impact on Healthcare Delivery and Patient Outcomes

The result would be that the blockchain-based health records would easily be shared with the patient's entire history by him or her with any provider. It would reduce medical errors, avoid duplicate tests, and improve treatment decisions in certain life emergencies. More significantly, if they are allowed to exercise more control over access and the use of health data, patients may become highly motivated and more involved in their healthcare. Consequently, it would result in better adherence to treatment plans and allow improvement in health outcomes. It can accelerate clinical trials and drug development by enabling secure data sharing of anonymized patient data, bringing new treatments faster and with less expense to market [51]. Together, blockchain and AI can enable more precise treatment plans, tailored to the genetic profile of a patient and medical history. Blockchain can also offer the advantage of real-time sharing of anonymized health data in a secure manner. This will, in turn, enable quicker and better responses by the officials in the fields of public health in case of any disease outbreak or other health-related calamities. By reducing fraud, administrative processes, and other wastages through blockchain, the overall cost of healthcare may be reduced, which can be transferred to the patients or reinvested in care. Blockchain can be used for making portable, secure health records for refugees and displaced persons. This could also guarantee a more balanced distribution of medical resources within less industrialized countries. The immutability of blockchain can bring greater confidence in healthcare systems and clinical research. This may boost participation in clinical trials and adherence to public health recommendations [52].

Of course, all these potential impacts are quite promising, but it has to be taken into account that all these potential impacts will have to be realized, and there are a number of challenges, as discussed earlier. Quite naturally, it is quite difficult to predict the timeline regarding wide-scale blockchain adoption in healthcare; this most probably will differ depending on the region or exact use case. Moreover, there might be some unintended consequences, as with any transformative technology, which is quite hard to predict. For example, more widespread data sharing could accelerate medical discovery but also create novel privacy hazards or even exacerbate health inequities if not done thoughtfully. The future of blockchain in health is more integrative than disruptive. Indeed, the early successes in niche applications may herald more broad-based adoption. This could be a path where, with time, blockchain continues to mature, and the stakeholders in healthcare get comfortable; it becomes integral to the infrastructure of healthcare, working quietly in the background to make it more efficient, secure, and patient-centred.

ETHICAL CONSIDERATIONS

Ethical issues are the most crucial in implementing blockchain technology into healthcare. Indeed, these two aspects you have identified are central: data ownership and control, and equity and access issues. Let me consider them in more detail:

Data Ownership and Control

While the potential to allow patients to be in full control over their health data is complementary to the ethical principle of respect for autonomy, blockchain-based tokenization can also advance informed consent by giving patients more granular choices about who may access and use their data, for what purpose. Tokenization may also allow the selling of personal health information, again raising a set of ethical issues relating to commodification. Economically precarious individuals may feel compelled to compromise their privacy, selling their data because they have little other choice. The "right to be forgotten" applicable under some privacy laws contrasts with the immutability of Blockchain. This presents a major ethical challenge in balancing data permanence with an individual's right to erasure of their data. There are also questions regarding what happens to an individual's blockchain-based health record after that person has died. This raises complex issues related to digital inheritance and privacy rights after death. Special considerations exist about handling and protecting the health data of children on a blockchain. This would include questions of when and how control of the data should transition from parent to child.

Equity and Access Issues

Blockchain-based healthcare systems run the very real risk of excluding those without reliable internet access, let alone the technical skills to navigate such systems. This can exacerbate existing health disparities, particularly for the elderly, rural, and poor populations. If blockchain increases the cost of healthcare, then access would be further reduced for economically poor classes. Conversely, if blockchain decreases healthcare costs, then access could improve. While blockchain will enhance the portability of health records among refugees and migrants, it also raises several questions relating to issues of data sovereignty and cross-border data regimes [53]. That would suggest that blockchain might have a better potential to make improvements in drug supply chains in developing countries, but it needs a considerable investment in infrastructure. If AI combined with blockchain for health data analysis is pursued, then there is a risk of perpetuation or amplification of the biases already existing in healthcare. The training datasets in such systems have to be representative of a diverse population. It means the blockchain interfaces need to be multilingual and culturally apt for equitable access. For blockchain health systems to be accessible, designs must be inclusive to avoid exclusion of people with disabilities. All users are entitled, as part of an ethical imperative, to appreciate how their data is used and stored on the blockchain; this will need huge investment in public education and clear communication strategies. While blockchain could increase democratization in medical research participation, on the other hand, it also raises concerns about the over- and underrepresentation of certain groups within the population. Other essential factors pertain to the equity of benefiting from the research outcome. These ethical considerations are best addressed from a multidisciplinary perspective that includes technologists, healthcare providers, ethicists, patient advocates, policymakers, and others representing diverse communities. Some possible strategies include the following:

- Developing robust governance frameworks, focusing on patient rights with data protection.
- Progressive data control features will evolve as individuals mature or as their circumstances change.
- Design education that improves digital literacy and blockchain understanding among different populations.
- Development of blockchain systems that inherently possess the features for accessibility and multilingual support.
- Ethics guidelines on using health data for research and commercial purposes.
- Blockchain implementations in healthcare must be governed with continuous ethical review and adjustment.

By carefully considering such ethical dimensions, we can work toward blockchain implementation in health that improves efficiency and security but also furthers equity, respects individual rights, and thereby contributes to better health for all. In the end, it is in improving patient outcomes, enhancing the healthcare experience, and making quality healthcare more accessible for all that the success of blockchain in healthcare will be truly measured. In spite of the major challenges, the potential benefits make blockchain a very attractive technology for the future of healthcare.

CONCLUSION

Blockchain can enable a myriad of advancements in some of the most overriding issues in modern healthcare: data security, interoperability, and patient-centric management of health information. Blockchain promises better integrity and traceability of medical records with its fundamentally decentralized, immutable ledger, smoother claims settlement processes, and easy sharing of research data securely. But scalability, regulations, and integration of these new systems will be challenges that one needs to overcome for broad-scale adoption. Over time, as these are surmounted and the technology matures, there is immense potential for blockchain to impact healthcare delivery in terms of improvement in patient outcomes and operational efficiency. Blockchain needs continuous research, pilots, and collaborations between various stakeholders to achieve its full potential in healthcare.

REFERENCES

[1] T. Benil, J. J. C. N. Jasper, 'Cloud based security on outsourcing using blockchain in E-health systems', Computer Networks 178 (2020): 107344, 2020. [http://dx.doi.org/10.1016/j.comnet.2020.107344]

[2] U. Chelladurai, and S. Pandian, "A novel blockchain based electronic health record automation system for healthcare", *J. Ambient Intell. Humaniz. Comput.*, pp. 1-11, 2021.

[3] J. Vora, A. Nayyar, S. Tanwar, S. Tyagi, N. Kumar, M.S Obaidat, J.J Rodrigues, 'BHEEM: A blockchain-based framework for securing electronic health records', In 2018 IEEE Globecom Workshops (GC Wkshps), pp. 1-6, IEEE, Dec., 2018. [http://dx.doi.org/10.1109/GLOCOMW.2018.8644088]

[4] D.C. Nguyen, P.N. Pathirana, M. Ding, and A. Seneviratne, "Blockchain for secure ehrs sharing of mobile cloud-based e-health systems", *IEEE Access,* vol. 7, pp. 66792-66806, 2019. [http://dx.doi.org/10.1109/ACCESS.2019.2917555]

[5] V. Jaiman, and V. Urovi, "A consent model for blockchain-based health data sharing platforms", *IEEE Access,* vol. 8, pp. 143734-143745, 2020. [http://dx.doi.org/10.1109/ACCESS.2020.3014565]

[6] A. Fernandes, V. Rocha, A.F da Conceição, F. Horita, 'Scalable Architecture for sharing EHR using the Hyperledger Blockchain', In 2020 IEEE International Conference on Software Architecture Companion (ICSA-C), pp. 130-138, IEEE, March 2020.

[7] F. Tang, S. Ma, Y. Xiang, and C. Lin, "An efficient authentication scheme for blockchain-based electronic health records", *IEEE Access,* vol. 7, pp. 41678-41689, 2019. [http://dx.doi.org/10.1109/ACCESS.2019.2904300]

[8] H. Guo, W. Li, E. Meamari, C. Shen, and M. Nejad, "Attribute-based multi- signature and encryption for ehr management: A blockchain-based solution", *2020 IEEE International Conference on Blockchain and Cryptocurrency (ICBC),* pp. 1-5, 2020. [http://dx.doi.org/10.1109/ICBC48266.2020.9169395]

[9] R. Guo, H. Shi, Q. Zhao, and D. Zheng, "'Secure attribute-based signature scheme with multiple authorities for blockchain in electronic health records systems", *IEEE Access,* vol. 6, pp. 11676-11686, 2018. [http://dx.doi.org/10.1109/ACCESS.2018.2801266]

[10] C. Priya, "Enabling the efficiency of Blockchain Technology in Tele- Healthcare with Enhanced EMR", *2020 International Conference on Computer Science, Engineering and Applications (ICCSEA),* IEEE, pp. 1-6, 2020.

[11] M. Antwi, A. Adnane, F. Ahmad, R. Hussain, M. H. ur Rehman, C. A. Kerrache, 'The Case of HyperLedger Fabric as a Blockchain Solution for Healthcare Applications', Blockchain: Research and Applications, 100012, March 2021.

[12] M. Zarour, M.T.J. Ansari, M. Alenezi, A.K. Sarkar, M. Faizan, A. Agrawal, R. Kumar, and R.A. Khan, "M, A. Agrawal, R. A. Khan, 'Evaluating the impact of blockchain models for secure and trustworthy electronic healthcare records'", *IEEE Access,* vol. 8, pp. 157959-157973, 2020. [http://dx.doi.org/10.1109/ACCESS.2020.3019829]

[13] Y. Zhuang, L.R. Sheets, Y.W. Chen, Z.Y. Shae, J.J.P. Tsai, and C.R. Shyu, "'A patient-centric health information exchange framework using blockchain technology'", *IEEE J. Biomed. Health Inform.,* vol. 24, no. 8, pp. 2169-2176, 2020. [http://dx.doi.org/10.1109/JBHI.2020.2993072] [PMID: 32396110]

[14] B. Sharma, R. Halder, and J. Singh, "Blockchain-based interoperable healthcare using zero-knowledge proofs and proxy re-encryption", *2020 International Conference on Communication Systems & Networks (COMSNETS),* pp. 1-6, 2020. [http://dx.doi.org/10.1109/COMSNETS48256.2020.9027413]

[15] Y. Wang, A. Zhang, P. Zhang, and H. Wang, "Cloud-assisted EHR sharing with security and privacy preservation via consortium blockchain", *IEEE Access,* vol. 7, pp. 136704-136719, 2019. [http://dx.doi.org/10.1109/ACCESS.2019.2943153]

[16] Y. Wang, M. He, 'CPDS: A Cross-Blockchain Based Privacy-Preserving Data Sharing for Electronic Health Records', In 2021 IEEE 6th International Conference on Cloud Computing and Big Data Analytics (ICCCBDA), pp. 90-99 IEEE, April 2021. [http://dx.doi.org/10.1109/ICCCBDA51879.2021.9442539]

[17] W. Jiamsawat, C. Choksuchat, S. Matayong, 'Blockchain-Based Electronic Medical Records Management of Hospital Emergency Ward', In 2021 International Conference on COMmunication Systems & NETworkS (COMSNETS), pp. 674-679, IEEE, January 2021. [http://dx.doi.org/10.1109/ICCCBDA51879.2021.9442539]

[18] Y. Wang, M. He, 'CPDS: A Cross-Blockchain Based Privacy-Preserving Data Sharing for Electronic Health Records', In 2021 IEEE 6th International Conference on Cloud Computing and Big Data Analytics (ICCCBDA), pp. 90-99 IEEE, April 2021. [http://dx.doi.org/10.1109/ICCCBDA51879.2021.9442539]

[19] P. Meier, J.H. Beinke, C. Fitte, J. Schulte to Brinke, and F. Teuteberg, "Generating design knowledge for blockchain-based access control to personal health records", *Inf. Syst. E-Bus. Manag.,* vol. 19, no. 1, pp. 13-41, 2021. [http://dx.doi.org/10.1007/s10257-020-00476-2]

[20] H.B. Mahajan, "Emergence of healthcare 4.0 and blockchain into secure cloud-based electronic health records systems: solutions, challenges, and future roadmap", *Wirel. Pers. Commun.,* vol. 126, no. 3, pp. 2425-2446, 2022.

[21] N. Sammeta, and L. Parthiban, "Hyperledger blockchain enabled secure medical record management with deep learning-based diagnosis model", *Complex Intell. Syst.,* pp. 1-16, 2021.

[22] A. Azaria, A. Ekblaw, T. Vieira, A. Lippman, 'Medrec: Using blockchain for medical data access and permission management', In 2016 2nd international conference on open and big data (OBD), pp. 25-30, IEEE, August 2016. [http://dx.doi.org/10.1109/OBD.2016.11]

[23] Ibrahim, F., Münscher, J. C., Daseking, M., & Telle, N. T. (2025). The technology acceptance model and adopter type analysis in the context of artificial intelligence. *Frontiers in Artificial Intelligence*, 7, 1496518.

[24] A.A. Omar, M.Z.A. Bhuiyan, A. Basu, S. Kiyomoto, and M.S. Rahman, "Privacy-friendly platform for healthcare data in cloud based on blockchain environment", *Future Gener. Comput. Syst.,* vol. 95, pp. 511-521, 2019. [http://dx.doi.org/10.1016/j.future.2018.12.044]

[25] J. Liu, X. Li, L. Ye, H. Zhang, X. Du, and M. Guizani, "BPDS: A blockchain based privacy-preserving datasharing for electronic medical records", *2018 IEEE Global Communications Conference (GLOBECOM),* pp. 1-6, 2018. [http://dx.doi.org/10.1109/GLOCOM.2018.8647713]

[26] A. Mehbodniya, J.L. Webber, R. Neware, F. Arslan, R.V. Pamba, and M. Shabaz, "Modified Lamport Merkle Digital Signature blockchain framework for authentication of internet of things healthcare data", *Expert Syst.,* vol. 39, no. 10, p. e12978, 2022.

[27] X. Liu, Z. Wang, C. Jin, F. Li, and G. Li, "A blockchain-based medical data sharing and protection scheme", *IEEE Access,* vol. 7, pp. 118943-118953, 2019. [http://dx.doi.org/10.1109/ACCESS.2019.2937685]

[28] Prabha, P., & Chatterjee, K. (2020, December). Securing telecare medical information system with blockchain technology. In *2020 2nd International Conference on Advances in Computing, Communication Control and Networking (ICACCCN)* (pp. 846-851). IEEE.

[29] H. Wang, and Y. Song, "Secure cloud-based EHR system using attribute- based cryptosystem and blockchain", *J. Med. Syst.,* vol. 42, no. 8, p. 152, 2018. [http://dx.doi.org/10.1007/s10916-018-0994-6] [PMID: 29974270]

[30] R.M.A. Latif, K. Hussain, N.Z. Jhanjhi, A. Nayyar, and O. Rizwan, "A remix IDE: smart contract-based framework for the healthcare sector by using Blockchain technology", *Multimedia Tools Appl.,* pp. 1-24, 2020.

[31] Rana, S. K., Rana, S. K., Rana, A. K., Nisar, K., Soomro, T. R., & Nisar, S. (2022, November). A survey on blockchain technology supported approaches for healthcare system, open issues and challenges. In 2022 14th International Conference on Mathematics, Actuarial Science, Computer Science and Statistics (MACS) (pp. 1-7). IEEE. [http://dx.doi.org/10.1109/MACS56771.2022.10023472]

[32] D. Singla, and S.K. Rana, "A Systematic Review on Blockchain-Based e-Healthcare for Collaborative Environment", *International Conference on Emergent Converging Technologies and Biomedical Systems,* pp. 361-376, 2022.Singapore

[33] D. Singla, and S. Rana, "Blockchain-Based Platform for Smart Tracking and Tracing the Pharmaceutical Drug Supply Chain", In: *Examining Multimedia Forensics and Content Integrity.* IGI Global, 2023, pp. 144-172. [http://dx.doi.org/10.4018/978-1-6684-6864-7.ch006]

[34] T. Singh, R. Vaid, and A. Sharma, "Security Issues in Blockchain Integrated WSN: Challenges and Concerns", *2022 International Conference on Innovative Computing, Intelligent Communication and Smart Electrical Systems (ICSES),* pp. 1-5, 2022. [http://dx.doi.org/10.1109/ICSES55317.2022.9914006]

[35] Tejbir Singh, Dr Rohit Vaid “Enigmas of various Techniques to implement Authentication and Integrity in Blockchain based Wireless Sensor Networks”, In Springer the Emergent Converging Technologies and Biomedical Systems (ETBS2022), Vol 1040, PP. 345-359 18 August 2023. [http://dx.doi.org/10.1007/978-981-2271-0-_29]

[36] Sakhare, A., Kshirsagar, A., & Pachghare, V. (2023, August). Survey on Data Privacy Preserving Techniques in Blockchain Applications. In 2023 9th International Conference on Smart Computing and Communications (ICSCC) (pp. 321-326). IEEE. [http://dx.doi.org/10.1109/ICSCC59169.2023.10335064]

[37] Zhang, G., Yang, Z., & Liu, W. (2022). Blockchain-based privacy preserving e-health system for healthcare data in cloud. *Computer Networks*, 203, 108586.

[38] Roehrs, A., da Costa, C. A., Righi, R. R., Mayer, A. H., da Silva, V. F., Goldim, J. R., & Schmidt, D. C. (2021). Integrating multiple blockchains to support distributed personal health records. *Health Informatics Journal*, 27(2), 14604582211007546.

[39] A. Al Omar, M.S. Rahman, A. Basu, and S. Kiyomoto, "Medibchain: A blockchain based privacy preserving platform for healthcare data", In: *International conference on security, privacy and anonymity in computation, communication and storage* Springer: Cham, 2017, pp. 534-543. [http://dx.doi.org/10.1007/978-3-319-72395-2_49]

[40] Rana, S. K., Rana, S. K., Nisar, K., Ag Ibrahim, A. A., Rana, A. K., Goyal, N., & Chawla, P. (2022). Blockchain technology and artificial intelligence based decentralized access control model to enable secure interoperability for healthcare. *Sustainability*, 14(15), 9471.

[41] H. Guo, W. Li, and C. Nejad, "C Shen, ‘Access control for electronic health records with hybrid blockchain-edge architecture", *2019 IEEE International Conference on Blockchain (Blockchain),* pp. 44-51, 2019. [http://dx.doi.org/10.1109/Blockchain.2019.00015]

[42] K. Shuaib, J. Abdella, F. Sallabi, M. A. Serhani, ‘Secure decentralized electronic health records sharing system based on blockchains’, Journal of King Saud UnYiversity-Computer and Information

Sciences, 2021.

[43] K.S. Alshudukhi, M.A. Khemakhem, F.E. Eassa, and K.M. Jambi, "An interoperable blockchain security frameworks based on microservices and smart contract in IoT environment", *Electronics (Basel),* vol. 12, no. 3, p. 776, 2023. [http://dx.doi.org/10.3390/electronics12030776]

[44] B. Nicolai, S. Tallarico, L. Pellegrini, L. Gastaldi, G. Vella, and S. Lazzini, "Blockchain for electronic medical record: assessing stakeholders' readiness for successful blockchain adoption in health-care", *Meas. Bus. Excell.,* vol. 27, no. 1, pp. 157-171, 2023. [http://dx.doi.org/10.1108/MBE-12-2021-0155]

[45] Kaur, A., Bansal, S., & Dattana, V. (2023). Blockchain in Healthcare: A Systematic Review and Future Perspectives. Deep Learning for Healthcare Decision Making, 211-243.

[46] G. De Novi, N. Sofia, I. Vasiliu-Feltes, C. Yan Zang, and F. Ricotta, "Blockchain Technology Predictions 2024: Transformations in Healthcare, Patient Identity, and Public Health", *Blockchain Healthc. Today,* vol. 6, p. 6, 2023. [PMID: 38187958]

[47] M.S. Rahman, I. Khalil, C.M.A. Pathum, A. Bouras, and X. Yi, "A novel architecture for tamper proof electronic health record management system using blockchain wrapper", *Proceedings of the 2019 ACM international symposium on blockchain and secure critical infrastructure,* pp. 97-105, 2019. [http://dx.doi.org/10.1145/3327960.3332392]

[48] D. Singla, S. Kumar, Y. Gulzar, M.S. Mir, D. Gupta, W. Jaziri, N. Sassi, and S. Arora, "Designing and implementing a resilient immutability mechanism for enhanced supply chain management in E-healthcare systems", *Frontiers in Sustainable Cities,* vol. 6, p. 1403809, 2024. [http://dx.doi.org/10.3389/frsc.2024.1403809]

[49] Rana, Sumit Kumar, Sanjeev Kumar Rana, Arun Kumar Rana, Kashif Nisar, Tariq Rahim Soomro, and Sana Nisar. "A survey on blockchain technology supported approaches for healthcare system, open issues and challenges." In 2022 14th International Conference on Mathematics, Actuarial Science, Computer Science and Statistics (MACS), pp. 1-7. IEEE, 2022. [http://dx.doi.org/10.1109/MACS56771.2022.10023472]

[50] Ghosh, P. K., A. Chakraborty, M. Hasan, K. Rashid and A. H. Siddique. "Blockchain Application in Healthcare Systems: A Review. Systems 2023, 11, 38." (2023).

[51] K. Vivekrabinson, D. Vijayakumar, S.R. Kumar, and R. Dhamodharan, "Medical data sharing using blockchain with secure patient/doctor interaction", *International Journal of System of Systems Engineering,* vol. 14, no. 2, pp. 145-158, 2024. [http://dx.doi.org/10.1504/IJSSE.2024.137060]

[52] H. Bodur, and I.F.T. Al Yaseen, "An Improved blockchain-based secure medical record sharing scheme", *Cluster Comput.,* vol. 27, no. 6, pp. 7981-8000, 2024. [http://dx.doi.org/10.1007/s10586-024-04414-6]

[53] S. Ait Bennacer, K. Sabiri, A. Aaroud, K. Akodadi, and B. Cherradi, "A comprehensive survey on blockchain-based healthcare industry: applications and challenges", *Indones. J. Electr. Eng. Comput. Sci.,* vol. 30, no. 3, pp. 1558-1571, 2023. [http://dx.doi.org/10.11591/ijeecs.v30.i3.pp1558-1571]

CHAPTER 5

Automation and Robotics in Healthcare: Transforming Patient Care

Vinod Kumar[1,*], Kanupriya Singh[2], Mandeep Kaur[3], Vikas Verma[4] and **Olivier Niyompuhwe[5]**

[1] *Department of Management, Gurugram University, Gurugram, Haryana, India*

[2] *Seth Jai Parkash Mukand Lal Institutions of Knowledge & Service, Radaur, Haryana, India*

[3] *Mittal School of Business, Lovely Professional University, Phagwara, Punjab, India*

[4] *MM Engineering College, Maharishi Markandeshwar (Deemed to be University), Mullana, Haryana, India*

[5] *Department of Forestry and Landscape Management, University of Rwanda, Kigali, Rwanda*

Abstract: The advent of robotics is changing the world economy. The World Health Organization (WHO) reports that more than 1 billion people live with some form of disability. In addition, changes around the world mean that patients are getting older and sicker, with many people living alone at home or in hospitals and relying on some form of aid to meet their specific needs. On the other hand, research and innovation in medical robotics have increased tremendously in recent years. Medical automation and robotics have the potential to deliver improved patient care, innovation, and safety for patients and physicians. This paper presents a systematic mapping study to understand the emerging role and the application of robotics in healthcare, and identifies existing and likely future challenges to maximize the benefits associated with robotics and related convergent technologies. This study employs a qualitative research technique. The methodology includes a comprehensive literature review on robotics in healthcare automation to gain qualitative insights. The research revealed significant improvements in healthcare efficiency and decision-making accuracy due to automation and robotics. The findings of this study offered valuable insights into the benefits and challenges of automation and robotics in healthcare.

Keywords: Ageing, Autonomous system, Automation, Healthcare, Health systems, Innovation, Imaging systems, Patient care, Robotics, Safety, Technologies, Wellbeing.

* **Corresponding author Vinod Kumar:** Department of Management, Gurugram University, Gurugram, Haryana, India; E-mail: gondi.vinod@gmail.com

Arun Kumar Rana, Mandeep Kaur & Sumit Kumar Rana (Eds.)

INTRODUCTION

Global health systems are struggling to combat rising costs and clearly improve medical, economic, and overall health outcomes. Robots are tangible systems that interact with their environment by sensing and responding through physical actions. Robots can differ in their design, sensory abilities, and levels of autonomy. With more than 10% of global Gross Domestic Product (GDP) spent on healthcare, digital innovation is becoming increasingly important for reducing costs and improving outcomes, and robotics is one area of digital innovation that could have a broad impact on healthcare. Robots are designed and configured to create changes in their environment. These systems use effectors to navigate within healthcare settings (locomotion) or to interact with and manipulate medical tools, equipment, or even patients. Typically, these robots rely on sensor data to make informed decisions, enhancing their ability to assist in medical tasks.

Around 20% of the global population faces challenges related to physical, cognitive, or sensory functioning, as well as mental or behavioral health. These challenges can be temporary or permanent, acute or chronic, and may evolve throughout a person's life. Among these individuals, 190 million experience significant difficulties in performing activities of daily living (ADLs). These ADLs range from basic physical tasks, such as grooming, feeding, and mobility, to more complex cognitive tasks, such as problem-solving, managing finances, and housekeeping. Further, for those who need help with ADL activities, this goal is difficult to achieve for several reasons: first, this level of care is extremely expensive, and second, there is a shortage of medical personnel; it is worth it. However, family and friends try to accommodate these programs, but they also have full-time jobs and other family responsibilities, and cannot perform as expected. Noteworthy progress has been made in adopting and expanding automation due to advancements in computing, information, and communication technologies.

Considered the most transformative technologies of our time, recent advances in Artificial Intelligence (AI) and Machine Learning (ML) have expanded to include electricity in place of traditional machines and industrial robots. These breakthroughs have expanded to areas such as knowledge-based work, healthcare, and many other industries [1]. The new era of robots is called the new robot. The word robot comes from the Czech word "robota," meaning servant, or servile. Robots are defined as artificial intelligence that can navigate their physical environment to perform complex tasks. More specifically, robots generally do three things autonomously or semi-autonomously: recognize the environment, perform calculations, make decisions, and work collaboratively in the physical environment. While the details of these three dimensions vary from robot to robot, most robots continue to iterate on Perception-Cognition-Function. Machines not only have to perform repetitive tasks every day in complex environments, but they also must collaborate with humans on various activities in unmanaged environments. Further, while automation has historically changed work, productivity, and business operations, the integration of AI and robotics into healthcare is creating an unprecedented revolution in the automation of care [2]. This shift is not just a competitive issue, but also a new moral and social issue. It is important to ensure that the great probable use of automation and AI is not only for economic benefit, but also for the betterment of people and improved health [3].

Workflow Automation in Healthcare

Automation is pursued by organizations for distinct reasons, including time savings, increased productivity, and improved work quality. For example, a business center is trying to reduce the time employees spend on job tasks, such as tracking activities and training employees, through automation [12]. If goals are not clearly defined and stakeholders affected by automation are not included in the process, automation goals will not be achieved. Reasons for not achieving these goals include choosing processes that are not suitable for automation, choosing tools that are not suitable for the job, not having the right tools, or not using the tools correctly. Continuous monitoring and analysis should be performed as job automation is implemented. This includes understanding how best to use technology to manage operations and analyzing how automation can be used to make needed changes in design or implementation. The industry-wide adoption of automation will require much collaboration, as in other industries. Although healthcare jobs are different from other industries and therefore the automation methods of other industries may not be directly applicable, the use of automation in the medical field requires several important considerations when deciding what work to do and when selecting levels of automation. First, where humans must review critical job decision points, make decisions, and reason "in the loop" to decide whether the job gets done, it requires low automation, semi-automation, or full automation. The literature suggests that poor job performance negatively affects job satisfaction and trust when compared to other industries (*e.g.*, manufacturing) where physicians, staff, and patients are committed to creating services that have commitment, communication, and coordination to the goals or situations needed for healthcare.

LITERATURE REVIEW

Many technologies are linked to the commitment to improving the public economy through digital services to support patients, make processes more efficient, and improve the work environment for health and wellness professionals [4]. Robots are gradually entering hospitals and other medical facilities due to the integration of human-robot collaboration technology and artificial intelligence [5]. Additionally, advances in machine learning hold significant promise that machines will be able to perform tasks common to humans, including problem solving, cognitive processing, relationships, and natural language use. The introduction of robotics into medicine is likely to increase due to technological advances, decreasing costs, and increasing pressure to control costs [6]. However, robots have the potential to disrupt innovation, so it is important to understand the challenges society will face when employing robots [7]. Some important studies show the integration of service robots with smart centers. This integration is transparent to users and provides services according to their profiles and needs [8]. Human-robot interaction is essential to obtain the best possible estimate between users and robots through voice commands, gestures, or other means of communication [9]. The Da Vinci Surgical System is a robotic-assisted surgery platform used in several hospitals across India. It allows surgeons to perform complex procedures with greater precision and control through minimally invasive techniques, improving patient outcomes and reducing recovery times [10]. Also, while not a robot, the Aarogya Setu app is a significant example of healthcare automation. It uses AI to trace COVID-19 contacts, check health statuses, and provide information, helping manage the pandemic effectively [11].

Robotics in Healthcare

The use of robotics in healthcare is often driven by the need for socialization, recognition, and satisfaction [12, 13]. The main reason for the use of robots in medicine is the ability to improve health by providing better and less expensive care to doctors in a prompt and efficient manner, and to provide the best possible care by improving care for caregivers. Reducing human error and reducing workplace injuries. There are two main drivers for robotics in healthcare: social and operational factors.

Societal Drivers

The motivation for using robotics in healthcare focuses on three primary areas: expanding healthcare services, reducing labor costs, and improving patient outcomes. It is expected that older people will experience more problems in these areas as they age, and that they are more likely to suffer from injuries, damage, and pain. In addition, according to research conducted in all age groups, approximately 90% of the world's population suffers from physical, mental, emotional, or behavioral problems. Although not yet definitive, the epidemic is linked to population growth and aging, which shows an increase in the number of people with diseases such as diabetes, obesity, and cancer.

Technological Drivers

This technological advancement is leading to the development of robotics in medical eyewear, which in turn is influencing other technological advances: lower costs, improved sensor performance, faster models, more storage capacity, more electronics and small electronics, more in batteries and communication technology, and accelerating advances in machine cognition (*i.e.* artificial intelligence), improved autonomy, and improved product development. In addition, robotics in healthcare involves physical interactions between nurses, patients, and technology. Human and robot interaction means the robot must be able to perceive, learn, and understand the environment to provide useful information to the human, or even the examiner or patient. Some examples of technology drivers include: The use of robots in healthcare has a physical impact on caregivers, patients, and products [6]. Human-machine interaction means that the robot must be able to understand and encompass its environment so that it can give useful advice to people, whether they are caregivers or patients. Some examples of technology drivers include:

Advanced Imaging Systems

Advanced imaging systems are pivotal in modern healthcare, providing detailed and accurate insights into the human body for diagnosis, treatment planning, and monitoring, like OCT (Optical Coherence Tomography) it is widely used in ophthalmology for imaging the retina and other eye structures, OCT provides high-resolution cross-sectional images that help diagnose and monitor conditions such as macular degeneration and glaucoma. OCT uses light waves to capture micrometer-resolution images, offering real-time, non-invasive visualization of tissue layers [14].

- **AI-Powered Diagnostics:** AI-powered diagnostics are transforming healthcare by using artificial intelligence to enhance the accuracy, efficiency, and speed of disease detection and diagnosis, like Medical Imaging Analysis, which includes IBM Watson, which uses AI to analyze medical images, such as MRIs, CT scans, and X-rays [15]. It helps radiologists find abnormalities, detect diseases earlier, and provide second opinions with high accuracy. Google Health's DeepMind- DeepMind's AI algorithms analyze retinal scans to diagnose conditions like diabetic retinopathy and age-related macular degeneration with high precision.
- **Enhanced Robotic Surgery Systems:** Enhanced robotic surgery systems are a significant advancement in the field of surgical technology, providing greater

precision, flexibility, and control during procedures [16]. The Da Vinci system is known for its robotic arms equipped with surgical instruments and a high-definition 3D camera. Surgeons control the robot through a console, allowing for minimally invasive procedures with enhanced dexterity and precision. It is used in various specialties, including urology, gynecology, cardiothoracic surgery, and general surgery. It improves outcomes for complex procedures like prostatectomies, hysterectomies, and cardiac valve repairs.

- **Wearable Health Technologies:** Wearable health technologies are transforming healthcare by providing continuous, real-time monitoring of various health metrics. These devices offer valuable insights into an individual's health, enabling early detection of potential issues and supporting preventive care. For instance, Continuous Glucose Monitors (CGMs) continuously track blood glucose levels throughout the day and night, providing real-time data to help manage diabetes. They include sensors placed under the skin that send data to a smartphone or dedicated device [17].
- **Autonomous Disinfection Robots:** Autonomous disinfection robots are innovative tools designed to enhance cleanliness and reduce the spread of infectious diseases in various environments, particularly in healthcare settings. For example, the Xenex Light Strike robot uses high-intensity UV-C light to disinfect surfaces and kill pathogens, including bacteria, viruses, and spores. It works autonomously and can be programmed to cover specific areas [18].

METHODOLOGY

This study's method thoroughly examines currently available secondary data sources such as journals, articles, and research reports about healthcare automation and robotics, including PubMed, Scopus, IEEE Xplore, Web of Science, and Google Scholar. Publications from 2015 to 2023 were included to capture the most recent developments in robotics and healthcare automation. The search for this information was done using search terms such as robots or automation, automation and patient care combined in health care, and treatment or cure. The peer-reviewed journal articles, book chapters, and systematic reviews focusing on the application of automation and robotics in the healthcare field were included, and conference abstracts without full text, studies unrelated to healthcare (*e.g.*, industrial robotics), and non-English publications were excluded. In total, around 105 articles were screened for the review. This has laid a foundation of knowledge in artificial intelligence, automation, health care, robotics, and their convergence in this research. This approach offered a comprehensive view of healthcare automation and robotics, addressing the benefits, limitations, challenges, and key factors for success.

Objectives of the Study

- The goal of the research is to understand the emerging role of robotics in health care.
- To find the existing challenges and future research directions
- To gain knowledge about how robotics is being applied in human care

APPLICATIONS OF ROBOTICS IN HEALTHCARE

Medical robots are diversified; these robots can provide physical and cognitive support. They can be involved in a variety of activities in the environment, from preventive measures to treatment, from short-term care to long-term care. In these tasks, robots can support hospital, administrative, and support staff.

Public Safety

In healthcare, robotics plays a pivotal role in enhancing operational efficiency, patient safety, and care delivery, like the diverse applications seen in public safety. For instance, the largest deployment of healthcare robots involves tasks such as patient monitoring and support, with robots being used in hospitals and clinics to ensure compliance with health protocols and help healthcare staff. These robots, often equipped with advanced sensors and communication tools, help detect patient needs, check vital signs, and ensure adherence to safety measures, significantly reducing the risk of human error and enhancing patient care [9]. Another critical application of robotics in healthcare is the disinfection of medical facilities, a practice that has become increasingly vital in the context of pandemic preparedness and infection control. Just as drones and ground robots have been adapted for disinfecting public spaces in urban environments, healthcare facilities employ autonomous robots to sanitize patient rooms, operating theaters, and other critical areas. These robots use UV-C light or disinfectant sprays to effectively end pathogens, thereby reducing the risk of hospital-acquired infections (HAIs) and protecting both patients and healthcare workers from exposure to harmful microorganisms.

In both scenarios, robotics improves efficiency and coverage and enhances safety by minimizing human exposure to potential hazards. These technologies are subject to healthcare regulations and standards, much like the aviation restrictions for small unmanned aerial systems in public safety, ensuring their deployment is both safe and effective in healthcare environments.

Clinical Care

In healthcare, the application of robotics has greatly expanded, particularly in clinical care, where robots are used to enhance patient diagnosis, treatment, and overall hospital operations [19]. The use of these robots affects healthcare workers, support staff, and small segments of the general population, including patients and their families. Robots in clinical care are typically employed within various hospital settings, such as waiting areas, treatment rooms, patient rooms, and even entrances and parking garages, where healthcare workers might be at risk of exposure. These applications are governed by public health regulations, insurance policies, and hospital-specific guidelines. If robots are classified as medical devices, they must follow more regulatory requirements. Furthermore, the financial viability of using robots in clinical care depends on whether the costs are reimbursable by insurers; without such reimbursement, hospitals may be less inclined to invest in robotic technology. The most significant use of robots in medicine is the introduction of medicine, where doctors and nurses use robots to interact with patients remotely to help diagnose and cure diseases while minimizing physical contact. Some robots can perform physical tasks, such as pressing sensors on patients, and a few have been developed for more invasive procedures, based on prior advancements in medical robotics. These robots are often commercially available or adapted from existing commercial models. Another critical application of robotics in clinical care is hospital disinfection. Robots equipped with UV-C light are employed to rapidly disinfect hospital environments, reducing the risk of hospital-acquired infections. These robots perform initial disinfection, which is then followed by manual cleaning to ensure thorough sanitization. The use of these robots has increased, particularly in response to the heightened need for infection control during pandemics. Further, robots have been used for the autonomous delivery of prescriptions and meals within hospitals [20]. These robotic carts navigate hospital corridors, delivering essential items to patients and allowing healthcare workers to focus more on direct patient care. This application has seen increased visibility as hospitals cope with surges in patient numbers, highlighting the role of robots in supporting healthcare staff.

Continuity of Work and Education

Robotics has also played a crucial role in keeping continuity of operations during challenging times, such as its application in other industries. Healthcare facilities have used ground robots primarily to ensure the continued delivery of services while protecting healthcare workers and patients [21]. In addition, robots have been employed in healthcare logistics, particularly in hospital warehouses, to manage inventory and distribute medical supplies efficiently. This use of robotics helps healthcare facilities cope with increased demand and workforce reductions due to illness, ensuring that essential supplies are available where and when they are needed. Furthermore, robots have been used in the construction of new healthcare facilities, helping in tasks that require precision and reducing the need for human labor in potentially hazardous environments. Additionally, robots have supported healthcare security and monitoring facilities to ensure safety and compliance with health regulations [22].

Overall, the integration of robotics into healthcare has allowed for the seamless continuation of essential services, safeguarding both healthcare workers and patients while keeping lofty standards of care and operational efficiency.

CLASSIFICATION OF ROBOTS IN HEALTHCARE

Nurse Robots in Hospitals

In Japan, nurse robots are increasingly being deployed in hospitals to support doctors in a manner similar to human nurses. This is particularly crucial given Japan's rapidly aging population, with the highest percentage of elderly individuals (those over 75 years) among OECD countries. The growing number of elderly patients presents significant challenges for the nation's medical facilities [23]. With a shortage of caregivers, many Japanese citizens find themselves needing to care for aging family members at home, often at the expense of their professional careers. Furthermore, healthcare workers in Japan face elevated levels of stress and exhaustion due to the heavy patient load. To address these challenges, the Japanese government is turning to technological innovations, such as nurse robots, to help manage the care of elderly patients and alleviate the burden on healthcare professionals. Robotic care, which offers low-cost, 24/7 service, is growing in popularity. Dinsow, for example, is a robot with specific features designed to help improve dementia symptoms for Alzheimer's patients by engaging them in cognitive activities. One exercise involves showing pictures of different people and having patients match each face to the correct name, improving memory and cognitive function.

Ambulance Robots

According to statistics, approximately 800,000 people suffer a heart attack in the EU each year, and the survival rate in these cases is only 8%. The high death toll is largely due to the slow response time of emergency services, which usually takes 10 minutes, and brain death occurs within 4 to 6 minutes of severe injury. Immediate treatment after an accident is important to prevent injuries from getting worse. Faster response times in emergencies can increase survival rates, especially in cases of drowning, cardiac arrest, shock, and respiratory problems [24]. Life-saving equipment such as emergency medicine, cardiopulmonary resuscitation (CPR), and automated external defibrillator (AED) devices are now designed to be light and compact enough to be carried directly on emergency drones. These drones are invaluable in providing emergency care to patients in mobile or remote areas, as they can deliver critical care with minimal delay. One example is a lightweight, small payload drone ambulance developed by Delft University of Technology in the Netherlands, designed to carry essential medical equipment, including a side-mounted external defibrillator (AED) to provide support after a heart attack. Saving lives in those critical minutes.

Assistive Robots

People with paraplegia experience significant difficulties in performing and supporting activities of daily living (ADL). In 2013, approximately 5.4 million individuals in the U.S. (1.7% of the population) were living with paralysis, with stroke being the leading cause, followed by Spinal Cord Injury (SCI), Multiple Sclerosis (MS), and Cerebral Palsy (CP) [25]. Recent advancements in robotics and Artificial Intelligence (AI) have led to the development of assistive robots, which can provide crucial support for ADLs at home and in the workplace. Various assistive robotic systems, such as those based on Wheelchair Mounted Robotic Arms (WARM), have been developed to aid individuals with physical impairments. One notable example is the FRIEND system, an intelligent wheelchair-mounted manipulator that has evolved through four generations. Early versions of FRIEND were focused on helping people with quadriplegia perform essential ADLs like drinking and eating. The fourth generation, FRIEND IV, expanded its capabilities to support users in real-world environments, such as aiding a quadriplegic librarian in cataloging books. The FRIEND IV system includes a seven-DOF robotic arm, a two-finger gripper, a hand camera, a chin joystick, and a head control interface, as well as a stereo-camera and laser scanner. It enabled the user to autonomously manipulate books, with speech recognition used for cataloging and an advanced Human-Machine Interface (HMI) for manual intervention when necessary, achieving a success rate of 95%. Beyond ADLs, assistive robots like the Jaco 2 robotic arm from Kinova have been widely used in research for manipulation tasks, such as drinking and eating. Assistive robots have also been applied to other ADLs, such as dressing, where systems like the Baxter humanoid robot have been used to help users with simulated upper-body impairments put on clothing. Similarly, robotic assistants have been developed for tasks like shoe fitting, beard shaving, hair brushing, and bathing, though these applications are still in the first stages of development and require further research to ensure they meet safety and acceptability standards.

Rehabilitation Robots

These are specialized robots with robotic technology designed to support individuals with physical impairments during their rehabilitation process. These robots are particularly valuable for patients affected by debilitating motor disabilities such as stroke, multiple sclerosis, head and spinal cord injuries, and spina bifida. Physiotherapy is a critical part of the recovery process for these patients, aiming to restore motor skills to their fullest potential. Rehabilitation programs are typically tailored by physiotherapists to enhance the patients' motor functions. Rehabilitation robots help physiotherapists by enabling patients to perform repetitive tasks, which are essential for regaining motor skills. These robots are equipped with sensors that collect data during therapy sessions, offering valuable insights that allow therapists to fine-tune the rehabilitation process based on the individual needs of each patient. This technology has been shown to improve gross motor skills more effectively than conventional therapy alone. Rehabilitation robots are categorized into two subgroups: upper-limb rehabilitation robots, which are designed to aid with impairments in the upper body, and lower-limb rehabilitation robots, which focus on aiding individuals with lower-body impairments. These robots play a crucial role in enhancing the effectiveness of rehabilitation by providing consistent, data-driven support throughout the recovery process.

Walking Assisting Robots

The Walking Assistant is intended to support humans with limited walking ability and to provide the necessary help in daily activities and rehabilitation. These devices vary according to the user's disability and special needs. For example, individuals with complete paralysis from spinal cord injuries or traumatic brain injuries may receive help from intelligent wheelchairs, while those with weakened lower limbs due to stroke or accidents might find wearable exoskeletons useful for rehabilitation. Additionally, advancements in intelligent prostheses are providing innovative solutions for amputees. Traditionally, the design of Intelligent Walking Assistants (IWAs) follows two main approaches: cane-based walkers and walking-frame-based walkers. IWAs are designed with standard functionalities that include obstacle avoidance, guidance, user intent prediction, gait estimation, velocity estimation, and fall detection and prevention. To achieve these capabilities, IWAs are equipped with a range of sensors, such as force-torque (FT) sensors, laser rangefinders (LRF), acoustic sensors, Charge-Coupled Device (CCD) cameras for localization, and RGB-Depth cameras. These sensors collectively enable the robot to effectively support and aid users in navigating their environment and performing daily activities. However, the recent advancements in assistive robotic systems have introduced innovative technologies and sensors. For example, the iWalk system [25] features an RGB-D RealSense camera for tracking gait, assessing gait stability, and evaluating mobility. The iWalk also incorporates an LRF sensor for estimating gait phases and uses microphones and speakers for speech recognition and voice feedback. Additionally, the system checks human activity during exercises and offers fall detection capabilities. However, it does not include mechanisms for fall prevention.

Cleaning Robots

Robots are used in hospitals to clean, sweep, and/or mop floors. Cleaning robots for use in hospitals seem to have the potential to deliver innovations that non-robot designers have long seen. Robots like these are important for hospital disinfection to eliminate bacteria and pesticides.

Surgical Robots

These robots can perform more minimally invasive surgeries (MIS) than human surgeons. Many distal operators are designed for distal procedures. The Da Vinci robotic surgical system from Intuitive Surgical Inc. is one such popular example; many other types of specialized surgical robots are in use for general endoscopic, cranial, and spine surgery as well as for biopsy. The clinical advantages are minimally invasive procedures, precision, and dexterity in confined anatomical spaces and reduced surgeon fatigue. A meta-analysis of research studies found robotic-assisted surgeries were associated with lower complication rates, faster recovery times, reduced blood loss, lower infection rates, and shorter recovery, though high costs are still a barrier. The LBR Med is a sensitive seven-axis lightweight robot; it is very flexible and easy to integrate into medical products for many surgical interventions. It is perfectly suited to applications in medical technology due to its responsive sensors, inclusive safety provisions, hygiene-optimized surfaces, and a controller intended for direct collaboration with the human operator.

CHALLENGES AND OPPORTUNITIES

While there are many benefits to robotics in healthcare, there are also issues that must be resolved before it can be widely used and successful. The following are some major obstacles:

Usability and Acceptability

Ensuring that robots are user-friendly and acceptable to both patients and healthcare providers is essential [26]. This involves designing intuitive interfaces and providing sufficient training to users. Robots that are challenging for primary stakeholders to use often face a substantial risk of abandonment, a trend well-documented in the Assistive Technology Community. For example, a 2010 study highlighted that up to 75% of hand rehabilitation robots were never tested with end users, resulting in their practical abandonment. A significant challenge is the low technology literacy among clinicians, even those who are highly skilled in their fields. If clinicians struggle with a robot's usability, their ability to train patients or caregivers to use the technology effectively is greatly reduced. This creates a barrier to the successful implementation and use of robotic systems in real-world settings.

Safety and Reliability

Robots must be engineered to run safely and reliably in healthcare settings. This includes rigorous testing to prevent malfunctions that could potentially harm patients or staff. When robots interact closely with individuals, ensuring safety and reliability becomes paramount. This is especially critical for patients, who may rely heavily on robots for physical or cognitive tasks and might struggle more to recover from robot failures compared to those without such dependencies. Despite its importance, information security in human-machine interaction is still an unexplored area. People with cognitive impairments and children are particularly vulnerable to fraud by robots [26]. Although some efforts have been made recently to address this issue, such as supporting design costs for manufacturers, more needs to be done. Important decisions include ensuring that the robot's face is reflected in its work (to prevent human manipulation), providing clarity on robot punishment, and protecting the privacy and reputation of the users.

Capability and Function

The robots' capabilities must align with their intended functions. They should be able to perform their designated tasks effectively and adapt to various clinical scenarios. Real, spontaneous, and robust thinking in human environments poses a major challenge for robots. While advances in computer vision have improved image recognition and camera stabilization performance, these algorithms often struggle to cope with the complexity of camera motion, people, and the environment. Problems such as data loss, sensor occlusion, and environmental clutter are common in human social environments, making it difficult for robots to effectively recognize, respond, and explore their environments. Recent progress has been made through multimodal sensing approaches in social signal processing and human-robot interaction, which contribute to more robust algorithms. Additionally, life-long learning and longitudinal experimental methods have helped address some of these perceptual challenges. Learning, too, is a challenge. This flexibility and accessibility make it difficult for manufacturers to compete and socialize. As we have already mentioned, simplicity is undoubtedly better; it helps limit the problem space and reduce the complexity of the system [27].

Cost Effectiveness

The financial implications of deploying healthcare robots must be considered. This includes not only the first investment but also maintenance costs and potential savings from improved efficiency and reduced human error. Robotics in healthcare often involves a large first investment for buying, installing, and integrating sophisticated robotic systems. For many healthcare facilities, especially those with limited budgets, these high upfront costs can be a major barrier. Beyond the first purchase, ongoing costs for maintenance, repairs, and software updates can be large. The need for specialized technical support and the potential for downtime can add to these expenses. Further, effective use of robotics requires training for healthcare staff and potentially for patients. These training programs can be time-consuming and costly, affecting overall cost-effectiveness. Addressing these cost-related challenges involves a combination of providing clear value through improved patient outcomes, exploring funding and reimbursement opportunities, and investing in cost-effective and scalable robotic solutions [28].

Clinical Effectiveness

This measures whether a robotic intervention achieves its intended outcomes, such as improving patient health or easing healthcare processes. The goal is to ensure that robotic technologies not only work in theory but also provide tangible benefits in practical, real-world scenarios. All consumer in vivo robots, and many in vivo robots, require regulatory approval before they can be marketed and sold, and as laws in society compete to obtain the technology, social robots can and should be included in clinical trials and robots in care.

LIMITATIONS

Healthcare robotics research has a lot of promise, but there are several obstacles in the way that could hinder its advancement and impact results. The chapter predominantly highlights the benefits and opportunities of health care automation and robotics, while it mentions challenges, the emphasis on positive outcomes may overshadow potential risks, limitations, and negative consequences. The chapter discusses various applications and types of robotics in health care. However, the findings may not be universally applicable due to the specific context and conditions of individual businesses or regions. Since marketing robots are rare and expensive, their availability is limited to organizations that can afford large purchases. Difficulty in gaining acceptance from the rehabilitant, their family members, and the caregivers, as the trusting relationship between a doctor and a patient is often considered an anthropogenic activity. With the rapid development of technology, the inability to manage and implement policy has led to serious problems in practice. Without roles and systems, many of the capabilities of robots can pose a threat to doctors and patients.

IMPLICATIONS

Although there is a large literature on the promise of robotics, it is limited to applications outside of healthcare or specific medical applications. Potential problems and unintended consequences of medical technology need to be explored visually. There is now a need for a management that is flexible, ethical, and innovative enough to adapt to the changing environment and the increase and integration of robotic resources [29]. This will require the training of a new generation of professionals specialized in high-risk areas such as healthcare, as current regulations will only make it possible to use technology voluntarily. Health robotics is a new field that needs national and international teams, as most of the roles are patient and staff-oriented and require the integration and coordination of humans and machines in high-risk environments.

CONCLUSION

This chapter provides an overview of the potential of robots in medicine and other fields. Although technological advances have been made in medical robotics, integrating robotics into healthcare may not be easy. Medical robotics is a new trend that can help everyone in many areas. There have been many developments in robotics in recent years that promise great benefits in the future. It is important for product developers to work with DRU to help bridge the gap between different technologies and set reasonable expectations. Most people have met robots through movies or media, and this rarely reflects reality. Robots are prone to making mistakes in the real world and will continue to do so soon. However, they still have the potential to make significant changes in healthcare. There are many opportunities for the design and operation of medical robots, such As Cyber-Physical Systems (CPS), optimization of renewable energy and energy management, and reliable and trustworthy control that ensures the safety and security of healthcare institutions.

Advancing automation in healthcare requires a strategic approach that considers which workflows to automate, the necessary instrumentation, and the development and implementation of effective solutions. Key stakeholders—including developers, informaticians, researchers, healthcare practitioners, and policymakers—must collaborate to evaluate workflows, define clear automation goals, and set up robust and transparent testing and evaluation methods. Automation solutions should include closed feedback loops for real-time performance monitoring and be supported by policies that promote advancement while safeguarding data and mitigating risks. As automation becomes more prevalent, it is essential to find, share, and implement best practices. This will require substantial investment in infrastructure and resources from all healthcare stakeholders to ensure the successful development, evaluation, and implementation of automation technologies.

To ensure the integration of robots into medical automation, efficiency, adaptability, and social impact must be considered. Reliability performance is important because the robot must and cannot be expected to work efficiently and safely in a medical environment without any problems. Customizable robots must perform a variety of tasks in a variety of situations while interacting with different users, including those who may not like live robots. The social influence of medical robots must also be carefully considered because they can affect the quality of patient care, the work of child caregivers, and special issues that arise. The challenges discussed in this article are not limited to medical robots; they are relevant to all robotic applications that involve human-robot interactions in the real world, such as manufacturing, marketing, transportation, and search and rescue. Our study should be seen as a steppingstone to encourage broader discussion of these challenges and may also help inform healthcare organizations and policymakers in important decisions about the purchase, development, and use of robotics.

REFERENCES

[1] Sharma, D., & Kumar, V. (2024). Enhancing Organizational Intelligence Integration of Artificial Intelligence and Knowledge Management: Frameworks in India. In Digital Technologies in Modeling and Management: Insights in Education and Industry (pp. 167-184). IGI Global.

[2] N. Vallès-Peris, O. Barat-Auleda, and M. Domènech, "Robots in Healthcare? What Patients Say", *Int. J. Environ. Res. Public Health,* vol. 18, no. 18, p. 9933, 2021. [http://dx.doi.org/10.3390/ijerph18189933] [PMID: 34574861]

[3] T. Zayas-Cabán, S.N. Haque, and N. Kemper, "Identifying Opportunities for Workflow Automation in Health Care: Lessons Learned from Other Industries", *Appl. Clin. Inform.,* vol. 12, no. 3, pp. 686-697, 2021. [http://dx.doi.org/10.1055/s-0041-1731744] [PMID: 34320683]

[4] Kumar, V., Sharma, D., & Chauhan, S. (2023). Role of Customer Experience-Driven Business Innovation Framework for Modern Enterprises. In Innovation, Strategy, and Transformation Frameworks for the Modern Enterprise (pp. 310-326). IGI Global. [http://dx.doi.org/10.4018/979-8-3693-0458-7.ch013]

[5] L.D. Riek, "Healthcare robotics", *Commun. ACM,* vol. 60, no. 11, pp. 68-78, 2017. [http://dx.doi.org/10.1145/3127874]

[6] N.B. Santos, R.S. Bavaresco, J.E.R. Tavares, G.O. Ramos, J.L.V. Barbosa, and J.L. Barbosa, "A systematic mapping study of robotics in human care", *Robot. Auton. Syst.,* vol. 144, p. 103833, 2021. [http://dx.doi.org/10.1016/j.robot.2021.103833]

[7] Choi, S., & Wan, L. C. (2021). The rise of service robots in the hospitality industry: Some actionable insights. Boston Hospitality Review, 1-11.

[8] J.A. Gonzalez-Aguirre, R. Osorio-Oliveros, K.L. Rodríguez-Hernández, J. Lizárraga-Iturralde, R. Morales Menendez, R.A. Ramírez-Mendoza, M.A. Ramírez-Moreno, and J.J. Lozoya-Santos, "Service

robots: Trends and technology", *Appl. Sci. (Basel),* vol. 11, no. 22, p. 10702, 2021.
[http://dx.doi.org/10.3390/app112210702]

[9] M. Chen, X. Wang, R. Law, and M. Zhang, "Research on the frontier and prospect of service robots in the tourism and hospitality industry based on International Core Journals: A Review", *Behav. Sci. (Basel),* vol. 13, no. 7, p. 560, 2023.
[http://dx.doi.org/10.3390/bs13070560] [PMID: 37504007]

[10] M. Kyrarini, F. Lygerakis, A. Rajavenkatanarayanan, C. Sevastopoulos, H.R. Nambiappan, K.K. Chaitanya, A.R. Babu, J. Mathew, and F. Makedon, "A Survey of Robots in Healthcare", *Technologies (Basel),* vol. 9, no. 1, p. 8, 2021.
[http://dx.doi.org/10.3390/technologies9010008]

[11] Murphy, R. R., Gandudi, V. B. M., & Adams, J. (2020). Applications of robots for COVID-19 response. arXiv preprint arXiv:2008.06976.

[12] J. Xu, A. Hsiao, S. Reid, and E. Ma, "Working with service robots? A systematic literature review of hospitality employees' perspectives", *Int. J. Hospit. Manag.,* vol. 113, p. 103523, 2023.
[http://dx.doi.org/10.1016/j.ijhm.2023.103523]

[13] B.H. Yang, and S. Rhee, "Development of the ring sensor for healthcare automation", *Robot. Auton. Syst.,* vol. 30, no. 3, pp. 273-281, 2000.
[http://dx.doi.org/10.1016/S0921-8890(99)00092-5]

[14] M.T. Thai, P.T. Phan, T.T. Hoang, S. Wong, N.H. Lovell, and T.N. Do, "Advanced intelligent systems for surgical robotics", *Adv. Intell. Syst.,* vol. 2, no. 8, p. 1900138, 2020.
[http://dx.doi.org/10.1002/aisy.201900138]

[15] N. Melarkode, K. Srinivasan, S.M. Qaisar, and P. Plawiak, "AI-powered diagnosis of skin cancer: a contemporary review, open challenges and future research directions", *Cancers (Basel),* vol. 15, no. 4, p. 1183, 2023.
[http://dx.doi.org/10.3390/cancers15041183] [PMID: 36831525]

[16] S.D. McCarus, "Senhance robotic platform system for gynecological surgery. JSLS", *Journal of the Society of Laparoscopic & Robotic Surgeons,* vol. 25, no. 1, 2021.

[17] C. Li, S.H. Lin, and A. Chib, "The state of wearable health technologies: a transdisciplinary literature review", *Mob. Media Commun.,* vol. 9, no. 2, pp. 353-376, 2021.
[http://dx.doi.org/10.1177/2050157920966023]

[18] I. Chio, K. Ruan, Z. Wu, K.I. Wong, L.M. Tam, and Q. Xu, "Design and autonomous navigation of a new indoor disinfection robot based on disinfection modeling", *IEEE Trans. Autom. Sci. Eng.,* vol. 20, no. 1, pp. 649-661, 2023.
[http://dx.doi.org/10.1109/TASE.2022.3165084]

[19] S. Adel, A. Zaher, N. El Harouni, A. Venugopal, P. Premjani, and N. Vaid, "Robotic applications in orthodontics: changing the face of contemporary clinical care", *BioMed Res. Int.,* vol. 2021, no. 1, p. 9954615, 2021.
[http://dx.doi.org/10.1155/2021/9954615] [PMID: 34222490]

[20] A.R. Alahmari, K.K. Alrabghi, and I.M. Dighriri, "An overview of the current state and perspectives of pharmacy robot and medication dispensing technology", *Cureus,* vol. 14, no. 8, p. e28642, 2022.
[http://dx.doi.org/10.7759/cureus.28642] [PMID: 36196333]

[21] D. Silvera-Tawil, "Robotics in Healthcare: A Survey", *SN Computer Science,* vol. 5, no. 1, p. 189, 2024.
[http://dx.doi.org/10.1007/s42979-023-02551-0]

[22] Javaid, M., Haleem, A., Singh, R. P., Rab, S., Suman, R., & Kumar, L. (2022). Utilization of robotics for healthcare: A scoping review. Journal of Industrial Integration and Management, 2250015

[23] Vänni, K. J., & Salin, S. E. (2017). A Need for Service Robots Among Health Care Professionals in Hospitals and Housing Services. In Lecture notes in computer science (pp. 178–187).

[http://dx.doi.org/10.1007/978-3-319-70022-9_18]

[24] C.Y. Yang, H. Samani, Z. Tang, and C. Li, "Implementation of extended kalman filter for localization of ambulance robot", *Int. J. Intell. Robot. Appl.,* vol. 8, no. 4, pp. 960-973, 2024. [http://dx.doi.org/10.1007/s41315-024-00352-z]

[25] Monowara, S. M., Shariar, M. A., Islam, M. S. U., & Jawad, M. J. N. (2020). IoT based brain-wave assistive system for paralyzed individuals (Doctoral dissertation, Brac University).

[26] K. Cresswell, S. Cunningham-Burley, and A. Sheikh, "Health Care Robotics: Qualitative Exploration of Key Challenges and Future Directions", *J. Med. Internet Res.,* vol. 20, no. 7, p. e10410, 2018. [http://dx.doi.org/10.2196/10410] [PMID: 29973336]

[27] Fosch-Villaronga, E., & Drukarch, H. (2021). On Healthcare Robots: Concepts, definitions, and considerations for healthcare robot governance. arXiv preprint arXiv:2106.03468.

[28] Z.H. Khan, A. Siddique, and C.W. Lee, "Robotics Utilization for Healthcare Digitization in Global COVID-19 Management", *Int. J. Environ. Res. Public Health,* vol. 17, no. 11, p. 3819, 2020. [http://dx.doi.org/10.3390/ijerph17113819] [PMID: 32481547]

[29] S. Gupta, P. Sharma, S. Chaudhary, V. Kumar, S.P. Singh, M. Lourens, and N. Beri, "Study on the Beneficial Impacts and Ethical Dimensions of Generative AI in Software Product Management", *International Journal of Intelligent Systems and Applications in Engineering,* vol. 12, pp. 251-264, 2024.

CHAPTER 6

Enhancing Healthcare Data Security and Privacy Using Blockchain Technology

Liz George[1,*] and **Jubilant J. Kizhakkethottam**[1]

[1] *Saintgits College of Engineering, APJ Abdul Kalam University, Indore, Madhya Pradesh, India*

Abstract: Technological advancements have paved the way for revolutionary transformations in the health care sector. A significant shift in patient care has been brought about by the development of technologies such as wearables, the Internet of Things, artificial intelligence, and the metaverse, which have made possible features like telemedicine and remote health monitoring. Incorporation of these technologies has resulted in more efficient and effective diagnosis, treatment, and nursing care. The digitization of health care data has paved the way for the easy handling and sharing of medical records. Meanwhile, there are various challenges specific to sensitive patient data involving security, privacy, and interoperability. Blockchain technology, with its unique attributes like immutability, decentralization, and security, became a key priority in developing applications in different sectors, ranging from financial to education. Blockchain's privacy feature has recently prompted its integration with numerous healthcare applications, reflecting the critical necessity to protect patients' private information. The cryptographic concepts in blockchain allow the encryption of medical data, prevent unauthorized access, and enable tamper-proof storage. This work focuses on the application of blockchain in various sectors of healthcare and examines how the integration of this technology has benefited those applications.

Keywords: Artificial intelligence, Blockchain, Big data, Confidentiality, Cryptography, Decentralization, Digitization, Data security, IoT, Interoperability, Metaverse, Privacy, Smart contracts, Transparency, Wearable devices.

INTRODUCTION

The information era witnessed the generation of an enormous volume of data and the development of new concepts like big data, cloud storage, and data analytics for secure data storage and analysis. The idea of digitized data gained popularity during this period, initiating the transformation of manual health records to electronic health records. This approach provides many advantages, such as improved healthcare services, reduced healthcare costs, and high availability of

* **Corresponding author Liz George:** Saintgits College of Engineering, APJ Abdul Kalam University, Indore, Madhya Pradesh, India; Tel: +9526611300; E-mail: lizgeorge.th@gmail.com

Arun Kumar Rana, Mandeep Kaur & Sumit Kumar Rana (Eds.)

data. The medical records are made easily accessible and can be under the shared control of patients and health care professionals. In the last decade, there has been a significant shift in healthcare applications, especially in patient healthcare. The traditional hospital-oriented consultation has been reformed, allowing patients to consult with medical practitioners from the convenience of their own homes. This was made possible by the integration of cutting-edge technologies such as IoT, AI, and wearable gadgets, which led to an improvement in treatment quality and cost management.

A safe and secure system is required for the efficient and effective handling of massive and diversified medical data while maintaining its privacy and integrity. Blockchain technology, with its unique qualities such as immutability, transparency, non-repudiation, and decentralization, has considerable prospects in tackling security concerns and data management challenges pertaining to medical data [1]. The cryptographic aspects of blockchain provide a guarantee regarding the privacy and safety of medical data [2]. In this work, an in-depth examination of the inadequacies of existing healthcare apps is conducted, and the viability of utilizing blockchain technology to overcome the highlighted drawbacks is investigated. A thorough literature analysis is undertaken to identify sectors in health care where blockchain can be efficiently implemented to increase data security and efficiency, while also considering the challenges.

Overview of Technological Advancements in Healthcare

The advent of the internet and the incorporation of digital technologies in the medical sector have helped in achieving goals like progressive improvement and prioritizing individual needs [3]. Effective data management became the key focus of digital healthcare, playing a major role in the delivery of health care services [4]. Healthcare data integration consolidates patient information into a storage system, allowing evaluation and sharing with stakeholders, as well as providing medical professionals with useful insights to improve medical outcomes. Currently, many giants in healthcare are promoting the integration of pioneering technologies like big data analytics, IoT, artificial intelligence, blockchain, and metaverse [5]. It represents the latest evolution in healthcare, enhancing the interconnection between cyber and physical aspects, with the aim of providing customized services to patients, medical practitioners, and medical institutions. These advancements transform healthcare from a hospital-centred paradigm to a patient-centred one, improving care by integrating new features like remote monitoring and telemedicine [6]. It delivers patient empowerment and strives to improve patient experience, health outcomes, and cost efficiency by providing flexible access to information and encouraging cross-departmental collaboration.

Importance of Data Management in Modern Healthcare

Data management in healthcare refers to the systematic collection, storage, and analysis of patient information and healthcare-related data. The proliferation of Electronic Health Records (EHRs), wearable health technologies, and telemedicine has generated vast amounts of data [7]. Electronic Health records include details about patients' past, present, and future health conditions, which allows for more personalized and evidence-based care. In the constantly shifting landscape of healthcare, efficient data management has emerged as a cornerstone for delivering high-quality patient care [8]. A multidisciplinary approach involving telecommunications, computer science, and instrumentation is required to manage e-health systems effectively, allowing the exchange of medical data across regions [9].

Enhancing Patient Outcome

Over the years, EHRs have evolved, empowering patients to take charge of their health care by compiling their medical history in a single, accessible database. Health care data management consolidates information from various sources, enabling caregivers to analyze and share data effectively to improve medical outcomes [10]. This integration enhances communication between patients and healthcare providers, allowing practitioners to monitor clinical parameters and provide customized treatments as necessary [11].

Improving Operational Efficiency

The healthcare system's operational efficiency is greatly enhanced by data management. Healthcare companies can reduce errors and increase productivity by using efficient data systems to streamline procedures like patient scheduling, invoicing, and inventory management [12].

Ensuring Compliance and Security

Effective data management is required to fulfill the strict regulations like HIPAA and GDPR introduced by different nations, to ensure medical data privacy. Strong data governance frameworks that incorporate security procedures, data privacy, and frequent audits must be put in place by organisations [13]. Proper data management not only safeguards patient information but also protects healthcare organizations from legal repercussions and financial penalties.

Facilitating Research and Innovation

The wealth of data generated within healthcare systems presents significant opportunities for research and innovation. Researchers can determine health patterns, evaluate the effectiveness of treatments, and create new cures and interventions by efficiently organising and analysing vast datasets. Collaborative data-sharing initiatives can further enhance research efforts, leading to breakthroughs in medicine and improved public health outcomes [14]. Different aspects of effective data management are shown in Fig. (**1**).

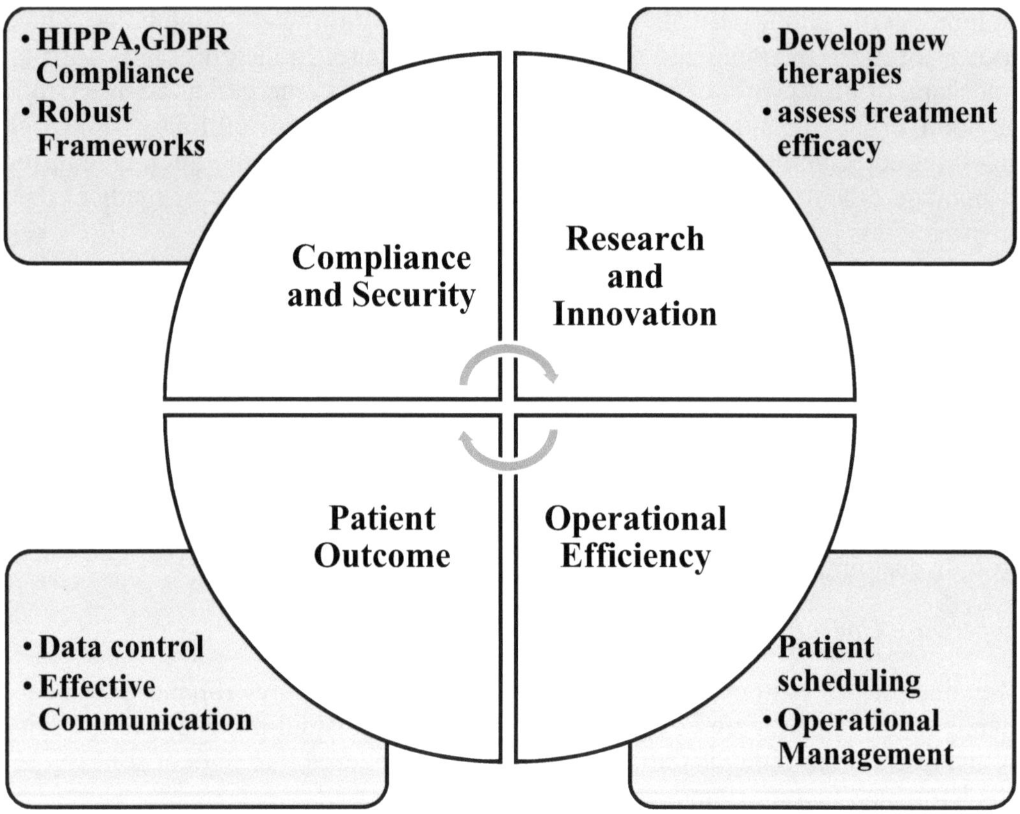

Fig. (1). Different aspects of effective data managemen.

TECHNOLOGIES TRANSFORMING HEALTHCARE

Life expectancy has increased dramatically in recent decades, making the older population a major source of concern. They frequently require assistance owing to mobility issues, dementia, or other medical conditions. In these circumstances, an independent, high-tech healthcare support system is helpful. By creating and developing effective, creative, state-of-the-art solutions in healthcare services that have a significant impact on clinicians and their patients as well as on health economies, emerging technologies like sensor technology, the Internet of Things (IoT), Artificial Intelligence (AI), big data, the metaverse, and others have completely changed the healthcare industry [15].

Wearable Devices and IoT

By enabling real-time data gathering and analysis through the connection of medical equipment to the internet, the Internet of Things (IoT) is revolutionising healthcare and providing deeper insights into patient behaviours, illness patterns, and treatment efficacy [16]. This revolution has been driven by advances in mobile computing, Near Field Communications (NFCs) like Bluetooth, RFID technology, and increased storage capacity [17]. IoT makes it possible to continuously monitor critical health data, giving patients more control over their treatments. When health measures diverge from typical ranges, this data is sent to healthcare providers, enabling prompt actions [18]. Health services based on IoT integrate resources into a unified system for tasks such as diagnosis, tracking, and virtual operations. Wearable gadgets such as smartwatches and fitness trackers are critical components of this system, monitoring health parameters such as heart rate, physical activity, blood pressure, sleep patterns, *etc.* [19]. These devices can communicate directly with healthcare providers, enabling real-time monitoring.

Wearable health gadgets do, however, come with inherent risks, such as the possibility of hacking and data breaches that jeopardize user security and privacy. Additionally, unclear user agreements, lack of robust privacy policies, and insufficient data protection legislation pose significant concerns [20]. These issues may deter widespread adoption of wearables. Furthermore, consumers often worry about the accuracy and reliability of the collected data, as well as the possible negative health repercussions of prolonged use of these devices. While wearable devices and IoT present transformative opportunities for healthcare, careful consideration of ethical and technical challenges is essential for their successful implementation.

Artificial Intelligence in Patient Care

Artificial Intelligence (AI) has the potential to significantly enhance healthcare by streamlining administrative tasks, reducing costs, and minimizing diagnostic errors [21]. It is revolutionizing modern healthcare through technologies that can predict, learn, and act, such as identifying new genetic relationships or assisting in robotic surgeries [22]. AI also aids pharmaceutical firms by accelerating drug discovery and automating target identification. AI systems manage vast amounts of healthcare data, eliminating time-consuming data monitoring tasks and producing accurate results, particularly in AI-assisted clinical trials. By analysing patient data, AI provides insights that improve patients' quality of life. AI assists doctors by providing current clinical and journal-based medical data to enhance patient care and reduce diagnostic and treatment mistakes [23]. Furthermore, AI can make inferences in real time for health risk alarms and outcome forecasts by using complex algorithms to find patterns in massive healthcare datasets. AI systems with Machine Learning (ML) components handle structured data, while Natural Language Processing (NLP) components mine unstructured texts. These systems, when trained on healthcare data, can effectively assist physicians with disease diagnosis and treatment recommendations [24]. Ultimately, AI enhances healthcare by offering precision, efficiency, and improved patient outcomes.

The incorporation of Artificial Intelligence (AI) in healthcare presents several drawbacks that hinder its effective implementation. These challenges encompass ethical, legal, and operational concerns that must be addressed to ensure safe and equitable use. AI introduces novel ethical dilemmas, including issues of patient autonomy and data privacy, which are not fully addressed by existing regulations [25]. AI systems frequently need access to enormous volumes of private patient data, which presents serious privacy concerns, making data interchange a big challenge. Personal health information may become unauthorized because of breaches.

The Role of the Metaverse in Healthcare

Metaverse integrates virtual and real-world interactions through immersive technologies like Virtual Reality (VR) and Augmented Reality (AR), offering personalized, efficient, and accessible healthcare solutions [26]. Blockchain, digital twins, and telepresence are the three main digital technologies upon which it is based [27]. Telepresence enables real-time remote engagements that allow doctors to communicate with patients in areas where access to healthcare is limited. By creating virtual versions of physical objects, digital twins make it possible for dynamic analysis, real-time monitoring, and accurate illness treatment [28]. Blockchain secures healthcare data in the metaverse, ensuring tamper-proof records and acting as a bridge, connecting the virtual and real worlds.

Medical Training and Education

The metaverse offers highly interactive and immersive environments for medical training. Medical practitioners and students can rehearse difficult procedures in lifelike, three-dimensional environments using virtual simulations without endangering real patients [29]. Augmented reality (AR) can overlay real-time data or instructional guides during training sessions, improving the learning process. This can also be used to train doctors in remote locations using digital twins and VR simulations.

Telemedicine

One of the key applications of the metaverse in healthcare is telemedicine, which allows healthcare professionals to provide remote medical services to patients. This enables healthcare providers to reach patients in remote or underserved areas, reducing the need for in-person visits and improving access to care [30]. Vital indications like blood sugar and pulse rate can be continuously monitored using real-time data provided by wearable devices combined with the metaverse, enabling the early identification of possible health problems [31].

Smart Surgery

Metaverse, when paired with robotic-assisted surgery and augmented reality, can improve smart operations by delivering real-time overlays of patient data, 3D models, and insights during procedures. Simulating multiple surgical situations to ascertain potential risks, recuperation time, and exposure to radiation facilitates preoperative risk assessment [32]. Surgeons can interact remotely using VR settings, sharing experience during live procedures or performing operations from faraway places, hence boosting surgical precision and results.

Medical Research

Drug development and medical research can be made more economical, safe, and efficient with the use of metaverse technology. It can assist in testing and enhancing therapies for illnesses linked to mobility and neurological issues [33]. Using digital twins, researchers may simulate human organs and medication interactions to evaluate proposed drugs' safety and efficacy prior to human trials.

Creating a metaverse environment for healthcare presents significant challenges, requiring high proficiency, resources, and seamless integration of technologies like VR, AR, and MR [34]. It is difficult to create dynamic and aesthetically pleasing virtual worlds, and the infrastructure must manage enormous volumes of data produced by millions of users. The user experience can be hampered by scalability problems, and implementation is made more difficult by VR systems' high price, mass, and immobility [35]. Inconsistency and interoperability across different platforms remain problematic, alongside concerns over privacy and security. The metaverse collects vast amounts of sensitive user data, making it a target for hackers, and existing real-world privacy laws may not apply in the virtual realm, necessitating the development of metaverse-specific privacy legislation [36].

Table **1** summarizes the merits and demerits related to the integration of modern technologies like Wearable Devices, IoT, AI, and the Metaverse in healthcare:

Table 1. Analysis of integration of modern technologies in healthcare.

Technologies	Merits	Demerits	Refs.
Wearable Devices and IoT	- Real-time health data monitoring. - Enables personalized treatment and early detection. - Enhances patient engagement.	- Security risks due to hacking and data breaches. - Unclear privacy policies and insufficient legislation. - Concerns over data accuracy and long-term health effects.	[16 - 20]
Artificial Intelligence (AI)	- Reduces diagnostic errors and administrative burdens. - Improves precision in treatment and surgery. - Accelerates drug discovery.	- Ethical issues regarding autonomy and privacy. - Requires large amounts of sensitive data. - Breaches could expose personal health information.	[21 - 25]
Metaverse	- Provides immersive medical training and remote surgeries. - Enhances telemedicine for remote patients. - Improves drug testing via digital twins.	- High cost and complexity of VR/AR technology. - Privacy and security concerns, especially with large data volumes. - Scalability and interoperability issues.	[26 - 36]

CHALLENGES IN HEALTHCARE DATA MANAGEMENT

Despite having unique regulatory regimes for each nation, health care systems in the entire globe are facing more or less the same challenges, ranging from changing needs of patients, care for the aging population, secure storage and sharing of data, to accurate diagnosis and treatment of chronic diseases [37]. Although the integration of modern technologies has paved the way for innovative practices in health care, there are many issues and challenges that need to be tackled to proceed further.

Security Concerns

However, the introduction of these new technologies and digitization has increased the vulnerability of patient records. Compromising the sensitive medical data has always been a major concern in the industry, which can result in potentially serious consequences [38]. Currently implemented security measures are weak with many drawbacks. The sharing of EHR has led to many security breaches, threatening the privacy of patients and the security and confidentiality of medical data. While security is the degree to which access to an individual's personal information is limited and permitted only to those who are authorized, privacy refers to the right of an individual to control when, how, and to what extent their personal information is transferred or shared by others [39].

Modification, alarm fabrication, denial of service, tracking user position and activity, physical device tampering, and jammer assaults are examples of violations pertaining to medical data security [40].

Privacy of Sensitive Patient Data

Managing the complex healthcare system with multiple entities and the categorization, as well as handling of the patient data represented using a versatile data structure, has always been a grave concern. Adding to that, with the advancement in technology, medical data is continually being targeted, and appropriate measures must be taken for the safekeeping of the data [41]. Considering the issues mentioned above, many nations have introduced strict privacy regulations like the Health Insurance Portability and Accountability Act (HIPAA) and General Data Protection Regulation (GDPR) regarding the handling and sharing of medical data to ensure privacy and confidentiality [42]. But all the privacy-related regulations introduced so far were more focused on protecting the healthcare data rather than assuring its responsible uses and disclosures. Advanced cryptographic algorithms for data encryption, secure communication lines for data transfer, and efficient authentication mechanisms are some of the actions that can be implemented to overcome the data security and privacy concerns.

Issues with Data Interoperability

Within the framework of contemporary healthcare, the issue of data interoperability presents considerable obstacles. Although significant technical progress has driven the healthcare sector towards a more unified and effective system, the smooth transfer and use of data among many platforms and stakeholders still present challenges [43]. The challenges related to data interoperability, as shown in Fig. (**2**), are of utmost priority as they directly affect the efficacy of patient care and the performance of healthcare operations.

Data Source Heterogeneity

Healthcare data comes from a variety of sources, including wearable technologies, laboratory findings, medical imaging, Electronic Health Records (EHRs), and Personal Health Records (PHRs). Disparate formats and standards employed by each source often provide challenges in the thorough aggregation and analysis of data [44]. The presence of this diversity limits the ability of medical professionals to fully comprehend a patient's state or to conduct in-depth analysis that can direct treatment interventions and health outcomes.

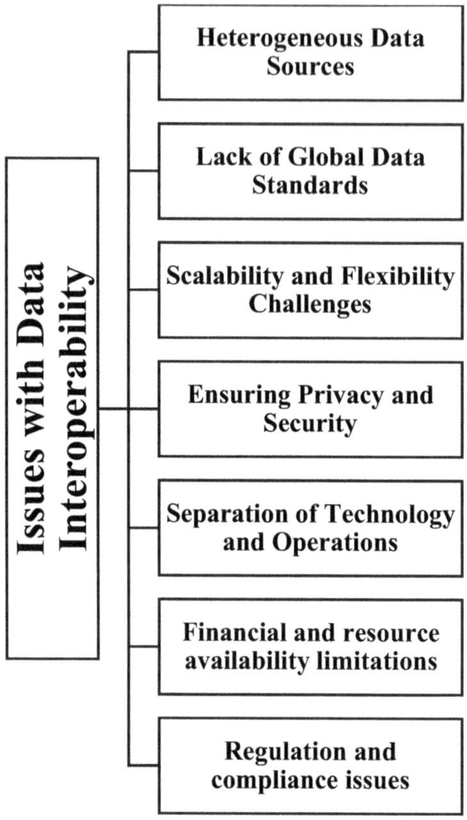

Fig. (2). Data interoperability issues.

Absence of Standardization

Universally accepted standards for data storage, retrieval, and interchange are currently absent. Disparate healthcare systems and providers frequently employ varied protocols and data formats, which hinder the efficient exchange of information [45]. The absence of such uniformity not only adds complexity to the integration of data but also heightens the likelihood of mistakes in medical treatment and administrative procedures.

Challenges with Scalability and Flexibility

With the continued exponential growth of healthcare data volumes, systems that were not originally built with interoperability in consideration are facing growing challenges in adapting and scaling. The absence of the necessary adaptability to integrate novel forms of data or to establish connections with developing technology sometimes results in inefficiencies and overlooked means of improving patient care.

Concerns Regarding Privacy and Security

Interoperability adds additional intricacy to the task of guaranteeing data privacy and security. The integration of different data systems requires the implementation of strong procedures to safeguard sensitive information and adhere to legal and regulatory obligations [46]. The task of ensuring the security of interoperable systems and preserving patient confidentiality is substantial, considering the growing number of access points and the diverse range of data handlers involved.

Separation of Technology and Operations

Healthcare organisations frequently function in isolated domains, where several departments use separate systems that lack the necessary capabilities to interact with one another [47]. The existence of these silos poses a significant obstacle to achieving interoperability, resulting in inefficiencies and a fragmented paradigm of healthcare delivery. Breaking down these barriers necessitates significant modifications in both the implementation of technology and the culture of the organization.

Limitations in Financial and Resource Availability

The development and upkeep of interoperable systems can incur significant expenses and require substantial resources. Poor EHR interoperability is s damaging to patient safety and costly for healthcare systems [48]. Numerous healthcare organizations encounter budgetary limitations that restrict their capacity to allocate resources towards essential technologies and personnel training. Achieving the necessary level of interoperability to enhance healthcare outcomes and operational efficiency might be difficult in the absence of sufficient resources.

Matters of Regulation and Compliance

Successfully navigating the intricate terrain of healthcare legislation presents an additional level of challenge in attaining interoperability. Regulatory compliance, such as HIPAA in the U.S. or GDPR in Europe, impacts the sharing and utilization of data between institutions and across borders. Achieving compliance while aiming for interoperability necessitates a careful equilibrium and frequently adds complexity to the integration endeavours [49].

BLOCKCHAIN TECHNOLOGY

Blockchain is a decentralized, distributed ledger technology that enhances the trust, security, and transparency of data across various sectors, including healthcare. Each block in the blockchain contains validated transaction data, a timestamp, and a cryptographic hash of the previous block, creating a secure and tamper-resistant chain [50]. The system operates without a central authority, relying on cryptographic methods like Merkle trees and nonce values for secure data storage and verification. This framework increases the dependability of healthcare procedures by guaranteeing that transactional data is recorded in an immutable and visible manner.

Fundamental Attributes of Blockchain

Node

Any user or system that participates in the blockchain network is referred to as a node. Every node can start or approve transactions and possesses a copy of the distributed ledger.

Transaction

Transactions are the basic units of operation within the blockchain. Generated by a node, transactions are added to a block only after being verified and validated by miners.

Block

A block is a data structure that stores validated transactions. Miners create blocks by verifying transactions, which are then linked together to form the blockchain.

Chain

The chain is a series of blocks connected via cryptography. To maintain the blockchain's integrity and order, each block includes a cryptographic hash of the one before it.

Miners

Specialized nodes called miners are in charge of transaction validation and verification. They contribute new blocks to the blockchain by resolving challenging mathematical riddles.

Merkle Tree

Also known as a Hash Tree, the Merkle Tree is a data structure used to efficiently and securely verify large amounts of data. It combines the hashes of several blocks of data to ensure accuracy and integrity.

Smart Contract

A smart contract is self-executing code that, when certain conditions are satisfied, automatically carries out particular activities. These contracts are resistant to tampering and are implemented through transactions that are cryptographically signed. Smart contracts facilitate process automation across a range of industries, including healthcare.

Cryptographic Security Mechanisms

Cryptography forms the foundation of blockchain's security, enabling secure, trustless, and tamper-resistant networks where data integrity and confidentiality are maintained without needing centralized authorities. In traditional systems, third-party intermediaries are often required to establish trust between parties, but blockchain uses cryptography to eliminate this need. Cryptographic techniques allow blockchain to create a secure environment where trusted records and transactions can occur between untrusted parties. Information is stored on the blockchain ledger using cryptographic methods, ensuring that data is secure, verified, and immutable [51].

Hashing Algorithms for Data Integrity

A core cryptographic technique employed in blockchain is the use of cryptographic hash functions. Hash algorithms take input data of any length and produce a fixed-length hash value. These algorithms have essential properties such as unidirectionality (making it impossible to reverse-engineer the original data from its hash), collision resistance (preventing different inputs from producing the same hash), and high sensitivity (even minor changes to the input result in entirely different hash values) [52]. Hashing plays a crucial role in ensuring data integrity by enabling the detection of even the smallest alterations to thc data.

Hashing techniques such as SHA-256 (Secure Hash Algorithm 256-bit) are frequently employed in blockchain technology to provide distinct hash outputs for every data block. Data immutability is ensured in large part by hash functions [53]. Any effort to change a transaction after it has been added to a block and recorded on the blockchain would produce a whole new hash value, which makes tampering simple to identify [54]. This maintains the integrity of the blockchain ledger by guaranteeing that transactions, once recorded, cannot be altered.

Hash functions can aid in linking blocks inside the network. A chain of cryptographically connected records is formed by each block containing the hash of the one before it. This structure greatly improves the distributed ledger's security and integrity by making it computationally impossible to change a block without also changing all following blocks [55].

Public-Key Cryptography for Authentication and Privacy

Another crucial blockchain mechanism is public-key cryptography, sometimes referred to as asymmetric encryption. Each user needs two keys: a private key for decryption and a public key for encryption. The private key is kept confidential, but the public key is freely exchanged. Users can securely sign transactions and authenticate themselves with this system without disclosing any personal information. Blockchain participants can safely demonstrate asset ownership and confirm the legitimacy of transactions using public-key cryptography [56].

A user's private key is used to generate digital signatures, which guarantee the legitimacy and non-repudiation of transactions [57]. A user uses their private key to sign a transaction when they start it. The user's public key can then be used by other blockchain network users to confirm the signature. Only the legitimate owner of the private key can approve transactions thanks to this procedure, and others can verify the legitimacy without having access to the private key itself [58].

Public-key cryptography also enhances privacy on blockchain networks. While transactions are publicly visible on blockchains like Bitcoin and Ethereum, users remain pseudonymous. Instead of revealing personal information, users are identified by their public key or blockchain address [59]. This approach balances transparency with privacy, allowing for secure transactions without compromising the identity of the participants.

Decentralization and Its Advantages

Decentralization in blockchain brings a multitude of advantages that revolutionize traditional systems by shifting control from centralized authorities to a distributed network of participants. One of the primary benefits is enhanced security. In a decentralized blockchain, data is stored across multiple nodes, making it highly resistant to cyberattacks and hacking attempts [60]. Without a single point of failure, it becomes exponentially more difficult for malicious actors to compromise the system, as they would need to control a majority of the network to alter or manipulate data. This security is further strengthened by blockchain's cryptographic algorithms, ensuring that transactions and records remain tamper-proof and immutable.

Transparency is yet another important benefit. Every transaction in decentralized blockchain networks is documented on a public ledger that is open to all users.

Because everyone can independently confirm the data's integrity and make sure no unauthorized changes have been made, this transparency promotes user trust [61]. This is especially helpful in sectors where responsibility and trust are crucial, such as supply chain management, healthcare, and finance. Additionally, decentralization removes the need for middlemen like banks or outside service providers, which lowers transaction costs and simplifies procedures [62]. Through direct user-to-user interactions, peer-to-peer networks can reduce the possible bottlenecks, costs, and delays that come with centralized systems.

Decentralization also makes the network more resilient. The entire system may be disrupted in a centralized system if the central authority fails or is compromised. A decentralized blockchain, on the other hand, is naturally fault-tolerant since the network may continue to function even if some nodes are compromised or go offline. Decentralization encourages democratization and inclusivity. It keeps power from being concentrated in the hands of a small number of entities by dispersing control throughout a large network of players. By using consensus techniques like proof of work or proof of stake, this guarantees that every user has an equal voice in network governance. By enabling members to collectively validate transactions and agree on the blockchain's current state, these methods promote cooperation and a sense of shared ownership.

APPLICATION OF BLOCKCHAIN IN HEALTHCARE

Blockchain, a distributed ledger technology, has shown promise in addressing the security issues that smart healthcare systems face. Blockchain is the perfect platform for safely storing and exchanging sensitive healthcare data because of its built-in features, which include immutability, decentralization, and cryptographic security. By guarding against illegal access, tampering, and data breaches, blockchain-based healthcare systems can guarantee the confidentiality and integrity of patient records.

Smart contracts are used in blockchain to implement application-specific logic. They can be effectively used in healthcare applications to evaluate patient data and provide customized services, to improve data transparency in clinical trials, and automate long and complex workflows [63]. Blockchain was successful in resolving major concerns regarding the secure storage and handling of data, the biggest hurdle faced in the medical sector.

Impact on Telemedicine and Remote Monitoring

Blockchain can also support the growing field of telemedicine and remote health monitoring, where data is shared between patients and healthcare providers through digital platforms. It offers a distributed architecture to manage and synchronize health records among various participants, ensuring the integrity and verification of data across all nodes. A study investigated the role of blockchain in improving the security of telemedicine platforms [64]. Their findings suggest that blockchain could enable secure real-time data sharing between patients and doctors while maintaining the privacy of medical consultations. Blockchain's decentralized, impenetrable storage of patient-generated data from wearable devices guarantees the security and dependability of the data in the context of remote health monitoring. Key issues, including tracking the whereabouts of sick patients, safeguarding remote consultation records, tracking down pharmaceuticals and medical test kits, confirming the legitimacy of doctors, and demonstrating the origin of defective test kits, are all addressed by this technology. A study investigated blockchain's potential application in wearable medical technology, pointing out that it might provide individuals more control over the use of their health information while guaranteeing that it is safely transmitted to the appropriate healthcare practitioners [65].

A study proposed HapiChain, a blockchain-based framework intended to enhance the security, scalability, and reliability of telemedicine workflows, offering telemonitoring and teleconsultation services [66]. It integrates blockchain technology, smart contracts, and the Interplanetary File System (IPFS) for secure and scalable data storage, while using the Ethereum blockchain as its decentralized platform. Another study introduced DBTMD, a Telemedicine Diagnosis privacy protection scheme using a double blockchain structure, comprising the user chain and the medical chain, to enable secure data interaction between users, doctors, and hospitals while allowing hospitals to supervise doctors [66]. The scheme incorporates an identity authentication chain for real-time verification of doctors' identities and has been shown to significantly reduce communication costs compared to existing solutions. The authors of a study suggested a blockchain-based architecture that uses Ethereum smart contracts to build a telemedicine healthcare system that is transparent, impenetrable, and guarantees the integrity of private patient data without the need for a central administrator. Patients are informed of all network transactions, and interactions between all parties are managed by the smart contracts.

Monitoring Drug Supply Chain Management

Counterfeit drugs are a global issue, leading to significant health risks and financial losses. Blockchain has shown promise in pharmaceutical supply chain management by providing traceability and transparency. A study exploring blockchain's use in drug supply chains to track the origin and movement of pharmaceuticals from manufacturers to consumers [69]. Their findings revealed that blockchain could effectively reduce counterfeit drugs by offering a transparent, tamper-proof ledger of every transaction. The study also emphasized the role of smart contracts in automating the verification process, ensuring that only authentic drugs are dispensed to patients. Another study further supported these findings, demonstrating that blockchain's decentralized nature makes it an ideal solution for monitoring pharmaceutical products in real-time, particularly in regions with weak regulatory oversight [70].

A study investigated pharmaceutical governance through the use of a Distributed Ledger Technology (DLT) that generates an immutable, transparent record of every transaction and a unique IoT-based blockchain system [71]. By enhancing drug governance throughout the supply chain, this system's implementation in the pharmaceutical business raises healthcare effectiveness and reliability. A paper introduced PharmaChain, decentralized Hyperledger fabric framework that enhances drug traceability in the pharmaceutical supply chain by leveraging confidentiality, accountability, and interoperability through secure, rapid transactions and smart contracts [72]. The system employs elliptic curve digital signatures, hash encryption, and protection against node attacks to prevent counterfeit pharmaceuticals and ensure public health. In another study, the proposed blockchain-based framework for the decentralized online sale of pharmaceuticals uses Ethereum smart contracts to monitor participant interactions, log transactions, and ensure secure payment dispersal without intermediaries like hospitals or pharmacies [73]. To guarantee the safe delivery of medications, smart contracts also monitor the condition of IoT containers, inform customers about their orders, and manage reimbursements in the event of contract violations.

Improving Diagnosis and Treatment

By tackling important issues like data security, interoperability, and transparency, blockchain technology has a great deal of promise to enhance healthcare diagnosis and treatment. It makes it possible for medical records to be shared and stored securely and decentralized, guaranteeing the integrity and correctness of patient data among various healthcare providers. Healthcare organizations may increase the speed and precision of diagnosis and treatment plans by utilizing blockchain technology to build a single, impenetrable database that offers real-time access to patient medical histories [74]. The application of smart contracts on blockchain platforms can further enhance medical workflows by automating processes like appointment scheduling, prescription management, and medical billing. This reduces administrative errors and ensures that all participants in the healthcare system, including patients, doctors, and insurance companies, are held accountable for their actions [75]. Blockchain's decentralized nature also eliminates the need for intermediaries, which can lower operational costs and increase efficiency in treatment delivery. Another paper proposed MedRec, a blockchain-based decentralized record management solution that gives patients safe, unchangeable access to their medical records across physicians and treatment facilities [76]. Interoperability is promoted by the system's smooth integration with current local data storage systems, which guarantees authentication, secrecy, and data exchange.

Additionally, blockchain can support precision medicine by securely integrating and analyzing large datasets from multiple sources, including genomic data, patient health records, and clinical trial results. This allows for more personalized treatment approaches based on individual patient profiles [77]. The technology also facilitates better collaboration in clinical trials by ensuring the transparency and integrity of trial data, which accelerates the discovery of new therapies and enhances patient safety [78]. Through the integration of blockchain with Artificial Intelligence (AI) and Machine Learning (ML) algorithms, healthcare providers can leverage vast datasets to identify patterns and predict outcomes. This data-driven approach can enhance personalized medicine by tailoring treatment plans to individual patient profiles based on comprehensive, real-time data.

Effective Handling of Medical Billing and Insurance Claims

Fraud in medical billing and insurance claims is a widespread issue that costs the healthcare industry billions of dollars each year. Blockchain's capacity to provide a clear, real-time record of transactions can significantly reduce fraudulent activities in this area. The authors of a study reviewed the impact of blockchain on healthcare billing systems, noting that the technology could automate claims processing by using smart contracts, which trigger payments once predefined conditions are met [74]. This ensures that payments are transparent and minimizes administrative costs. Another study supported these findings by showcasing how blockchain-enabled insurance claims systems could verify transactions and reduce the time spent on claims processing [79]. Their research emphasized how blockchain could help healthcare providers and insurers create more efficient, secure systems for managing claims.

A paper proposed B-SAHIC, designed using Hyperledger Fabric, that automates and secures health insurance claims processing through a smart contract and provides a web-based portal for user interaction [80]. It incorporates CouchDB for off-chain data storage and ensures client data privacy through unique encryption keys for each submission. Performance studies indicate that B-SAHIC is fast and scalable, and has minimal resource consumption, making it a viable model for automation in other insurance sectors. The authors of a study explored how blockchain technology's decentralized and immutable ledger can be used to eliminate fraud, mistakes, and inefficiencies in conventional healthcare billing [81]. It examines blockchain's potential to enhance transparency, improve claim processing, reduce errors, and increase data security and overall competence in healthcare billing systems. The study concludes that blockchain offers significant benefits for transforming healthcare billing practices. A study focused on using blockchain and Ethereum smart contracts to manage medical records for insurance claims, creating a tamper-proof and transparent system without a central administrator [81]. It ensures data integrity and keeps patients informed while leveraging Machine Learning techniques like Random Forest Classifier and Support Vector Machines to prevent fraudulent claims. The integration of ML with blockchain enhances the precision and reliability of the insurance claim process. Table **2** shows different applications of blockchain and their key features.

Table 2. Different applications of blockchain and their key features.

Applications of Blockchain	Key Points	Refs.
Telemedicine and Remote Monitoring	▪ Blockchain ensures secure real-time data sharing between patients and healthcare providers, improving the privacy and integrity of medical consultations. ▪ Supports telemedicine by securing patient data from wearable devices in a decentralized, tamper-proof system. ▪ Proposals like HapiChain and DBTMD enhance telemedicine security through smart contracts and decentralized platforms.	[63 - 68]
Drug Supply Chain Management	▪ Blockchain provides traceability and transparency, reducing the risk of counterfeit drugs. ▪ Smart contracts automate the verification process for authentic drugs. ▪ Frameworks like PharmaChain improve drug governance, security, and scalability.	[69 - 73]
Diagnosis and Treatment	▪ Blockchain improves diagnosis accuracy by creating a unified, tamper-proof database for patient records. ▪ Enhances transparency and interoperability across healthcare providers. ▪ Platforms like MedRec allow secure access to medical histories, supporting precision medicine.	[74 - 78]
Medical Billing and Insurance Claims	▪ Reduces fraud in medical billing and claims processing by using transparent, real-time records. ▪ Smart contracts automate claims processing, reducing errors and costs. ▪ Solutions like B-SAHIC leverage blockchain to improve efficiency, scalability, and security in insurance claims.	[79 - 82]

BENEFITS OF BLOCKCHAIN INTEGRATION

Enhancing Privacy and Security

Blockchain technology plays a pivotal role in enhancing privacy and security in healthcare by transforming the traditional centralized structure of Electronic Health Records (EHRs) into a decentralized network [83]. This shift reduces reliance on third parties, improving the overall health management infrastructure, including storage management, data access, and the confidentiality of personal information. The decentralized approach mitigates security concerns by ensuring that data integrity and access are maintained without a central authority.

New cryptosystems that combine blockchain technology with Identity-Based Encryption (IBE) and Attribute-Based Encryption (ABE) have been introduced recently [84]. By providing total control over access to cloud-backed medical data, these solutions improve confidentiality, authentication, and the integrity of medical information. Additionally, blockchain's consent function optimizes the consensus algorithm governing the access, storage, and distribution of medical data within the EHR network. Decisions must be approved by all network participants, ensuring a high level of certainty before any data modifications are permitted. Privacy concerns in blockchain-based healthcare systems focus on maintaining the confidentiality of sensitive medical information. Researchers have explored various methods to address these concerns, including user authentication and access control mechanisms [85]. In terms of information protection, blockchain research has primarily concentrated on preventing illegal access and safeguarding data from unauthorized manipulation. Techniques such as multiple identities, biometric authentication [86], and effective user identification have been proposed to secure data. However, there is a notable lack of focus on defending against external threats like sensor data attacks, transactional assaults, and conspiracies, which remain critical areas for further investigation.

Blockchain technology provides a robust framework for enhancing privacy and security in healthcare by leveraging its decentralized nature and advanced cryptographic methods. This approach addresses key challenges related to data integrity, access control, and protection against unauthorized access, contributing to a more secure and efficient healthcare system.

Streamlining Data Sharing and Accessibility

Blockchain technology has emerged as a transformative solution for streamlining data sharing and accessibility in the healthcare sector, particularly in managing sensitive patient information. One of the early applications of blockchain in healthcare involves enhancing the sharing of health data, which is inherently sensitive and requires rigorous protection. Different research works have highlighted blockchain's role in the administration of medical information and electronic private records, recognizing its potential to manage and secure vast amounts of data efficiently.

Blockchain offers a robust framework for creating effective data ecosystems by integrating Patient Health Records (PHRs) from various sources. The proposed integration allows for a comprehensive and unified view of patient data, which can significantly reduce the time required for treatment [87]. By facilitating easier access to accurate and up-to-date patient information, blockchain enables physicians to quickly identify symptoms and make informed decisions, thereby improving the quality of care. Blockchain can legally and ethically manage healthcare information, addressing concerns related to data processing, distribution, and compliance [88]. Studies have emphasized the importance of preserving the authenticity and integrity of medical information, with blockchain providing solutions to prevent data theft, avoid duplication of storage costs [89], and ensure the permanence of data retention. As blockchain adoption grows, attention has also shifted towards improving data protection from medical equipment and ensuring secure inter-institutional information exchange [90].

Blockchain technology streamlines data sharing and accessibility in healthcare by creating a secure, decentralized system that integrates and manages patient information effectively [91 - 93]. It enhances the speed and accuracy of data retrieval, supports compliance with legal and ethical standards, and facilitates secure data exchange between institutions, ultimately leading to better patient care and operational efficiency in healthcare systems.

Fostering Trust and Transparency

Blockchain technology plays a pivotal role in fostering trust and transparency in healthcare by handling key problems related to fraud, data manipulation, and resource mismanagement. Its inherent features, such as an immutable ledger and decentralized verification, provide a robust framework for ensuring transparency across various sectors of healthcare.

In pharmaceutical supply chains, blockchain enhances transparency by creating an auditable trail of every transaction. As noted in another study, this technology enables the recording and verification of every process involved in the drug supply chain, ensuring the authenticity of medications and preventing counterfeit drugs from entering the market [94]. In addition to protecting patients' privacy, it also strengthens trust in the pharmaceutical industry. In clinical trials, blockchain addresses issues of data integrity and reliability. Traditional trials often face problems like selective reporting and data manipulation. The authors of a study highlight that blockchain can record all trial data transparently and immutably, ensuring that the data remains unaltered and accessible to relevant parties [95]. This transparency improves the credibility of research findings and fosters greater trust in medical research outcomes. Blockchain also enhances trust in telemedicine and remote consultations, which have become increasingly important, especially during the COVID-19 pandemic. Concerns about data security and the authenticity of remote interactions are prevalent. Blockchain technology secures telemedicine platforms by encrypting patient-doctor communications and using smart contracts to log and verify interactions [96]. Specifies the role of blockchain to provide a transparent, trustworthy system for remote consultations, ensuring confidentiality and reliability.

BLOCKCHAIN IN THE HEALTH CARE SECTOR- CHALLENGES

Blockchain technology offers immense potential to transform healthcare data management by enhancing security, transparency, and integrity, but its integration faces several challenges. One major issue is scalability, as healthcare systems generate massive volumes of data, including electronic health records, medical images, and real-time streams from wearable devices [97]. Most blockchain platforms struggle to handle such large-scale data efficiently due to limitations in transaction throughput, latency, and block size, hindering real-time decision-making. Data privacy and regulatory compliance also pose difficulties. The immutable nature of Blockchain can conflict with regulations like HIPAA and GDPR that require data modification or deletion, such as the "right to be forgotten," necessitating advanced cryptographic and selective disclosure solutions [98].

Interoperability further complicates adoption, as healthcare systems rely on diverse legacy infrastructures and standards. Ensuring seamless data exchange and compatibility with protocols like HL7 and FHIR remains a significant obstacle. Additionally, blockchain is not suited for storing large datasets directly on-chain, requiring off-chain storage solutions that increase complexity and cost. Deploying and maintaining permissioned networks can also be expensive, limiting adoption by resource-constrained organizations [99].

Governance, legal uncertainties, and organizational readiness present additional barriers. Establishing clear policies, defining access control, and ensuring accountability across multiple stakeholders are challenging. The absence of comprehensive legal frameworks, lack of technical expertise, and resistance to change further slow adoption. Overcoming these challenges will require collaborative efforts among healthcare providers, technologists, policymakers, and regulators to ensure blockchain's successful integration and unlock its transformative potential for secure, efficient, and interoperable healthcare systems.

FUTURE PROSPECTS AND CONCLUSION

Blockchain adoption in the healthcare sector is still nascent and limited. To fully realize its potential, future developments should focus on creating Lightweight Blockchain Models that that incorporate optimized cryptographic primitives and efficient consensus algorithms such as Proof-of-Authority (PoA) or Delegated Proof-of-Stake (DPoS), resulting in reduced computational overhead, a decrease in energy consumption, and faster transaction processing. Given the large size and sensitivity of healthcare data, particularly medical imaging and genomic data, it is neither practical nor efficient to store all information directly on the blockchain. Hybrid architectures that combine blockchain's immutability and access control capabilities with off-chain storage solutions can be incorporated, allowing blockchain to manage metadata, patient consent, and access permissions, while large data sets are securely stored and retrieved from external storage. This approach enhances scalability, performance, and cost-effectiveness while maintaining robust data integrity and traceability.

Development of interoperability frameworks and cross-platform standards that facilitate seamless communication and data sharing while complying with healthcare regulations such as HIPAA, GDPR, and FHIR is highly recommended. Efforts in this area should also include the creation of standardized APIs and middleware solutions that enable legacy healthcare systems to integrate with blockchain-based infrastructures without extensive reengineering. Furthermore, the combination of blockchain with Internet of Things (IoT) and Artificial Intelligence (AI) technologies presents an exciting avenue for advancement. Integrating AI, such as Federated Learning, into blockchain-based IoT healthcare systems can enhance data analysis and decision-making processes, improving patient care efficiency and privacy.

In conclusion, while blockchain technology holds transformative potential for healthcare, its successful implementation will depend on advancing lightweight models, integrating AI, and leveraging quantum computing. These innovations will help address current limitations and fully exploit the capabilities of blockchain to improve healthcare services and patient outcomes.

REFERENCES

[1] D. Cagigas, J. Clifton, D. Diaz-Fuentes, and M. Fernández-Gutiérrez, "Blockchain for Public Services: A Systematic Literature Review", *IEEE Access,* vol. 9, pp. 13904-13921, 2021. [http://dx.doi.org/10.1109/ACCESS.2021.3052019]

[2] A.C.M.H. Pranto Kumar Ghosh, "KRAHS. Blockchain Application in Healthcare Systems: A

Review", *Systems (Basel),* vol. 11, no. 1, 2023.

[3] V.V. Popov, E.V. Kudryavtseva, N. Kumar Katiyar, A. Shishkin, S.I. Stepanov, and S. Goel, "KEV,KKN,SA,SSI,GS. Industry 4.0 and digitalisation in healthcare", *Materials (Basel),* vol. 15, no. 6, p. 2140, 2022.
[http://dx.doi.org/10.3390/ma15062140] [PMID: 35329592]

[4] M. Paul, L. Maglaras, M.A. Ferrag, and I. Almomani, "Digitization of healthcare sector: A study on privacy and security concerns", *ICT Express,* vol. 9, no. 4, pp. 571-588, 2023.
[http://dx.doi.org/10.1016/j.icte.2023.02.007]

[5] A. Gupta, and A. Singh, "Healthcare 4.0: recent advancements and futuristic research directions", *Wirel. Pers. Commun.,* vol. 129, no. 2, pp. 933-952, 2023.
[http://dx.doi.org/10.1007/s11277-022-10164-8] [PMID: 36594000]

[6] C.B. Christoph Thuemmler, "Health 4.0: Application of Industry 4.0 Design Principles in Future Asthma Management", In: *Health 4.0: How Virtualization and Big Data are Revolutionizing Healthcare.* Springer, 2017, pp. 23-37.
[http://dx.doi.org/10.1007/978-3-319-47617-9_2]

[7] E.K. Achampong, "Electronic Health Record (EHR) and Cloud Security: The Current Issues", *International Journal of Cloud Computing and Services Science (IJ-CLOSER),* vol. 2, no. 6, pp. 417-420, 2014.
[http://dx.doi.org/10.11591/closer.v2i6.5343]

[8] Naresh Kasoju NSRRSSSBSCKCVMPRHV&SB. Digital health: trends, opportunities and challenges in medical devices, pharma and bio-technology. CSI Transactions on ICT. 2023; 11: 11-30.

[9] M.L.M. Kiah, B.B. Zaidan, A.A. Zaidan, M. Nabi, and R. Ibraheem, "MIRASS: medical informatics research activity support system using information mashup network", *J. Med. Syst.,* vol. 38, no. 4, p. 37, 2014.
[http://dx.doi.org/10.1007/s10916-014-0037-x] [PMID: 24700079]

[10] J. Pawelek, K. Baca-Motes, J.A. Pandit, B.B. Berk, and E. Ramos, "The Power of Patient Engagement With Electronic Health Records as Research Participants", *JMIR Med. Inform.,* vol. 10, no. 7, p. e39145, 2022.
[http://dx.doi.org/10.2196/39145] [PMID: 35802410]

[11] M. Hussain, A. Al-Haiqi, A.A. Zaidan, B.B. Zaidan, M.L.M. Kiah, N.B. Anuar, and M. Abdulnabi, "The landscape of research on smartphone medical apps: Coherent taxonomy, motivations, open challenges and recommendations", *Comput. Methods Programs Biomed.,* vol. 122, no. 3, pp. 393-408, 2015.
[http://dx.doi.org/10.1016/j.cmpb.2015.08.015] [PMID: 26412009]

[12] D. Bhati, M.S. Deogade, and D. Kanyal, "Improving Patient Outcomes Through Effective Hospital Administration: A Comprehensive Review", *Cureus,* vol. 15, no. 10, p. e47731, 2023.
[http://dx.doi.org/10.7759/cureus.47731] [PMID: 38021686]

[13] S.A.F.A.B.J. Javad Pool, "A systematic analysis of failures in protecting personal health data: A scoping review", *Int. J. Inf. Manage.,* p. 74, 2024.

[14] S.K.S.M.S. Sabyasachi Dash, "K. Big data in healthcare: management, analysis and future prospects", *J. Big Data,* 2019.

[15] S.G. Swati Sikdar, "Advancements of Healthcare Technologies: Paradigm Towards Smart Healthcare Systems", In: *Recent Trends in Image and Signal Processing in Computer Vision.* Springer, 2020, pp. 113-132.
[http://dx.doi.org/10.1007/978-981-15-2740-1_9]

[16] P.S. C v, and D.S.K.M. Bargavi, "IoT for Healthcare Data Analytics", *International Journal of Research Publication and Reviews,* vol. 5, no. 5, pp. 6365-6369, 2024.
[http://dx.doi.org/10.55248/gengpi.5.0524.1421]

[17] S.P. Dash, "S.P. D. The impact of IoT in healthcare: global technological change & the roadmap to a networked architecture in India", *J. Indian Inst. Sci.,* vol. 100, no. 4, pp. 773-785, 2020. [http://dx.doi.org/10.1007/s41745-020-00208-y] [PMID: 33162693]

[18] P.S.S.S.G. Pon Harshavardhanan, "IoT as Wearable Device in Smart Healthcare Systems: A New Paradigm", In: *Technologies for Sustainable Healthcare Development.* IGI Global, 2024. [http://dx.doi.org/10.4018/979-8-3693-2901-6.ch005]

[19] V.P.P. Giuseppe Aceto, "Industry 4.0 and Health: Internet of Things, Big Data, and Cloud Computing for Healthcare 4.0", *J. Ind. Inf. Integr.,* p. 18, 2020.

[20] A. Marakhimov, and J. Joo, "Consumer adaptation and infusion of wearable devices for healthcare", *Comput. Human Behav.,* vol. 76, pp. 135-148, 2017. [http://dx.doi.org/10.1016/j.chb.2017.07.016]

[21] Isha Anand Bhagat, "KGWNAK,DAS. Artificial Intelligence in Healthcare: A Review", *Int. J. Sci. Res. Sci. Eng. Technol.,* vol. 11, no. 4, 2024.

[22] S. Polevikov, "Advancing AI in healthcare: A comprehensive review of best practices", *Clin. Chim. Acta,* vol. 548, p. 117519, 2023. [http://dx.doi.org/10.1016/j.cca.2023.117519] [PMID: 37595864]

[23] S.E. Dilsizian, and E.L. Siegel, "Artificial intelligence in medicine and cardiac imaging: harnessing big data and advanced computing to provide personalized medical diagnosis and treatment", *Curr. Cardiol. Rep.,* vol. 16, no. 1, p. 441, 2014. [http://dx.doi.org/10.1007/s11886-013-0441-8] [PMID: 24338557]

[24] Almasri IA. The Power of Artificial Intelligence for Improved Patient Outcomes, Ethical Practices and Overcoming Challenges. IgMin research. 2024; 2(7): 597-600.

[25] R.J.E.J.T. Angela Aristidoua, *Bridging the chasm between AI and clinical implementation.* The Lancet Journal, 2022, p. 399.

[26] S.M. Park, and Y.G. Kim, "A Metaverse: Taxonomy, Components, Applications, and Open Challenges", *IEEE Access,* vol. 10, no. 10, pp. 4209-4251, 2022. [http://dx.doi.org/10.1109/ACCESS.2021.3140175]

[27] R. Chengoden, N. Victor, T. Huynh-The, G. Yenduri, R.H. Jhaveri, M. Alazab, S. Bhattacharya, P. Hegde, P.K.R. Maddikunta, and T.R. Gadekallu, "Metaverse for Healthcare: A Survey on Potential Applications, Challenges and Future Directions", *IEEE Access,* vol. 11, pp. 12765-12795, 2023. [http://dx.doi.org/10.1109/ACCESS.2023.3241628]

[28] T. Sun, X. He, and Z. Li, "Digital twin in healthcare: Recent updates and challenges", *Digit. Health,* vol. 9, p. 20552076221149651, 2023. [http://dx.doi.org/10.1177/20552076221149651] [PMID: 36636729]

[29] S. Sinem, "Ovunc MBYSEME,SC. Using immersive technologies to develop medical Education Materials", *Cureus,* p. 13, 2021.

[30] G. Bansal, K. Rajgopal, V. Chamola, Z. Xiong, and D. Niyato, "Healthcare in Metaverse: A Survey on Current Metaverse Applications in Healthcare", *IEEE Access,* vol. 10, pp. 119914-119946, 2022. [http://dx.doi.org/10.1109/ACCESS.2022.3219845]

[31] Rachmad YE. MediVerse: Challenges And Development Of Digital Health Transformation Towards Metaverse in Medicine. Journal of Engineering, Electrical and Informatics. 2022; 2.

[32] G. Badiali, V. Ferrari, F. Cutolo, C. Freschi, D. Caramella, A. Bianchi, and C. Marchetti, "Augmented reality as an aid in maxillofacial surgery: Validation of a wearable system allowing maxillary repositioning", *J. Craniomaxillofac. Surg.,* vol. 42, no. 8, pp. 1970-1976, 2014. [http://dx.doi.org/10.1016/j.jcms.2014.09.001] [PMID: 25441867]

[33] K. Subramanian, "Digital twin for drug discovery and development – the virtual liver", *J. Indian Inst. Sci.,* vol. 100, no. 4, pp. 653-662, 2020.

[http://dx.doi.org/10.1007/s41745-020-00185-2]

[34] S. Ali, Abdullah, T.P.T. Armand, A. Athar, A. Hussain, M. Ali, M. Yaseen, M.I. Joo, and H.C. Kim, "Metaverse in Healthcare Integrated with Explainable AI and Blockchain: Enabling Immersiveness, Ensuring Trust, and Providing Patient Data Security", *Sensors (Basel),* vol. 23, no. 2, p. 565, 2023. [http://dx.doi.org/10.3390/s23020565] [PMID: 36679361]

[35] J.J.K. Liz George, "Unleashing the Future of Healthcare in the Metaverse: The Pivotal Role of Blockchain in Data Privacy", In: *Examining the Metaverse in Healthcare: Opportunities, Challenges, and Future Directions.* IGI Global, 2024. [http://dx.doi.org/10.4018/979-8-3693-1515-6.ch004]

[36] Y. Canbay, A. Utku, and P. Canbay, "Privacy Concerns and Measures in Metaverse: A Review", *15th International Conference on Information Security and Cryptography,* 2022. [http://dx.doi.org/10.1109/ISCTURKEY56345.2022.9931866]

[37] S.B.A.A. Maryam Etemadi, "A systematic review of healthcare recommender systems: Open issues, challenges, and techniques", *Expert Syst. Appl.,* p. 213, 2023.

[38] W.S. Khin Than Win, "M. Personal health record systems and their security protection", *J. Med. Syst.,* pp. 309-315, 2006.

[39] I. Keshta, and A. Odeh, "Security and privacy of electronic health records: Concerns and challenges", *Egyptian Informatics Journal,* vol. 22, no. 2, pp. 177-183, 2021. [http://dx.doi.org/10.1016/j.eij.2020.07.003]

[40] F. Kargl, E. Lawrence, M. Fischer, and Y.Y. Lim, "Security, privacy and legal issues in pervasive ehealth monitoring systems", *7th International Conference on Mobile Buisness,* 2008. [http://dx.doi.org/10.1109/ICMB.2008.31]

[41] M. Steven, and V.P. Williamson, "Balancing Privacy and Progress: A Review of Privacy Challenges, Systemic Oversight, and Patient Perceptions in AI-Driven Healthcare", *Appl. Sci. (Basel),* vol. 12, no. 4, 2024.

[42] S.M. Shah, and R.A. Khan, "Secondary Use of Electronic Health Record: Opportunities and Challenges", *IEEE Access,* vol. 8, pp. 136947-136965, 2020. [http://dx.doi.org/10.1109/ACCESS.2020.3011099]

[43] "Daniel M Walker cWLTPJ. Perspectives on Challenges and Opportunities for Interoperability: Findings From Key Informant Interviews With Stakeholders in Ohio", *JMIR Med. Inform.,* 2023.

[44] Vera Ehrenstein HKHL. Obtaining Data From Electronic Health Records. In Tools and Technologies for Registry Interoperability, Registries for Evaluating Patient Outcomes: A User's Guide.: AHQR; 2019.

[45] A. Szarfman, J.G. Levine, J.M. Tonning, F. Weichold, J.C. Bloom, J.M. Soreth, M. Geanacopoulos, L. Callahan, M. Spotnitz, Q. Ryan, M. Pease-Fye, J.S. Brownstein, W. Ed Hammond, C. Reich, and R.B. Altman, "Recommendations for achieving interoperable and shareable medical data in the USA", *Commun. Med.,* vol. 2, no. 1, p. 86, 2022. [http://dx.doi.org/10.1038/s43856-022-00148-x] [PMID: 35865358]

[46] A.A. Boxwala, M. Dierks, M. Keenan, S. Jackson, R. Hanscom, D.W. Bates, and L. Sato, "Organization and representation of patient safety data: current status and issues around generalizability and scalability", *J. Am. Med. Inform. Assoc.,* vol. 11, no. 6, pp. 468-478, 2004. [http://dx.doi.org/10.1197/jamia.M1317] [PMID: 15298992]

[47] S. Hempel, D. Ganz, S. Saluja, M. Bolshakova, T. Kim, C. Turvey, K. Cordasco, A. Basu, T. Page, R. Mahmood, A. Motala, J. Barnard, M. Wong, N. Fu, and I.M. Miake-Lye, "Care coordination across healthcare systems: development of a research agenda, implications for practice, and recommendations for policy based on a modified Delphi panel", *BMJ Open,* vol. 13, no. 5, p. e060232, 2023. [http://dx.doi.org/10.1136/bmjopen-2021-060232] [PMID: 37197809]

[48] M.P. Thompson, and I. Graetz, "Hospital adoption of interoperability functions", *Healthc. (Amst.),* vol.

7, no. 3, p. 100347, 2019.
[PMID: 30595558]

[49] E. Conley, and M. Pocs, "GDPR Compliance Challenges for for interoperable health information exchanges (HIEs) and trustworthy research environments", *Eur. J. Biomed. Inform. (Praha),* vol. 14, no. 3, pp. 48-61, 2018.
[http://dx.doi.org/10.24105/ejbi.2018.14.3.7]

[50] Z. Tian, M. Li, M. Qiu, Y. Sun, and S. Su, "Block-DEF: A secure digital evidence framework using blockchain", *Inf. Sci.,* vol. 491, pp. 151-165, 2019.
[http://dx.doi.org/10.1016/j.ins.2019.04.011]

[51] R.X.L.L. Rui Zhang, "Security and Privacy on Blockchain", *ACM Comput. Surv.,* vol. 52, no. 3, 2019.

[52] Y.Y.J.L.C.Q.J.Z. Sheping Zhai, "Research on the Application of Cryptography on the Blockchain", *J. Phys. Conf. Ser.,* vol. 1168, no. 3, 2019.

[53] D.A.R.A. Muhammad Rehan Anwar, "Hash Algorithm", In: *Verification Of Certificate Data Integrity And Security.* Aptisi Transactions on Technopreneurship, 2021, p. 3.

[54] A.S.G.S.B. Virinder Kumar Singla, "Navigating blockchain-based clinical data sharing: An interoperability review", In: *Applied Data Science and Smart Systems.* Taylor & Francis, 2024.
[http://dx.doi.org/10.1201/9781003471059-52]

[55] B. Nadji, "(. Data Security, Integrity, and Protection", In: *Data, Security, and Trust in Smart Cities.* Springer, 2024, pp. 59-83.
[http://dx.doi.org/10.1007/978-3-031-61117-9_4]

[56] J. Bonneau, "AMJC, AN, JAK. SoK: Research Perspectives and Challenges for Bitcoin and Cryptocurrencies", *2015 IEEE Symposium on Security and Privacy,* 2015.San Jose
[http://dx.doi.org/10.1109/SP.2015.14]

[57] Weidong Fang WCWZJPWG,GW. Digital signature scheme for information non-repudiation in blockchain: a state of the art review. EURASIP Journal on Wireless Communications and Networking. 2020; 2020.

[58] M.T. Hammi, B. Hammi, P. Bellot, and A. Serhrouchni, "Bubbles of Trust: A decentralized blockchain-based authentication system for IoT", *Comput. Secur.,* vol. 78, pp. 126-142, 2018.
[http://dx.doi.org/10.1016/j.cose.2018.06.004]

[59] J. Bernal Bernabe, J.L. Canovas, J.L. Hernandez-Ramos, R. Torres Moreno, and A. Skarmeta, "Privacy-Preserving Solutions for Blockchain: Review and Challenges", *IEEE Access,* vol. 7, pp. 164908-164940, 2019.
[http://dx.doi.org/10.1109/ACCESS.2019.2950872]

[60] S.B.G.B. Anthony Ugochukwu Nwosu, "Blockchain Transforming Cyber-Attacks: Healthcare Industry", *11th International Conference on Innovations in Bio-Inspired Computing and Applications,* 2020.

[61] B.A. Vehbi Neziri, "Blockchain for Open Information Governance: A New Era of Data", *2023 UBT International Conference,* 2023.

[62] Cheng-Te Tseng SSCS. Exploring the Sustainability of the Intermediary Role in Blockchain. Sustainability 2021. 2021; 13(4).

[63] P.C.E.R. Roberto Cerchione, "Blockchain's coming to hospital to digitalize healthcare services: Designing a distributed electronic health record ecosystem", *Technovation,* p. 120, 2023.

[64] S. Angraal, H.M. Krumholz, and W.L. Schulz, "Blockchain Technology", *Circ. Cardiovasc. Qual. Outcomes,* vol. 10, no. 9, p. e003800, 2017.
[http://dx.doi.org/10.1161/CIRCOUTCOMES.117.003800] [PMID: 28912202]

[65] P.R.C.K.S.A.R.A. Sanjeev Kumar Dwivedi, "Blockchain-Based Internet of Things and Industrial IoT: A Comprehensive Survey", *Secur. Commun. Netw.,* 2021.

[66] H. Kordestani, K. Barkaoui, and W. Zahran, "HapiChain: A Blockchain-based Framework for Patient-Centric Telemedicine", *IEEE 8th International Conference on Serious Games and Applications for Health.* [http://dx.doi.org/10.1109/SeGAH49190.2020.9201726]

[67] Wei Wang LWZ. A privacy protection scheme for telemedicine diagnosis based on double blockchain. Journal of Information Security and Applications. 2021; 61. [http://dx.doi.org/10.1016/j.jisa.2021.102845]

[68] A. Abugabah, N. Nizamuddin, and A.A. Alzubi, "Decentralized Telemedicine Framework for a Smart Healthcare Ecosystem", *IEEE Access,* vol. 8, pp. 166575-166588, 2020. [http://dx.doi.org/10.1109/ACCESS.2020.3021823]

[69] J.H. Tseng, Y.C. Liao, B. Chong, and S. Liao, "Governance on the Drug Supply Chain via Gcoin Blockchain", *Int. J. Environ. Res. Public Health,* vol. 15, no. 6, p. 1055, 2018. [http://dx.doi.org/10.3390/ijerph15061055] [PMID: 29882861]

[70] M.K.L.S. Sara Saberi, "Blockchain technology and its relationships to sustainable supply chain management", *Int. J. Prod. Res.,* pp. 2117-2135, 2018.

[71] Ahmadi V, Benjelloun S, Kik ME, Sharma T, Chi H. Drug Governance: IoT-based Blockchain Implementation in the Pharmaceutical Supply Chain. In Sixth International Conference on Mobile And Secure Services; 2020; Miami.

[72] S.S. Gomasta, A. Dhali, T. Tahlil, M.M. Anwar, and A.B.M.S. Ali, "PharmaChain: Blockchain-based drug supply chain provenance verification system", *Heliyon,* vol. 9, no. 7, p. e17957, 2023. [http://dx.doi.org/10.1016/j.heliyon.2023.e17957] [PMID: 37483827]

[73] S. Abdallah, and N. Nizamuddin, "Blockchain-based solution for Pharma Supply Chain Industry", *Comput. Ind. Eng.,* vol. 177, p. 108997, 2023. [http://dx.doi.org/10.1016/j.cie.2023.108997]

[74] C. Cornelius, "Agbo QHMJME. Blockchain Technology in Healthcare: A Systematic Review", *Health Care (Don Mills),* vol. 7, no. 2, 2019.

[75] Y. Zhuang, L.R. Sheets, Y.W. Chen, Z.Y. Shae, J.J.P. Tsai, and C.R. Shyu, "A Patient-Centric Health Information Exchange Framework Using Blockchain Technology", *IEEE J. Biomed. Health Inform.,* vol. 24, no. 8, pp. 2169-2176, 2020. [http://dx.doi.org/10.1109/JBHI.2020.2993072] [PMID: 32396110]

[76] A. Azaria, A. Ekblaw, and T. Vieira, "MedRec: Using Blockchain for Medical Data Access and Permission Management", *2nd International Conference on Open and Big Data,* 2016. [http://dx.doi.org/10.1109/OBD.2016.11]

[77] V. Patel, "A framework for secure and decentralized sharing of medical imaging data via blockchain consensus", *Health Informatics J.,* vol. 25, no. 4, pp. 1398-1411, 2019. [http://dx.doi.org/10.1177/1460458218769699] [PMID: 29692204]

[78] P.R. Mehdi Benchoufi, *Blockchain technology for improving clinical research quality.* Trails, 2017, p. 18.

[79] L. Zhou, L. Wang, and Y. Sun, "MIStore: a Blockchain-Based Medical Insurance Storage System", *J. Med. Syst.,* vol. 42, no. 8, p. 149, 2018. [http://dx.doi.org/10.1007/s10916-018-0996-4] [PMID: 29968202]

[80] R.A.I.S.I. Mahafujaa Khatun, "B-SAHIC: A blockchain based secured and automated health insurance claim processing system", *J. Intell. Fuzzy Syst.,* vol. 44, no. 3, 2023.

[81] "Dr. Saloni Sharma RC. Blockchain Technology in Healthcare Billing: Enhancing Transparency and Security", *International Journal for Research Publication and Seminar.,* vol. 10, no. 2, pp. 106-117, 2017.

[82] K. Alnavar, and C.N. Babu, "Blockchain-based Smart Contract with Machine Learning for Insurance

Claim Verification", *5th International Conference on Electrical, Electronics, Communication, Computer Technologies and Optimization Techniques,* 2021.Mysuru
[http://dx.doi.org/10.1109/ICEECCOT52851.2021.9707964]

[83] P.P. Ray, B. Chowhan, N. Kumar, and A. Almogren, "BIoTHR: Electronic Health Record Servicing Scheme in IoT-Blockchain Ecosystem", *IEEE Internet Things J.,* vol. 8, no. 13, pp. 10857-10872, 2021.
[http://dx.doi.org/10.1109/JIOT.2021.3050703]

[84] F. Li, K. Liu, L. Zhang, S. Huang, and Q. Wu, "EHRChain: A Blockchain-Based EHR System Using Attribute-Based and Homomorphic Cryptosystem", *IEEE Trans. Serv. Comput.,* vol. 15, no. 5, pp. 2755-2765, 2022.
[http://dx.doi.org/10.1109/TSC.2021.3078119]

[85] D.D. Taralunga, and B.C. Florea, "A blockchain-enabled framework for mhealth systems", *Sensors (Basel),* vol. 21, no. 8, p. 2828, 2021.
[http://dx.doi.org/10.3390/s21082828] [PMID: 33923842]

[86] A. Haleem, M. Javaid, R.P. Singh, R. Suman, and S. Rab, "Blockchain technology applications in healthcare: An overview", *International Journal of Intelligent Networks,* vol. 2, pp. 130-139, 2021.
[http://dx.doi.org/10.1016/j.ijin.2021.09.005]

[87] P. Tagde, S. Tagde, T. Bhattacharya, P. Tagde, H. Chopra, R. Akter, D. Kaushik, and M.H. Rahman, "Blockchain and artificial intelligence technology in e-Health", *Environ. Sci. Pollut. Res. Int.,* vol. 28, no. 38, pp. 52810-52831, 2021.
[http://dx.doi.org/10.1007/s11356-021-16223-0] [PMID: 34476701]

[88] A.H. Allam, I. Gomaa, H.H. Zayed, and M. Taha, "IoT-based eHealth using blockchain technology: a survey", *Cluster Comput.,* vol. 27, no. 6, pp. 7083-7110, 2024.
[http://dx.doi.org/10.1007/s10586-024-04357-y]

[89] Ajay Kumar Shrestha JVD. A Blockchain Platform for User Data Sharing Ensuring User Control and Incentives. Frontiers in Blockchain. 2020; 3.

[90] Z.A.Z. Remya Siva, "Security and privacy in cloud-based e-health system", *Symmetry (Basel),* vol. 13, no. 5, 2021.

[91] M. Uddin, "Blockchain Medledger: Hyperledger fabric enabled drug traceability system for counterfeit drugs in pharmaceutical industry", *Int. J. Pharm.,* vol. 597, p. 120235, 2021.
[http://dx.doi.org/10.1016/j.ijpharm.2021.120235] [PMID: 33549813]

[92] M. David, "Maslover JKKBPM. Using Blockchain Technology to Manage Clinical Trials Data: A Proof-of-Concept Study", *JMIR Med. Inform.,* vol. 6, no. 4, 2018.

[93] Y.T. Shen, L. Chen, W.W. Yue, and H.X. Xu, "Digital Technology-Based Telemedicine for the COVID-19 Pandemic", *Front. Med. (Lausanne),* vol. 8, p. 646506, 2021.
[http://dx.doi.org/10.3389/fmed.2021.646506] [PMID: 34295908]

[94] N.Z. Bawany, T. Qamar, H. Tariq, and S. Adnan, "Integrating Healthcare Services Using Blockchain-Based Telehealth Framework", *IEEE Access,* vol. 10, pp. 36505-36517, 2022.
[http://dx.doi.org/10.1109/ACCESS.2022.3161944]

[95] A. Ali, H. Ali, A. Saeed, A. Ahmed Khan, T.T. Tin, M. Assam, Y.Y. Ghadi, and H.G. Mohamed, "Mohamed H.G. Blockchain-powered healthcare systems: enhancing scalability and security with hybrid deep learning", *Sensors (Basel),* vol. 23, no. 18, p. 7740, 2023.
[http://dx.doi.org/10.3390/s23187740] [PMID: 37765797]

[96] J. Andrew, and K. Deva Priya Isravel, "Martin Sagayam, Bharat Bhushan, Yuichi Sei, and Jennifer Eunice. Blockchain for healthcare systems: Architecture, security challenges, trends and future directions", *J. Netw. Comput. Appl.,* p. 103633, 2023.

[97] Mohammed Abdul, *Shezon Saleem. Navigating blockchain's twin challenges: Scalability and regulatory compliance.* Blockchains, 2024, pp. 265-298.

[98] D. Stefanescu, L. Montalvillo, P. Galán-García, J. Unzilla, and A. Urbieta, "A Systematic Literature Review of Lightweight Blockchain for IoT", *IEEE Access,* vol. 10, pp. 123138-123159, 2022. [http://dx.doi.org/10.1109/ACCESS.2022.3224222]

[99] F.A. Reegu, H. Abas, Y. Gulzar, Q. Xin, A.A. Alwan, A. Jabbari, R.G. Sonkamble, and R.A. Dziyauddin, "Blockchain-Based Framework for Interoperable Electronic Health Records for an Improved Healthcare System", *Sustainability (Basel),* vol. 15, no. 8, p. 6337, 2023. [http://dx.doi.org/10.3390/su15086337]

CHAPTER 7

Wearable Technology and Smart Medical Devices

Heena Dhiman[1,*], **Sachin Dhiman**[2], **Gurpreet Singh**[1] and **Arun Kumar Rana**[3]

[1] *MM Engineering College, Maharishi Markandeshwar (Deemed to be University), Mullana, Haryana, India*

[2] *Chitkara College of Pharmacy, Chitkara University, Rajpura, Punjab, India*

[3] *Department of Electronics and Communication Engineering, Galgotias College of Engineering and Technology, Greater Noida, Uttar Pradesh, India*

Abstract: The health care sector has seen an evolution due to rapid advancements in wearable technology and smart medical devices, which have fundamentally transformed patient monitoring, diagnosis, and treatment. This chapter focuses on how these technologies are emerging and how they might enhance personalized therapy, remote patient management, and preventive healthcare. This chapter covers a range of wearable devices, such as fitness trackers, smartwatches, and medical-grade sensors, and assesses how well they can continually monitor vital signs and gather data in real-time. Future developments in this rapidly growing field are also explored, along with related concerns including user adoption, data security, and regulatory challenges. This chapter aims to offer an in-depth primer on wearable technology, smart medical devices, and their revolutionary role in current healthcare delivery.

Keywords: Artificial intelligence, Healthcare, Smart medical device, Wearable device.

INTRODUCTION

Amidst the tremendous advancements in medical devices, clinical trials, data analytics, and information technology. Since healthcare costs constitute nearly 20% of the US GDP, the latest developments in digital health technologies—such as wearables, health monitoring, and electronic health records—have the potential to significantly affect the socioeconomic landscape in addition to revolutionizing healthcare processes and enhancing the security of patients and the quality of care. The historical evolution of the healthcare industry is shown in Fig. (**1**).

In addition to creating significant obstacles for the delivery of healthcare, technological developments like these have additionally opened up new avenues

* **Corresponding author Heena Dhiman:** MM Engineering College, Maharishi Markandeshwar (Deemed to be University), Mullana, Haryana, India; E-mail: dr.sangeeta.patil@rungta.ac.in

for development and are providing opportunities for healthcare technology to expand outside its conventional purview, such as optimization of processes and adoption of technology. Information technology, systems engineering techniques, and organizational innovations are being more recognized as vital components for dealing with the interconnected productivity and quality issues that health care organizations worldwide are facing [1]. Starting in the eighteenth century and extending into the mid- and late nineteenth century, Industry 1.0 is the first industrial revolution. A mechanization revolution helped society transition from agriculture to industrialization, in addition to the creation of the steam engine, sewing machines, railroads, and the steel sector. Because electricity consumption is crucial, Industry 2.0 brought about a paradigm shift from individual or small-scale manufacturing to large-volume mass production. The Henry Ford assembly lines revolutionized industrial processes by facilitating the efficient and systematic allocation and connection of multiple tasks and machines.

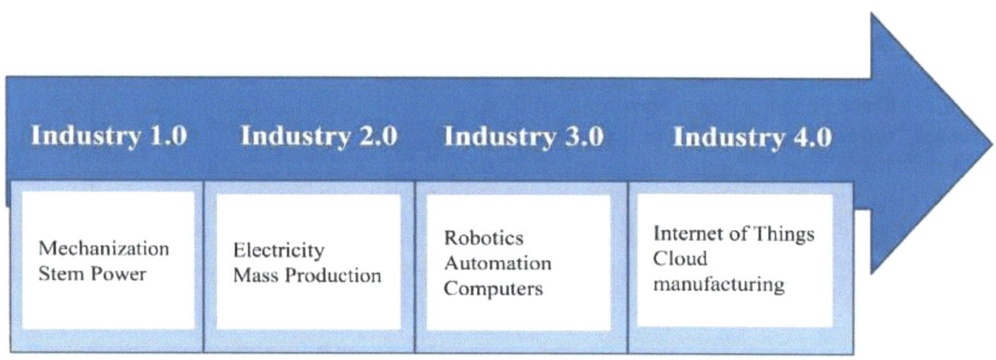

Fig. (1). Historical evolution of healthcare.

Massive applications of automation technologies, characterized by the electronic recording and connectivity of business operations and manufacturing processes, stemmed from the explosive development of electronics, computers, and robotic technology during the latter few decades of the 20th century. Industry 3.0, or the third wave of the industrial revolution, was brought in by the widespread implementation of computer-integrated and flexible manufacturing systems, manufacturing executive systems, material resource planning, and enterprise resource planning. This additionally marked the beginning of the fourth revolution. Entering the twenty-first century, Industry 4.0 is the fourth revolution in manufacturing, with the intention of fusing information, process, equipment, and operation technologies with cyber-physical networks [2].

In order to increase operational efficiency and safety, the Industrial Internet of Things (IIoT) links people, machines, and other devices to collect and analyze data. Among the most promising technologies for the next few years is the Internet of Things (IoT). With the advancement of this technology, healthcare and well-being will reap enormous rewards. The Internet of Health Things, or IoHT, is a term used to describe the Internet of Things (IoT) and the methods that it provides for healthcare and ambient supported living. The review is based on the latest publications and products that the industry has to offer for this market. Devices worn by people are called wearables. Wearable technology could help in private tracking and treatment in the field of medicine [3]. Indeed, health systems worldwide have acknowledged the promise of wearable technology to support healthcare. Wearable technology isn't just for specialized medical equipment that patients utilize, though. Prominent IT giants, such as Apple, have been investigating wearable health technology's potential for consumers who are health-conscious.

Role of Wearable Technology in Healthcare

By facilitating ongoing, real-time patient monitoring, augmenting preventive treatment, and strengthening chronic disease management, wearable technology is revolutionizing the field of medicine. With their advanced detectors and software, these instruments capture vital health information that can be reviewed and examined to improve outcomes for patients, monitor medical problems, and optimize treatment [4]. The role of wearable systems is divided into two major parts in healthcare, as shown in Fig. (**2**).

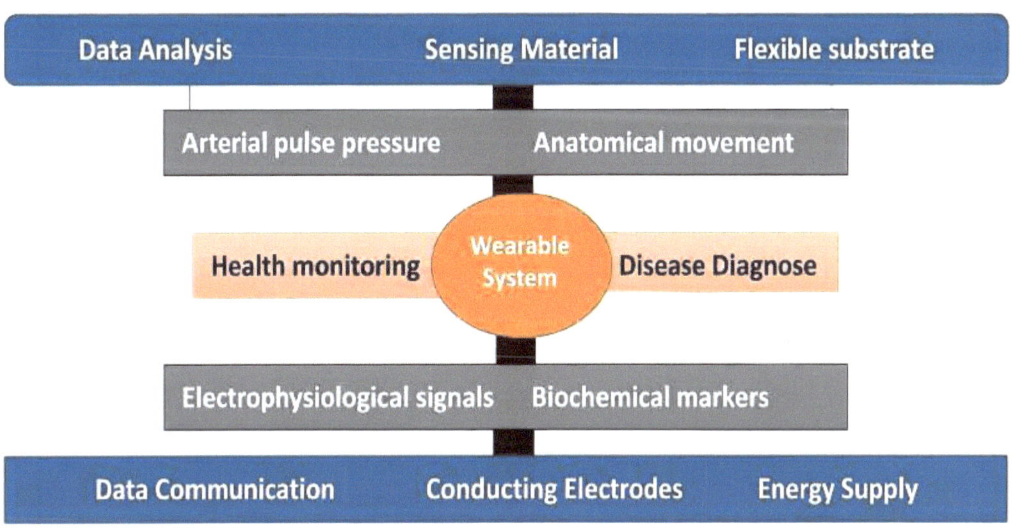

Fig. (2). Industrial wearable system in healthcare.

The integration of materials science, electronics, sensors, and analytics in a wearable system to create a closed-loop structure that can diagnose diseases and monitor health in real time. By connecting technical enablers (top and bottom layers) with physiological signal gathering (middle layer), it creates a full bio-integrated monitoring platform. The main functions of wearable technology in contemporary healthcare are explored below:

- **Early Health Issue Detection:** Cardiovascular parameters, saturation of oxygen, exercise levels, and the state of sleep are among the many physiological markers that wearable technology can monitor. It is possible to identify possible health problems early thanks to this real-time data [5].
- **Remote Patient Monitoring (RPM)**: Wearable devices allow individuals who have long-term ailments such as heart disease, Type 2 diabetes, or breathing problems to be tracked remotely while outside of healthcare facilities. This eliminates the need for frequent in-person visits and enables medical professionals to continually assess a patient's condition and adjust therapy as appropriate. By using closer monitoring and prompt interventions, RPM improves patient outcomes while lessening the burden on healthcare facilities.
- **Customized Medical Records:** The ability to customize treatment regimens and lifestyle recommendations depending on individual needs has been rendered possible by wearables, which are vital in the personalization of healthcare. Health care practitioners and patients are empowered to make data-driven decisions thanks to wearables' constant flow of health data.
- **Tailored Care Programs:** Medical professionals may develop individualized therapies using the data collected by wearable technology. Continuous Glucose Monitors (CGMs), for instance, offer real-time blood sugar measurement that enables accurate modifications to the amount of insulin used in the management of diabetes [6].
- **Patient Engagement and Self-Management:** Through giving individuals convenient access to their healthcare measurements, wearables empower patients to actively manage their own health. Through these gadgets, patients are able to monitor their adherence to therapy regimens, keep an eye on their progress, and get feedback.
- **Promotion of Active Lives:** Physical activity levels, like steps walked, calories burned, and hours of exercise, are monitored by fitness trackers and smartphones. They assist users in reaching daily fitness objectives and promote consistent physical activity by giving them real-time feedback.

SMART WEARABLE DEVICES IN KEY AREAS OF HEALTHCARE

Modern healthcare is being revolutionized by smart medical gadgets, which are changing the way both patients and doctors monitor, diagnose, and treat a wide range of medical conditions. Real-time data gathering, monitoring, and communication with healthcare practitioners are made feasible by these devices' superior computational powers, Bluetooth connectivity, and sensor capabilities. By enabling more proactive and accurate medical procedures, smart medical devices support the expanding trend of personalized, remote, and preventative healthcare. Modern technology is used in the creation of smart medical devices, which help with health status monitoring, diagnosis, and therapy. To gather and send health data, individuals utilize wireless technologies, microprocessors, and sensors.

These gadgets frequently have integrations with cloud-based platforms or smartphone apps, allowing for remote monitoring, real-time analysis, and patient-provider contact. Types of intelligent medical devices:

- Wearable Technology: A class of wearable devices that measure heart rate, sleep habits, and physical activity, such as fitness trackers and smartwatches.
- Implantable Devices: These include drug delivery devices, pacemakers, and neurostimulators that offer continuous internal treatment or monitoring [7].
- Connected Medical Devices: For improved functionality, devices such as insulin pumps, smart thermometers, or smart inhalers can be linked to mobile applications or other platforms.
- Diagnostic Devices: Wise instruments that offer diagnostic information, which include handheld ultrasound machines or digital stethoscopes.

Physical Fitness and Health Prevention

Wearables provide users with tailored data that enables them to better understand their own fitness requirements and health habits. Wearables provide recommendations based on an individual's fitness level, lifestyle, and health objectives by examining patterns in activity, sleep, and health measurements. Users are empowered to make well-informed decisions regarding their fitness and health according to individual feedback. The ability to deliver real-time feedback on fitness and health activities is one of wearables' main advantages [8]. Real-time data helps users make quick behavioral adjustments that improve results, whether it's heart rate monitoring during an exercise, movement reminders, or notifications for increased anxiety levels, as shown in Fig. (**3**). Various features are as follows:

- Distance tracking: This helps with goal-setting for activities involving long distances by tracking how far users have run or walked.
- Step Counting: This application monitors daily steps, promoting physical activity and assisting users in achieving predetermined activity objectives.
- Real-time data: It allows for measuring the intensity of workouts by continuously tracking heart rate during activity or throughout the day.

- Sleep Quality: Tracks time spent sleeping as well as the depth, brightness, and Rapid Eye Movement (REM) phases of sleep.
- Calories Burned: The calculator aids in weight management by estimating the number of calories burned during the day and during activities.
- The Daily Goals feature enables users to set up fitness objectives such as steps, calories, and activity minutes, and it sends out reminders to ensure that they are met.
- Progress tracking: Shows users' accomplishments over time so they can see them in visual form.
- Sedentary Alerts: These notifications can help people remain physically healthier by encouraging them to get up from a prolonged period of sitting.

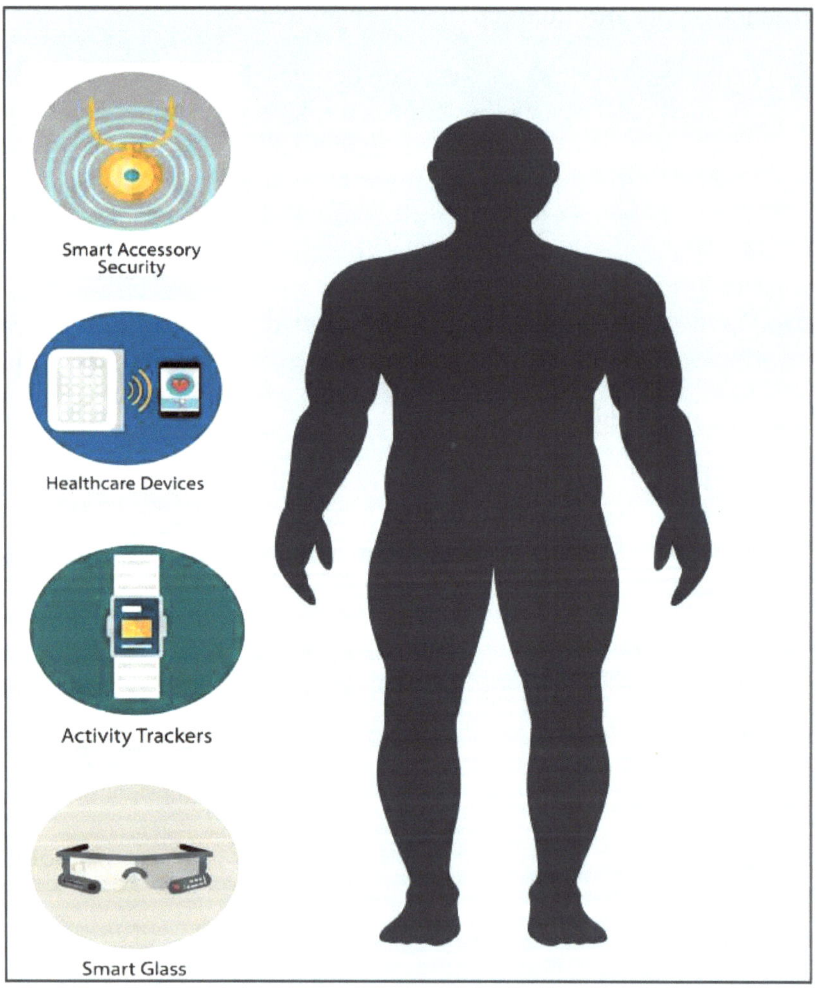

Fig. (3). Smart wearable devices.

Remote Patient Monitoring (RPM)

In telemedicine and personal wellness medicine, smart wearable health monitoring technologies are desperately needed. These devices facilitate the long-term, comfortable, and portable detection, monitoring, and recording of biosignals, as shown in Fig. (**4**). The number of high-performance wearable systems has been steadily rising in recent years, with the development and optimization of wearable health-monitoring systems centered on advanced materials and system integration, as shown in Fig. (**5**). But there are still a lot of obstacles to overcome in these areas, like weighing the trade-off between stretchability and flexibility, sensor accuracy, and system resilience. Because of this, further evolution is needed to encourage the creation of wearable health monitoring devices [9].

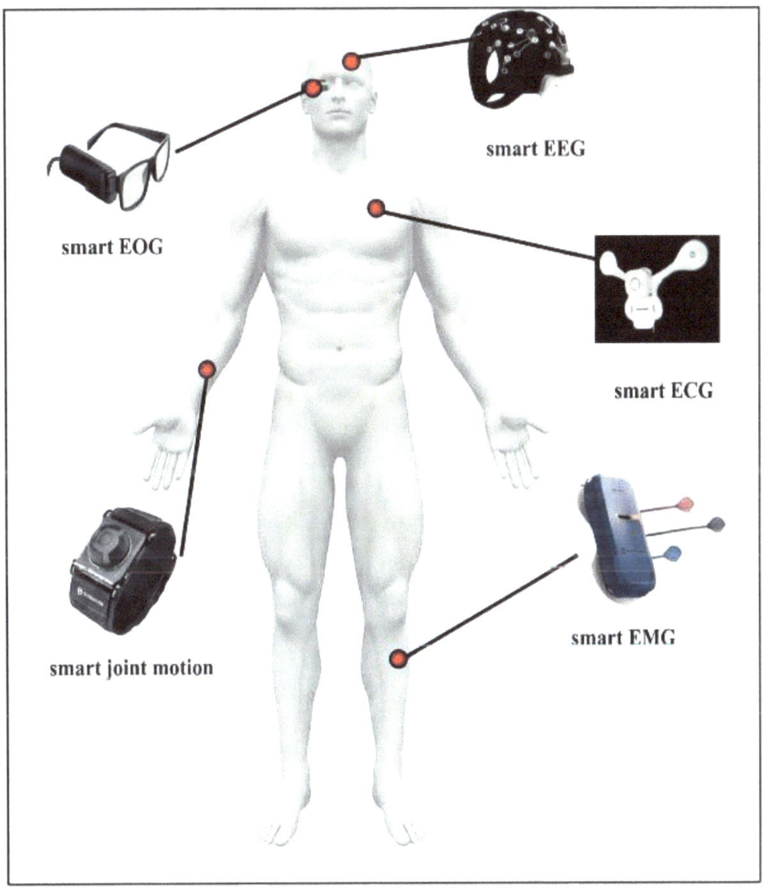

Fig. (4). Remote Patient Monitoring system.

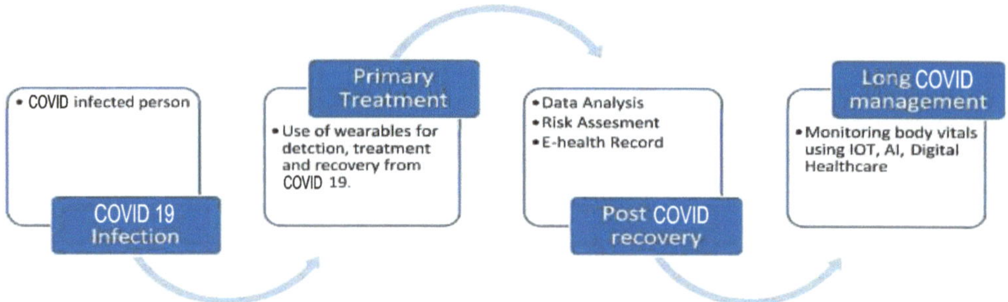

Fig. (5). Smart wearable sensors for frequent monitoring of biometrics Post-COVID.

Human basic physiological signs, including blood pressure, heart rate, oxygen saturation, and wrist pulse, are currently widely monitored via wearable technology. Wearable technology has been shown to offer a lot of promise for drug administration, therapy, and illness diagnosis, among other uses. Wearable systems can monitor anatomical body movements and collect electrophysiology signals, such as the electrocardiograph (ECG), electroencephalograph (EEG), electromyography (EMG), and electrooculogram (EOG), via epidermal electronic devices. These gadgets additionally offer visual information for examinations and the management of cardiovascular and cerebrovascular diseases [10].

Furthermore, wearable (bio)chemical sensing systems have been developed, manufactured, and employed to diagnose conditions like diabetes mellitus, cancer, and other illnesses.

The application of (bio)chemical biomarkers in the bloodstream and breath as diagnostic information to analyze the physiological function of the human body is a promising approach. Given their painless, affordable, and portable nature, wearable diagnosis, monitoring, and therapy systems can be used in place of more complex, large-scale technology for early illness detection and monitoring [11]. Patients in underserved or distant locations can obtain high-quality care without having to travel great distances.

Chronic Disease Management

Enhancing the quality of life and managing health for individuals with long-term, persistent diseases is the goal of the integrated strategy known as chronic disease management. It entails a variety of tactics and procedures meant to manage symptoms, stop complications, and improve general health.

- Enhanced Symptom Management: Tailored interventions and routine monitoring aid in managing symptoms and lowering the chance of problems.

- Lessening of Exacerbations: Early intervention can stop flare-ups and the illness from getting worse.
- Symptom Relief: Pain and suffering brought on by chronic illnesses can be reduced with effective care.
- Enhanced Functions: Assists in preserving or enhancing mental and physical abilities, making it easier for patients to carry out everyday tasks.
- Preventing Hospitalizations: Good management lowers the demand for urgent medical attention and hospital stays.
- Reduced Treatment Costs: Individuals may minimize the costs of costly interventions and repercussions by controlling the condition early on.
- Tailored Treatment Plans: Allow customized care plans that accommodate the requirements, preferences, and treatment reactions of individual patients.
- Increased Autonomy: Patients no longer need to rely on medical professionals for routine care because they are better able to manage their health problems on their own [12].

Precision in Disease Diagnostics

Significantly more complex medical data may be analyzed by machine learning algorithms than by humans. These algorithms can recognize patterns that might be too subtle for a human to see since they have been trained on huge databases of photos, clinical studies, and medical records.

To enhance the interpretation of images such as X-rays, CT scans, MRIs, and mammograms, radiology, pathology, and dermatology use machine learning models, especially those that are based on deep learning. In many cases, these models are more accurate than humans at diagnosing anomalies like cancers, fractures, or even early indicators of Alzheimer's disease. Machine learning algorithms are highly proficient in discovering patterns among diagnostic data. This includes pinpointing minute variations in a patient's vital signs or spotting anomalies in blood tests that may serve as early symptoms of disease.

Diagnostic procedures can now be automated thanks to machine learning, which considerably cuts the amount of time and effort required to perform examinations by hand. When resources are scarce and there may be a shortage of professionals, this can be especially helpful. By processing medical pictures automatically, AI-powered solutions lighten the burden on pathologists and radiologists. When appropriate, these innovations may detect areas of concern and mark photos for additional human evaluation. Through the use of algorithms based on machine learning, potential medical conditions can be identified before symptoms appear. Using patterns found in a patient's medical records, predictive models, for example, can evaluate risk factors for diabetes or heart disease and recommend early therapies [13].

Personalized Examinations

Personalized diagnosis is made possible by machine learning, which analyzes patient data to provide more individualized diagnostic insights based on individual traits, including genetics, medical history, and lifestyle.

- **Genomic Data Analysis:** To detect mutations or genetic markers linked to certain diseases, machine learning models process and interpret genomic data. This may result in the early detection of uncommon genetic illnesses or specific cancers that are hereditary.
- **Tailored Diagnostic Algorithms:** Machine learning-powered personalized diagnostic tools are able to adapt to the unique health profile of each user. These systems, for instance, can monitor individualized health baselines and identify changes that can indicate the development of a disease [14].

For instance, COVID-19 challenges the requirement to perform frequent biometric information tracking and indicates that wearable device technologies may be able to address this issue for disease diagnosis and treatment follow-up. Smart wearable sensors for frequent monitoring of biometrics, PostCOVID, are shown in Fig. (**5**).

Detecting diseases early on can greatly improve patient outcomes, making machine learning's function in diagnostics one of its most important applications.

IMPACT OF AI AND DATA ANALYTICS IN WEARABLES

With the use of AI algorithms, medical professionals will be able to make informed decisions with regard to patient care, anticipate health outcomes, and detect connections in the enormous quantities of data that wearable devices capture. Healthcare providers can be empowered to implement preventive steps through the use of AI algorithms that evaluate an individual's heart rate, sleep cycles, and level of physical activity to predict the risk of heart attacks or strokes. Healthcare professionals need wearable sensors to provide highly accurate, individualized monitoring of the user's physiological and chemical characteristics. These types of sensors come in a variety of forms, including textile-based, mouthguards, contact lenses, microfluidic patches, and pressure sensors.

The electronic readers needed to decipher these signals and send the information to mobile apps, which presents a difficulty, though. For these devices to effectively record a person's physiological information over an extended period of time, continuous data reading is required. In order to maintain continuous data reading, wearable gadget electronic readers need to have long-lasting batteries [15]. It is necessary to strike a careful balance between the realistic constraints of batteries and the sophisticated processing requirements of AI algorithms for data processing, as the constant execution of these algorithms can reduce battery life. Due to the need for exact sensor calibration, interference reduction, and accounting for changes in user activity and physiology, the precision and dependability of the data gathered by these wearables are vital. To maintain data fidelity, calibration and validation procedures are essential. Safety and confidentiality are critical issues when it comes to AI-based data collection for physiological data concerning humans. Traditional healthcare services usually have limited accuracy and are costly when it comes to disease diagnosis and monitoring. Flexible electronics-based wearable health technology has generated a lot of interest recently for patient health monitoring due to its appealing features, which include reduced medical expenses, rapid access to patient health data, the capacity to function and transmit data in challenging environments, room temperature storage, non-invasive implementation, mass scaling, *etc*. Fig. (**6**) shows the comparison among centralized, wearable, and AI-based wearable sensors.

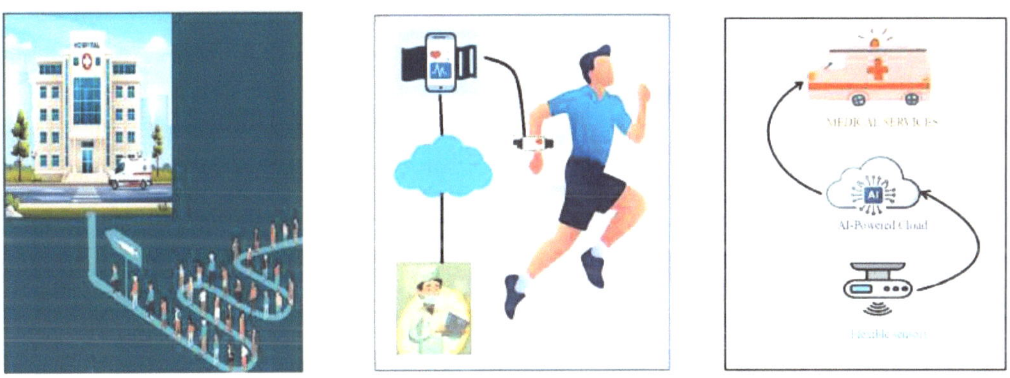

Fig. (6). Comparison among centralized, wearable, and AI based wearable sensors.

With the use of this technology, diseases can be identified early and treated right away [16]. By precisely detecting physiological conditions and biochemical signals, wearable sensors have created new opportunities for individualized health monitoring.

BENEFITS OF WEARABLE SMART MEDICAL DEVICES

Smart medical gadgets have a number of advantages that improve patient care, diagnosis, treatment, and overall health results drastically. Real-time collection, monitoring, and transmission of patient data is made possible by these devices' sophisticated sensors, data analytics, and connection characteristics. Key health advantages of smart medical devices are listed below:

- **Remote Patient Monitoring:** The utilization of smart medical equipment enables remote patient monitoring, which lowers the need for unnecessary hospital stays and allows for home-based care. Blood pressure monitors and smart scales, for example, can notify healthcare professionals of any issues before they get worse.
- **Post-Operative Care:** By confirming that patients are recuperating as anticipated, intelligent technologies contribute to monitoring recuperation, identifying issues early on, and lowering readmission rates.
- **Precision Medicine:** High-precision health parameter detection, accurate medicine administration, manual error-free data recording and interpretation, and elimination of mistakes made by humans are all possible with smart medical devices.
- **Process Automation:** Electronic devices like medication dispensers and smart infusion pumps automate drug distribution, avoiding human error by ensuring exact amounts are given at the right moments [17].
- **Wearable Diagnostics:** Tools such as biosensors, smart watches, and wearable ECG monitors may constantly gather medical information, which can aid in the prompt identification of illnesses such as sleep apnea, arrhythmias, or even faint symptoms associated with stroke [6].
- **Advanced Data Processing and Diagnostic Imaging:** Several smart gadgets improve diagnostic imaging, permitting radiologists and pathologists to diagnose patients more rapidly and effectively.
- **Telemedicine Compatibility:** Physicians may monitor patients remotely and conduct consultations without in-person visits as a result of smart device integration with telehealth platforms.
- **Global Reach:** By enabling doctors to remotely evaluate and keep an eye on patients across long distances, smart gadgets can improve care in locations in which access to healthcare is scarce [18].
- **Interactive Health Apps:** These software applications, which can be downloaded on a number of smart devices, encourage individuals to actively interact with their health information through features such as schedule monitoring, exercise, and medicine reminders.

- **Gamification and feedback:** Certain gadgets, such as ones that remind users to take their prescribed medicines or establish daily exercise goals, employ gamification or rewards programs to boost adherence to treatment plans [19].
- **Big Data and Predictive Analytics:** It can be done to examine the constant data produced by smart devices to spot patterns and anticipate potential threats to health. This allows healthcare professionals to take a proactive approach to patient treatment.
- **Better Clinical Decision-Making:** Possessing quicker access to real-time data empowers healthcare professionals to arrive at more informed decisions, ultimately increasing the standard of care given.

POTENTIAL RISKS

- **Data fragmentation:** Considering an abundance of mobile device technology runs on commercial platforms, it's possible that data from those gadgets won't interface effectively with other medical facilities or Electronic Health Records (EHRs). This may result in inadequate knowledge for healthcare providers or make it more difficult to use the information wisely when making decisions.
- **Interoperability Problems:** Exploitation and inaccurate comprehension of the data in different medical environments may result from a lack of standardization among various devices and platforms.
- **Non-Adherence:** Although smartwatches provide numerous advantages, not all users regularly maintain the suggested dosage or style [20]. Patient abandonment of the device could result in insufficient or inconsistent data collection if it is uncomfortable, cumbersome, or too complex to operate.
- **User-incorrect Data Interpretation:** A great deal of technological devices deliver information to the consumer directly, and consumers might not be medical professionals or comprehend how to correctly decode it. In the absence of medical advice, this may cause uncertainty, needless anxiety, or even poor health decisions.
- **Regulatory Gaps:** There are currently inadequacies in supervision while wearable technology continues to evolve faster than established regulatory frameworks. It is concerning for their safety, effectiveness, and dependability because some gadgets are not subjected to the same stringent testing or approval procedures as conventional medical devices.
- **Liability Issues:** It could not always be evident who is at fault when a wearable gadget produces inaccurate information that causes harm [21].
- **Informed Consent:** It's possible that certain individuals are unaware of the entire scope of data collection, usage, and risks associated with wearing these devices. Getting users to give informed authorization and understand the consequences is a major ethical challenge.

CONCLUSION

By facilitating continuous monitoring, strengthening the involvement of patients, managing chronic diseases better, and advocating preventive treatment, wearables have transformed the healthcare industry. They enable real-time data to empower patients and healthcare professionals, resulting in more efficient, timely, and customized care. In order to make healthcare more proactive, patient-centered, and more economical, wearable technology will continue to be essential as technology develops. AI data analytics technologies, which provide sophisticated insights, predictive modeling, and automation, are revolutionizing the way enterprises and sectors handle massive amounts of data. Resources such as Tableau and RapidMiner help users see and interpret data efficiently, while platforms like TensorFlow, IBM Watson, Microsoft Azure ML, and Google Cloud AI offer reliable circumstances for creating advanced AI models. Organizations can now make data-driven, well-informed decisions more quickly than previously possible thanks to the integration of computational intelligence and data analytics.

REFERENCES

[1] J. Li, and P. Carayon, "Health Care 4.0: A vision for smart and connected health care", *IISE Trans. Healthc. Syst. Eng.,* vol. 11, no. 3, pp. 1-10, 2021.
[http://dx.doi.org/10.1080/24725579.2021.1884627] [PMID: 34497970]

[2] M.M. Ahsan, and Z. Siddique, "Industry 4.0 in Healthcare: A systematic review", *International Journal of Information Management Data Insights,* vol. 2, no. 1, p. 100079, 2022.
[http://dx.doi.org/10.1016/j.jjimei.2022.100079]

[3] S.J. Kline, *Conceptual foundations for multidisciplinary thinking.* Stanford University Press, 1995.

[4] J. Rodrigues, D. Segundo, and A. Junqueira, *Heres & Sabino, Murilo & Prince, Rafael & Al-Muhtadi, Jalal & Albuquerque, Victor.* Enabling Technologies for the Internet of Health Things. IEEE Access. PP, 2018, pp. 1-1.
[http://dx.doi.org/10.1109/ACCESS.2017.2789329]

[5] M. Holko, T.R. Litwin, F. Munoz, K.I. Theisz, L. Salgin, N.P. Jenks, B.W. Holmes, P. Watson-McGee, E. Winford, and Y. Sharma, "Wearable fitness tracker use in federally qualified health center patients: strategies to improve the health of all of us using digital health devices", *NPJ Digit. Med.,* vol. 5, no. 1, p. 53, 2022.
[http://dx.doi.org/10.1038/s41746-022-00593-x] [PMID: 35469045]

[6] J. Sliwa,Chapter 9 - Reuse of data from smart medical devices for quality control and evidence-based medicine,Editor(s): Ciprian Dobre, Fatos Xhafa,In Intelligent Data-Centric Systems,Pervasive Computing,Academic Press,2016,Pages 255-297,ISBN 780128036631.
[http://dx.doi.org/10.1016/B978-0-12-803663-1.00009-7]

[7] E.P. Adeghe, C.A. Okolo, and O.T. Ojeyinka, "A review of wearable technology in healthcare: Monitoring patient health and enhancing outcomes", *OARJ of Multidisciplinary Studies,* vol. 7, no. 01, pp. 142-148, 2024.

[8] M.H. Iqbal, A. Aydin, O. Brunckhorst, P. Dasgupta, and K. Ahmed, "A review of wearable technology in medicine", *J. R. Soc. Med.,* vol. 109, no. 10, pp. 372-380, 2016.
[http://dx.doi.org/10.1177/0141076816663560] [PMID: 27729595]

[9] M. Zhang, M. Luo, R. Nie, and Y. Zhang, "Technical attributes, health attribute, consumer attributes and their roles in adoption intention of healthcare wearable technology", *Int. J. Med. Inform.,* vol. 108, pp. 97-109, 2017.
[http://dx.doi.org/10.1016/j.ijmedinf.2017.09.016] [PMID: 29132639]

[10] A. Vegesna, M. Tran, M. Angelaccio, and S. Arcona, "Remote patient monitoring via non-invasive digital technologies: a systematic review", *Telemed. J. E Health,* vol. 23, no. 1, pp. 3-17, 2017.
[http://dx.doi.org/10.1089/tmj.2016.0051] [PMID: 27116181]

[11] N. Nakamura, T. Koga, and H. Iseki, "A meta-analysis of remote patient monitoring for chronic heart failure patients", *J. Telemed. Telecare,* vol. 20, no. 1, pp. 11-17, 2014.
[http://dx.doi.org/10.1177/1357633X13517352] [PMID: 24352899]

[12] H. Dhiman and R. Kumar, "A Systematic Review on Role of AI and IOT in Prediction and Rehabilitation Model for Brain Stroke," 2023 6th International Conference on Contemporary Computing and Informatics (IC3I), Gautam Buddha Nagar, India, 2023, pp. 2301-2307.
[http://dx.doi.org/10.1109/IC3I59117.2023.10398094]

[13] N. Gillani, and T. Arslan, "Intelligent sensing technologies for the diagnosis, monitoring and therapy of Alzheimer's disease: a systematic review", *Sensors (Basel),* vol. 21, no. 12, p. 4249, 2021.
[http://dx.doi.org/10.3390/s21124249] [PMID: 34205793]

[14] J.H. Kim, and E. Kang, "The Role of Wearable Devices for the Success of the Healthcare Business: Verification from PRISMA Approach", *Journal of Economics Marketing, and Management,* vol. 10, no. 4, pp. 13-24, 2022.

[15] E. Bruno, S. Simblett, A. Lang, A. Biondi, C. Odoi, A. Schulze-Bonhage, T. Wykes, and M.P. Richardson, "Wearable technology in epilepsy: The views of patients, caregivers, and healthcare professionals", *Epilepsy Behav.,* vol. 85, pp. 141-149, 2018.
[http://dx.doi.org/10.1016/j.yebeh.2018.05.044] [PMID: 29940377]

[16] S. Shajari, K. Kuruvinashetti, A. Komeili, and U. Sundararaj, "The Emergence of AI-Based Wearable Sensors for Digital Health Technology: A Review", *Sensors (Basel),* vol. 23, no. 23, p. 9498, 2023.
[http://dx.doi.org/10.3390/s23239498] [PMID: 38067871]

[17] H. Dhiman, R. Kumar and P. Rani, "A Hybrid Model for Early Prediction of Stroke Disease," 2022 10th International Conference on Reliability, Infocom Technologies and Optimization (Trends and Future Directions) (ICRITO), Noida, India, 2022, pp. 1-6.
[http://dx.doi.org/10.1109/ICRITO56286.2022.9965122]

[18] M. Joshi, H. Ashrafian, L. Aufegger, S. Khan, S. Arora, G. Cooke, and A. Darzi, "Wearable sensors to improve detection of patient deterioration", *Expert Rev. Med. Devices,* vol. 16, no. 2, pp. 145-154, 2019.
[http://dx.doi.org/10.1080/17434440.2019.1563480] [PMID: 30580650]

[19] Sungmee Park, and S. Jayaraman, "Enhancing the quality of life through wearable technology", *IEEE Eng. Med. Biol. Mag.,* vol. 22, no. 3, pp. 41-48, 2003.
[http://dx.doi.org/10.1109/MEMB.2003.1213625] [PMID: 12845818]

[20] D. Jin, H. Adams, A.M. Cocco, W.G. Martin, and S. Palmer, "Smartphones and wearable technology: benefits and concerns in cardiology", *Med. J. Aust.,* vol. 212, no. 2, pp. 54-56.e1, 2020.
[http://dx.doi.org/10.5694/mja2.50446] [PMID: 31851375]

[21] I. Pavón, L. Sigcha, P. Arezes, N. Costa, G. Arcas, and J.M. López, "Wearable technology for occupational risk assessment: Potential avenues for applications", In: *Occupational safety and hygiene VI.* CRC Press, 2018, pp. 447-452.
[http://dx.doi.org/10.1201/9781351008884-79]

CHAPTER 8

AI in Healthcare: Analyzing Adoption Drivers Using Fuzzy AHP

Ashwarya Kapoor[1,*] and **Rajiv Sindwani**[2]

[1] *School of Commerce, Manav Rachna International Institute of Research and Studies, Faridabad, Haryana, India*

[2] *Department of Management Studies, J.C. Bose University of Science and Technology, YMCA, Faridabad, Haryana, India*

Abstract: The purpose of the present study is to comprehend the significance of artificial intelligence adoption in healthcare services and identify the drivers that are critical in investigating healthcare professionalsƒ?(tm) intention to adopt artificial intelligence in healthcare services. A comprehensive review of the literature and expert opinion was carried out to identify the critical drivers to the adoption of artificial intelligence in healthcare services. A total of five critical drivers for adopting artificial intelligence relevant in the context of healthcare services have been proposed. The proposed critical drivers were prioritized using a multi-criterion decision-making (MCDM) technique known as the fuzzy Analytic Hierarchy Process (Fuzzy AHP). This study is among the pioneering studies in exploring and prioritizing the critical drivers influencing artificial intelligence adoption in healthcare services. The findings of the present study will be fruitful for both the industry and academics. It will apprise artificial intelligence-based healthcare services providers about the critical drivers that need to be prioritized to boost user adoption.

Keywords: Artificial intelligence, Expert opinion, Fuzzy AHP, Healthcare services, Multi-criteria decision making, Prioritization.

INTRODUCTION

An enormous and consistent technological development has occurred in production since the Industrial Revolution. Technological innovations in machinery have replaced labour-intensive tasks, contributing to human progress. Beyond supporting physical labour, artificial intelligence has emerged as a critical technological advancement. It enables individuals to supersede manual tasks with enhanced mental capabilities and expertise across various industries. Artificial Intelligence (AI) is "a field of science and technology which allows computer

* **Corresponding author Ashwarya Kapoor:** School of Commerce, Manav Rachna International Institute of Research and Studies, Faridabad, Haryana, India; Tel: 7982480291; E-mail: ashwaryakapoor.soc@mriu.edu.in

Arun Kumar Rana, Mandeep Kaur & Sumit Kumar Rana (Eds.)

programs and intelligent computers to perform activities conventionally requiring human intelligence" [1]. As a result, a major appeal of artificial intelligence lies in its ability to execute a range of human-like tasks, learning from past experience and adjusting to inputs and new settings [2]. Nowadays, AI has evolved swiftly and has been implemented to facilitate numerous advantages across diverse fields, including the crucial healthcare sector. Advancements in artificial intelligence technologies like machine learning applications, big data, and robotics are used to detect, monitor, and assess risks and advantages in the healthcare industry [3]. Applying the artificial intelligence technology to the problem of medical diagnosis is expected to assist physicians in their routine work to improve the diagnostic level and alleviate their work pressure significantly. Thus, adopting artificial intelligence technology in healthcare services offers an insightful solution for barriers faced by several healthcare systems globally [4]. Artificial intelligence technology is now being applied in different fields such as surgery, gynecology, radiology, ophthalmology, radiotherapy, cardiology, and oncology [5]. If adopted on a wider scale, medical artificial intelligence has the power to disrupt the spread of infection, offer secure diagnosis, and therefore alleviate the pressure on testing laboratories globally [6]. The adoption of artificial intelligence in healthcare services in India has not yet reached full scale. Despite its transformative potential, AI adoption in healthcare remains challenging, especially among healthcare professionals. For instance, radiologists in India have shown hesitation in using AI-based diagnostic imaging tools, citing concerns over accuracy and potential liability in case of errors. Similarly, in cardiology and oncology, physicians often view AI as an aid but not a replacement, leading to cautious rather than full adoption. Barriers extend beyond clinical skepticism. Many doctors report a lack of trust in algorithms due to limited transparency ("black-box" decision-making) and concerns regarding patient data privacy. Moreover, integrating AI systems into existing hospital workflows often requires significant training and adaptation, which increases resistance among busy practitioners. A 2023 study highlighted that while AI solutions were introduced in several Indian hospitals for COVID-19 diagnosis, the majority of professionals continued to rely on conventional methods due to unfamiliarity with AI tools and fear of misdiagnosis. These instances demonstrate that while AI offers efficiency and accuracy, healthcare professionals' acceptance is not straightforward.

Therefore, identifying the key factors influencing artificial intelligence acceptance among healthcare professionals requires significant attention [7]. Furthermore, studies about factors driving artificial intelligence adoption in healthcare services in India remain in their early stages, with much of the existing literature focusing on developed countries [8]. Thus, in the healthcare sector, examining artificial intelligence adoption and identifying the determinants of its success still presents a significant research gap. Several researchers have underscored the necessity for further research on the adoption of artificial intelligence by healthcare professionals [9 - 13].

To fill the existing gap, the present study proposed critical drivers to the adoption of AI in healthcare services and prioritized them employing a novel MCDM technique known as fuzzy AHP. This study has the following objectives:

- To propose critical drivers to the adoption of AI in healthcare services using a review of the literature and expert opinion.
- To prioritize proposed critical drivers to the adoption of AI in healthcare services using the fuzzy analytic hierarchy process.

The remaining paper is arranged as follows. Section 2 comprises an extensive review of the literature. This section proposes the critical drivers for adopting AI in healthcare services. Further, Section 3 talks about the methodology employed in the research. Subsequently, in Section 4, the focus shifts to the examination and analysis of the data. Finally, the discussion and implications, conclusions, limitations, and future research directions are presented in Sections 5, 6, and 7, respectively.

IDENTIFICATION OF CRITICAL DRIVERS TO AI ADOPTION IN HEALTHCARE SERVICES

The authors used an extensive literature review to propose the critical drivers to AI adoption in healthcare services. To achieve this, the authors consulted a range of journals indexed in reputable databases, including Science Direct, Emerald Insight, Sage, Wiley, Springer, and Taylor & Francis. A Systematic search was meticulously performed across these databases to retrieve relevant articles. Keywords utilised for the search were ('adopt*' OR 'accept*') AND ('critical' OR 'key') AND ('drivers' OR 'factors' OR 'dimensions') AND ('artificial intelligence' OR 'AI') AND ('healthcare' OR 'healthcare professionals' OR 'healthcare services'). Initially, a large pool of research articles was identified. Amongst these, pilot studies, opinions, articles in languages other than English, conference reports, editorials, discussion papers, grey literature, and commentaries were eliminated. This process narrowed down the selection to 384 articles from esteemed journals. Furthermore, elimination of articles was performed by utilising the “Tollgate Approach” as shown in Fig. (**1**). To begin with, the authors performed the abstract and title screening. Articles where artificial intelligence adoption among healthcare professionals was not the key theme were excluded, resulting in the elimination of 297 articles. The leftover 87 articles underwent elimination based on the introduction and conclusion sections. Articles having objectives that did not align with the motive of the current research were removed. It resulted in the deletion of 9 articles. Among the remaining 78 articles, the authors identified high-quality papers through full-text reading. It was characterized by a clearly described problem statement, a robust research design, precise data analysis, and well-articulated findings. This rigorous process further resulted in the elimination of 29 articles. It ultimately led to a final set of 49 articles. The authors read these 49 articles in depth and identified various drivers to the adoption of artificial intelligence relevant in the context of healthcare services. The drivers identified from the literature review were thoroughly discussed with an academician. After detailed deliberation, five critical drivers to the adoption of artificial intelligence in healthcare services were proposed. The proposed drivers have been presented in Fig. (**2**) and are briefed below:

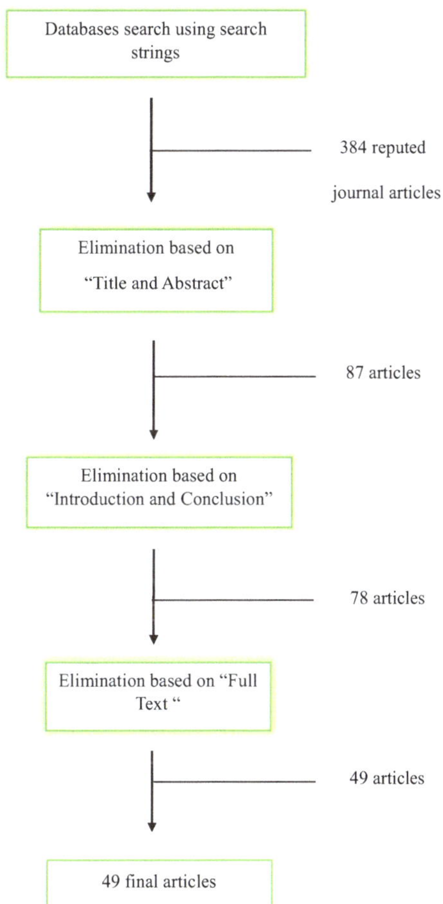

Fig. (1). Tollgate approach.

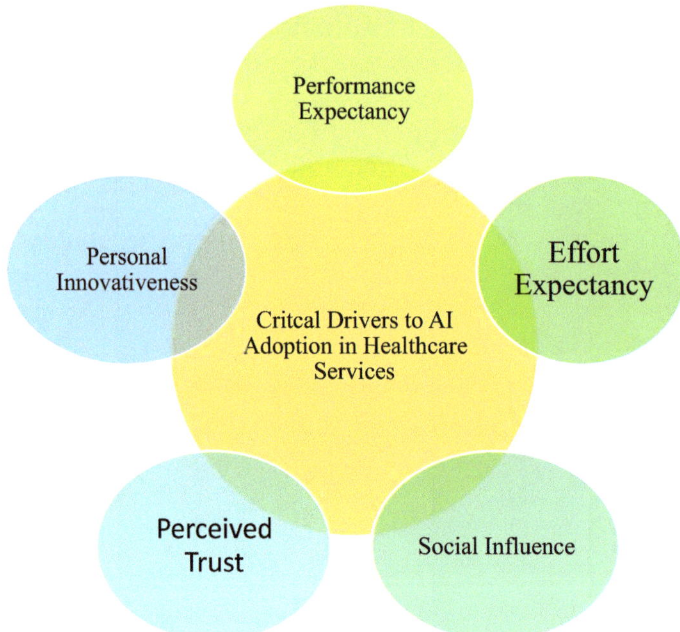

Fig. (2). Critical drivers to ai adoption in healthcare services.

Performance Expectancy (PE)

PE is "the extent to which an individual believes that using a particular system will improve their job performance" [14]. Professionals in the healthcare sector are usually more concerned than other technology adopters about selecting the most effective technologies for delivering high-quality healthcare services. A key factor in trust in an artificial intelligence in a healthcare system is an individual's belief in the system's capabilities, which is closely linked to factors such as error margins, input data quality, and algorithms used in making decisions [15 - 18]. McKnight characterized trust in technology as beliefs regarding its capability, independent of underlying motives.

Effort Expectancy (EE)

EE refers to "the degree of ease associated with the use of the system, stemming from the concept of perceived ease of use introduced in the original Technology Acceptance Model (TAM)." Numerous researchers have demonstrated the positive effect of EE on adoption intention in the context of novel IT systems, like mobile wallets, internet banking, and electronic medical record systems [19]. The simpler the operation of a new IT system, the more likely individuals are to engage with it. Therefore, it is crucial for healthcare professionals to perceive convenience while interacting with AI-based medical diagnosis support systems, as a lack of this perception could reduce their motivation to adopt technology [20 - 23].

Social Influence (SI)

SI is "the degree to which an individual perceives that important others believe they should use the new system" [24]. Users are often influenced by close ones, including superiors, friends, or relatives. The positive or negative views and behaviours of these individuals can strongly impact one's decision to adopt a new system. Existing researchers have outlined social influence as a key dimension in the adoption of m-health technologies, including cloud computing and electronic government services [25 - 28]. Therefore, it is likely that doctors*f*?(tm) intention to use artificial intelligence in healthcare services will be influenced by significant people in their social networks.

Perceived Trust (PT)

McKnight characterized trust as "beliefs about a technology's capabilities, independent of its underlying motives or intent." PE and trust as significant dimensions affecting the intention to adopt artificial intelligence in healthcare. Despite trends suggesting that performance expectancy often has the greatest impact, trust has shown substantial potential effects. The authors of a study found that professionals in the healthcare sector are not much inclined to use digital technologies if they do not understand the motive behind their use and believe that these technologies will improve the quality of care provided [29]. The authors of another study sought to investigate the scientific literature on the conceptualization of PT in AI within the domain of healthcare implementation and to identify the factors influencing trust in artificial intelligence in this setting [30].

Personal Innovativeness (PI)

PI is "an individual's willingness to experiment with new innovations." According to the Diffusion of Innovation theory, people exhibit varying levels of readiness to adopt new innovations based on their inherent tendencies [31]. Individuals with a higher level of innovativeness in information technology can effectively manage and adopt new technologies compared to others. They typically perceive new technologies as less complex and challenging to use [32]. Recent literature has highlighted personal innovativeness as a key dimension in technology adoption, such as mobile health and fitness apps. Another study emphasized the positive relationship between personal innovativeness and the adoption of artificial intelligence by healthcare providers [33].

RESEARCH METHODOLOGY

Fuzzy AHP

The Analytic Hierarchy Process technique breaks down complex decisions with multi-criteria issues into a hierarchy [34]. It enables decision makers to rank options and choose the best option. Researchers across the world have widely applied this technique for choosing alternatives, prioritizing barriers, allocating resources, and conducting cost-benefit analysis. However, AHP is less effective when it is used for diminishing the imprecision and inherent ambiguity associated with mapping decision-makers' perspectives to precise numbers [35]. Thus, fuzzy logic has been used to resolve issues related to the ambiguity of data. Fuzzy set theory was developed in 1965 by Zadeh. It aims to select limited options by evaluating a set of predefined criteria. A linguistic variable is a "variable whose values are presented in natural language words" [36-39]. "Fuzzy Weight," for instance, is a linguistic variable having values of "Very High," "High," "Medium," "Low," "Very Low," *etc*. In the present study, linguistic variables have been defined by a Triangular Fuzzy Scale (TFS). It has been exhibited in Table **1**. It has been utilised for analyzing criteria. Membership function transform component x in X to a real number having a value between 0 and 1 (Equation 1 and Fig. **3**).

The identified drivers to the adoption of artificial intelligence in healthcare services must be prioritized. The following steps are employed to prioritize the identified drivers [40 - 46].

Step 1: Linguistic terms, as shown in Table **1**, are utilised for creating a pairwise comparison matrix for identified criteria (eq. 2 and 3).

Table 1. "Fuzzy pairwise linguistic scale".

"Linguistic Scale"	"Inverse of Fuzzy AHP Scale"	"AHP Scale"	"TFN (l, m, u)."
"Equally Important"	"(1, 1, 1)"	"1"	"(1, 1, 1)"
"Weakly Important"	"(1/4, 1/3, 1/2)"	"3"	"(2, 3, 4)"
"Fairly Important"	"(1/6, 1/5, 1/4)"	"5"	"(4, 5, 6)"
"Strongly Important"	"(1/8, 1/7, 1/6)"	"7"	"(6, 7, 8)"
"Absolutely Important"	"(1/9, 1/9, 1/9)"	"9"	"(9, 9, 9)"
"The intermittent values between two adjacent scales"	"(1/3, 1/2, 1)"	"2"	"(1, 2, 3)"
-	"(1/5, 1/4, 1/3)"	"4"	"(3, 4, 5)"
-	"(1/7, 1/6, 1/5)"	"6"	"(5, 6, 7)"

(Table 1) cont.....

"Linguistic Scale"	"Inverse of Fuzzy AHP Scale"	"AHP Scale"	"TFN (l, m, u)."
-	"(1/9, 1/8, 1/7)"	"8"	"(7, 8, 9)"

Source: [15].

$$\mu_{\tilde{A}(x)} = \begin{cases} 0, x < l \\ \dfrac{(x-l)}{(m-l)}, if\, l \le x \le m \\ \dfrac{(u-x)}{(u-m)}, if\, m \le x \le u \\ 0, x > u \end{cases} \quad (1)$$

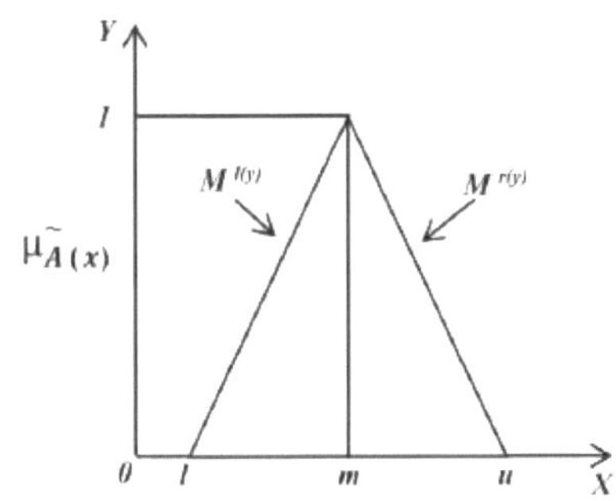

Fig. (3). Triangular fuzzy number.

$$\tilde{P} = \begin{bmatrix} 1 & \tilde{a}12 & \cdots & \tilde{a}1n \\ \vdots & 1 & \ddots & \vdots \\ \tilde{a}31 & \tilde{a}32 & 1 & \tilde{a}3n \\ \tilde{a}n1 & \tilde{a}n2 & \cdots & 1 \end{bmatrix} = \begin{bmatrix} 1 & \tilde{a}12 & \cdots & \tilde{a}1n \\ \vdots & 1 & \ddots & \vdots \\ \dfrac{1}{\tilde{a}31} & \dfrac{1}{\tilde{a}32} & 1 & \tilde{a}3n \\ \dfrac{1}{\tilde{a}n1} & \dfrac{1}{\tilde{a}n1} & \cdots & 1 \end{bmatrix} \quad (2)$$

$$\tilde{a}_{ij} = \begin{cases} \tilde{1},\tilde{3},\tilde{5},\tilde{7},\tilde{9}\ \textit{Criteria 'i' is of relative importance to criteria 'j'} \\ 1 i = j \\ \tilde{1}^{-1},\tilde{3}^{-1},\tilde{5}^{-1},\tilde{7}^{-1},\tilde{9}^{-1} \textit{Criteria 'j' is of relative importance to criteria 'i'} \end{cases} \quad (3)$$

Step 2: To ensure the consistency in preferences of decision makers, the matrix's consistency has been quantified utilising a standard equation of Consistency Index (CI) and Consistency Ratio (CR) (as shown in Equations 4 and 5, respectively). Matrix is deemed consistent if CR is 0.1 or lower, and perfectly consistent if CR is zero [47 - 51].

$$ConsistencyIndex(CI) = \frac{\lambda \max - n}{n-1} \quad (4)$$

Where λmax represents the greatest eigenvalue of the comparison matrix and "n" exhibits its component. CR is computed using the equation given below:

$$ConsistencyRatio(CR) = \frac{CI}{RI} \quad (5)$$

Where "CI = Consistency Index"

"RI = Random Index"

Step 3: Geometric mean approaches have been used for combining the opinions of the group (Equations 6 and 7).

$$l_{ij} = \left(\prod_{k=1}^{k} l_{ijk}\right)^{1/k}, m_{ij} = \left(\prod_{k=1}^{k} m_{ijk}\right)^{1/k}, u_{ij} = \left(\prod_{k=1}^{k} u_{ijk}\right)^{1/k} \quad (6)$$

$$\tilde{r}_i = (\tilde{a}_{i1} * \tilde{a}_{i2} * \tilde{a}_{i3} * .... * \tilde{a}_{in})^{1/n} \quad (7)$$

Step 4: Eq. 8 is used for computing the fuzzy weight for each criterion.

$$\tilde{w}_i = \tilde{r}_i * \left(\tilde{r}_1 + \tilde{r}_2 + \tilde{r}_3 + ... + \tilde{r}_n\right)^{-1} \quad (8)$$

$\tilde{w}_i$ exhibit fuzzy weights of identified criteria (*lwi*, *mwi*, *nwi*).

Where *lwi* represents a lower fuzzy weight, *mwi* represents a middle fuzzy weight, and *nwi* represents the fuzzy weight's upper value.

Step 5: The centre of area approach was employed to select the best non-fuzzy performance (Eq. 9)

$$w_i = \frac{(u_{wi} - l_{wi})}{3} + \frac{(m_{wi} - l_{wi})}{3} + l_{wi} \quad (9)$$

Step 6: The matrix w_i was transformed into a matrix N w_i for normalising the w_i matrix (Eq. 10).

$$Nw_i = \frac{w_i}{\sum^{n} w_i} \quad (10)$$

Table **2** signifies the pairwise judgment matrix of drivers. Further, Table **3** shows normalised weights of its criteria.

Table 2. Fuzzy pairwise judgment matrix of critical drivers to AI adoption in healthcare services.

Main Criteria	"Performance Expectancy"	"Efforts Expectancy"	"Social Influence"	"Perceived Trust"	"Personal Innovativeness"
"Performance Expectancy"	1,1,1	8.14,8.59,9	6.19,7.19,8.19	2.55,3.57,4.57	4.37,5.38,6.38
"Efforts Expectancy"	0.11,0.12.0.12	1,1,1	0.22,0.28,0.39	0.11,0.13,0.15	0.16.0.19,0.24
"Social Influence"	0.12,0.14,0.16	2.55,3.57,4.57	1,1,1	0.13,0.15,0.18	0.19,0.23,0.30
"Perceived Trust"	0.22,0.28,0.39	6.79,7.79,8.79	5.58,6.58,7.58	1,1,1	3.37,4.37,5.38
"Personal Innovativeness"	0.16,0.19,0.23	4.13,5.38,6.38	3.37,4.37,5.38	0.19,0.23,0.30	1,1,1

Source: The authors.

Table 3. Normalised weights and ranking of critical drivers to AI adoption in healthcare services.

Critical Factors	Normalised weights of the factors	Ranking
Performance Expectancy	0.5202	1
Efforts Expectancy	0.0309	5
Social Influence	0.0570	4
Perceived Trust	0.2935	2
Personal Innovativeness	0.1281	3
CR= 0.094. 0.094 < 0.10		

Source: The authors.

ANALYSIS

Proposed critical drivers to the adoption of artificial intelligence in healthcare services were allocated weights utilising fuzzy AHP. A pairwise-based questionnaire was sent to five domain experts. The panel included two practicing clinicians (one radiologist and one cardiologist) with over 10 years of clinical experience, one hospital IT administrator specializing in digital health implementation, one healthcare management professional with experience in policy and operations, and one academic researcher in healthcare technology adoption. Their combined expertise provided a balanced perspective, ensuring both practical and theoretical rigor in the pairwise evaluation process. They were requested to compare the proposed driver pairs using TFS as presented in Table **1**. Then, an average judgmental pairwise comparison of each criterion in relation to other criteria has been formulated. It has been exhibited in Table **2**. Table **3** presents the final results. As shown in Table **3**, fuzzy AHP determined the priority and ranking of each criterion along with the CR. The greater weight value represents the higher significance of proposed critical drivers that are sequenced as performance expectancy, perceived trust, personal innovativeness, social influence, and effort expectancy, respectively. Further, CR for proposed critical drivers was found to be less than the maximum admissible value, *i.e.*, 0.1.

DISCUSSION AND IMPLICATIONS

The current study proposed and prioritized the critical drivers to AI adoption in healthcare services. Results revealed PE as the topmost factor. Service providers must emphasize displaying operational efficiency and measurable improvements in clinical outcomes using artificial intelligence tools. This could be attained through running pilot programs, showcasing case studies, and providing simulations where the direct effect on patient care can be witnessed by the healthcare professionals. Training on regular intervals and updates regarding how AI could refine diagnosis, administrative tasks, and treatment will assist professionals in perceiving its performance value. Perceived trust has been ranked as the second most critical driver in encouraging adoption. To build perceived trust, service providers should focus on the privacy and security of the patient's data and the artificial intelligence system's reliability. Providing transparency regarding the working of artificial intelligence algorithms, performing audits at regular intervals, and ensuring artificial intelligence solutions comply with healthcare regulations could reduce concerns. Service providers can also collaborate with various healthcare institutions to validate the safety of artificial intelligence technology. Personal innovativeness ranked third in promoting the adoption of artificial intelligence in healthcare services. Innovative culture can be fostered for embracing artificial intelligence among healthcare professionals. It includes innovation challenges, organizing workshops, and knowledge-sharing platforms that enable healthcare professionals to experiment with artificial intelligence tools. Moreover, providing professional development programs on a regular basis that integrate artificial intelligence usage will promote a mindset of adaptability and innovation among healthcare professionals. Social influence was prioritized as the fourth catalyst facilitating adoption. Service providers must harness the impact of major opinion leaders, including healthcare administrators and doctors, to advocate for artificial intelligence adoption. By encouraging peer discussions, collaborative forums, and testimonials where early adopters can share success stories, artificial intelligence solutions will become more appealing to those influenced by the professional community. Networking conferences and events showcasing artificial intelligence in action will also foster social endorsement. Although effort expectancy influences the adoption of artificial intelligence among health care professionals, this factor was ranked lower in the present study. Simplifying the user interface and making artificial intelligence tools easy to integrate into existing workflows is key. Service providers should emphasize designing solutions that require minimal training and could be seamlessly incorporated into daily routines. Providing 24/7 technical support, accessible resources, and tutorials will reduce the perceived effort required to use artificial intelligence technologies, making adoption smoother for healthcare professionals.

CONCLUSION

The purpose of the current research was to prioritize the critical drivers of AI adoption in the domain of healthcare services. The in-depth review of the literature, along with the opinion of a domain expert, assisted in proposing a total of 5 critical drivers to artificial intelligence adoption in healthcare services. Then, fuzzy AHP was applied, and the weights for each driver were computed to attain the precise result. On the basis of the weights obtained by employing fuzzy AHP, the ranking for drivers was analyzed and exhibited in Table **3**. It could be confirmed with weights of the criterion, *i.e.*, performance expectancy (0.5202) > perceived trust (0.2935) > personal innovativeness (0.1281) > social influence (0.0570) > effort expectancy (0.0309). Prioritization assisted in assessing the relative importance of the proposed drivers, guiding service providers in building strategies for enhancing artificial intelligence adoption in healthcare services. "Performance expectancy" has emerged as the most essential driver for focusing on enhancing adoption, followed by perceived trust, personal innovativeness, social influence, and effort expectancy. This research contributed remarkably to the industry and academia by developing a structure to assess and rank critical adoption drivers to artificial intelligence in healthcare services using fuzzy AHP.

LIMITATIONS AND FUTURE SCOPE

While the research has achieved its objectives, there are several limitations that need to be addressed. A larger group of domain experts might be consulted for assessing the critical drivers to artificial intelligence adoption in healthcare services. It will assist in attaining holistic results. The opinion given by the domain expert might be biased. To address this issue, the findings should be compared with secondary data in the healthcare industry. Furthermore, research could be conducted to rank the critical adoption drivers by taking sub-factors of all proposed drivers. The fuzzy AHP prioritizes the proposed drivers but cannot evaluate the interrelationship between them. Future studies can use modern operations research methods such as DEMATEL and ANP to assess the interrelationship among the proposed drivers. Other MCDM approaches, such as

VIKOR, TOPSIS, PROMETHEE, and BWM, can be used to rank the proposed drivers, and the findings obtained can be compared with the findings of the current study.

REFERENCES

[1] W. Afzal, R. Torkar, and R. Feldt, "A systematic review of search-based testing for non-functional system properties", *Inf. Softw. Technol.,* vol. 51, no. 6, pp. 957-976, 2009. [http://dx.doi.org/10.1016/j.infsof.2008.12.005]

[2] R. Agarwal, and J. Prasad, "A conceptual and operational definition of personal innovativeness in the domain of information technology", *Inf. Syst. Res.,* vol. 9, no. 2, pp. 204-215, 1998. [http://dx.doi.org/10.1287/isre.9.2.204]

[3] R.M. Aiken, and R.G. Epstein, "Ethical guidelines for AI in education: Starting a conversation", *Int. J. Artif. Intell. Educ.,* vol. 11, no. 2, pp. 163-176, 2000.

[4] Alharbi ST. Trust and acceptance of cloud computing: A revised UTAUT model. In2014 international conference on computational science and computational intelligence 2014 Mar 10 (Vol. 2, pp. 131-134).

[5] O. Ali, W. Abdelbaki, A. Shrestha, E. Elbasi, M.A.A. Alryalat, and Y.K. Dwivedi, "A systematic literature review of artificial intelligence in the healthcare sector: Benefits, challenges, methodologies, and functionalities", *Journal of Innovation & Knowledge,* vol. 8, no. 1, p. 100333, 2023. [http://dx.doi.org/10.1016/j.jik.2023.100333]

[6] A. Almarzouqi, A. Aburayya, and S.A. Salloum, "Determinants predicting the electronic medical record adoption in healthcare: A SEM-Artificial Neural Network approach", *PLoS One,* vol. 17, no. 8, p. e0272735, 2022. [http://dx.doi.org/10.1371/journal.pone.0272735] [PMID: 35972979]

[7] M.A. Alsalem, A.H. Alamoodi, O.S. Albahri, A.S. Albahri, L. MartA-nez, R. Yera, A.M. Duhaim, and I.M. Sharaf, "Evaluation of trustworthy artificial intelligent healthcare applications using multi-criteria decision-making approach", *Expert Syst. Appl.,* vol. 246, p. 123066, 2024. [http://dx.doi.org/10.1016/j.eswa.2023.123066]

[8] Alshehri M, Drew S, AlGhamdi R. Analysis of citizens acceptance for e-government services: applying the UTAUT model. arXiv preprint arXiv:1304.3157. 2013 Apr 10.

[9] J. Chen, "Adoption of M-learning apps: A sequential mediation analysis and the moderating role of personal innovativeness in information technology", *Computers in Human Behavior Reports,* vol. 8, p. 100237, 2022. [http://dx.doi.org/10.1016/j.chbr.2022.100237]

[10] Dharani N. ANN based COVID-19 prediction and symptoms relevance survey and analysis. In2021 5th international conference on computing methodologies and communication (ICCMC) 2021 Apr 8 (pp. 1805-1808).

[11] W. Fan, J. Liu, S. Zhu, and P.M. Pardalos, "Investigating the impacting factors for the healthcare professionals to adopt artificial intelligence-based medical diagnosis support system (AIMDSS)", *Ann. Oper. Res.,* vol. 294, no. 1-2, pp. 567-592, 2020. [http://dx.doi.org/10.1007/s10479-018-2818-y]

[12] D.A. Frank, C.T. ElbAÝk, C.K. BA,rsting, P. Mitkidis, T. Otterbring, and S. Borau, "Drivers and social implications of Artificial Intelligence adoption in healthcare during the COVID-19 pandemic", *PLoS One,* vol. 16, no. 11, p. e0259928, 2021. [http://dx.doi.org/10.1371/journal.pone.0259928] [PMID: 34807907]

[13] B.M.Z. Hameed, N. Naik, S. Ibrahim, N.S. Tatkar, M.J. Shah, D. Prasad, P. Hegde, P. Chlosta, B.P. Rai, and B.K. Somani, "Breaking barriers: Unveiling factors influencing the adoption of artificial intelligence by healthcare providers", *Big Data and Cognitive Computing,* vol. 7, no. 2, p. 105, 2023.

[http://dx.doi.org/10.3390/bdcc7020105]

[14] S. Hindocha, K. Zucker, R. Jena, K. Banfill, K. Mackay, G. Price, D. Pudney, J. Wang, and A. Taylor, "Artificial intelligence for radiotherapy auto-contouring: Current use, perceptions of and barriers to implementation", *Clin. Oncol. (R. Coll. Radiol.),* vol. 35, no. 4, pp. 219-226, 2023. [http://dx.doi.org/10.1016/j.clon.2023.01.014] [PMID: 36725406]

[15] J. Jain, N. Walia, S. Gupta, K. Aggarwal, and S. Singh, "A fuzzy analytical hierarchy process framework for stock selection in the Indian stock market", *J. Public Aff.,* vol. 22, no. 4, p. e2710, 2022. [http://dx.doi.org/10.1002/pa.2710]

[16] A. Kapoor, R. Sindwani, and M. Goel, "Prioritizing the key factors influencing the adoption of mobile wallets: an Indian perspective in covid-19 era", *J. Inf. Technol. Manage.,* vol. 13, no. 4, pp. 161-182, 2021.

[17] A. Kapoor, R. Sindwani, and M. Goel, "Evaluating mobile wallet acceptance factors using best worst method", *International Journal of Process Management and Benchmarking,* vol. 13, no. 4, pp. 449-469, 2023. [http://dx.doi.org/10.1504/IJPMB.2023.129822]

[18] Kapoor A, Sindwani R, Goel M. A novel framework for understanding the interplay between the mobile wallet service quality dimensions and loyalty intention. The TQM Journal. 2024 Jul 22.

[19] A. Kapoor, R. Sindwani, and M. Goel, "Decoding the conundrum: exploring complex interlinkages between mobile wallet adoption inhibitors among unorganised retailers", *J. Financ. Serv. Mark.,* vol. 29, no. 4, pp. 1487-1502, 2024. [http://dx.doi.org/10.1057/s41264-024-00277-5]

[20] A. Kapoor, R. Sindwani, M. Goel, and A. Shankar, "Mobile wallet adoption intention amid COVID-19 pandemic outbreak: A novel conceptual framework", *Comput. Ind. Eng.,* vol. 172, p. 108646, 2022. [http://dx.doi.org/10.1016/j.cie.2022.108646] [PMID: 36118531]

[21] S. Kaur, and S. Arora, "Understanding customersƒ?(tm) usage behavior towards online banking services: an integrated riskƒ?"benefit framework", *J. Financ. Serv. Mark.,* vol. 28, no. 1, pp. 74-98, 2023. [http://dx.doi.org/10.1057/s41264-022-00140-5]

[22] A.A. Khanfar, R. Kiani Mavi, M. Iranmanesh, and D. Gengatharen, "Determinants of artificial intelligence adoption: research themes and future directions", *Inf. Technol. Manage.,* vol. ƒ?›ƒ?›ƒ?›, pp. 1-21, 2024. [http://dx.doi.org/10.1007/s10799-024-00435-0]

[23] F. Ibrahim, J.C. Münscher, M. Daseking, and N.T. Telle, "The technology acceptance model and adopter type analysis in the context of artificial intelligence", *Front. Artif. Intell.,* vol. 7, p. 1496518, 2025.

[24] A. Khanijahani, S. Iezadi, S. Dudley, M. Goettler, P. Kroetsch, and J. Wise, "Organizational, professional, and patient characteristics associated with artificial intelligence adoption in healthcare: A systematic review", *Health Policy Technol.,* vol. 11, no. 1, p. 100602, 2022. [http://dx.doi.org/10.1016/j.hlpt.2022.100602]

[25] S. Kim, K.H. Lee, H. Hwang, and S. Yoo, "Analysis of the factors influencing healthcare professionalsƒ?(tm) adoption of mobile electronic medical record (EMR) using the unified theory of acceptance and use of technology (UTAUT) in a tertiary hospital", *BMC Med. Inform. Decis. Mak.,* vol. 16, no. 1, p. 12, 2015. [http://dx.doi.org/10.1186/s12911-016-0249-8] [PMID: 26831123]

[26] Y.J. Kim, J.H. Choi, and G.M.N. Fotso, "Medical professionalsƒ?(tm) adoption of AI-based medical devices: UTAUT model with trust mediation", *J. Open Innov.,* vol. 10, no. 1, p. 100220, 2024. [http://dx.doi.org/10.1016/j.joitmc.2024.100220]

[27] P. Kumar, S.K. Sharma, and V. Dutot, "Artificial intelligence (AI)-enabled CRM capability in

healthcare: The impact on service innovation", *Int. J. Inf. Manage.*, vol. 69, p. 102598, 2023. [http://dx.doi.org/10.1016/j.ijinfomgt.2022.102598]

[28] McKnight DH. Trust in information technology. The Blackwell encyclopedia of management. 2005; 7: 329-31.

[29] F. Ibrahim, J.C. Münscher, M. Daseking & N.T. Telle. "The technology acceptance model and adopter type analysis in the context of artificial intelligence", *Frontiers in Artificial Intelligence*, 2025, Vol. 7, 1496518.

[30] S. Nakrem, M. SolbjA,r, I.N. Pettersen, and H.H. Kleiven, "Care relationships at stake? Home healthcare professionals*f*?(tm) experiences with digital medicine dispensers *f*?" a qualitative study", *BMC Health Serv. Res.*, vol. 18, no. 1, p. 26, 2018. [http://dx.doi.org/10.1186/s12913-018-2835-1] [PMID: 29334953]

[31] O. Neumann, K. Guirguis, and R. Steiner, "Exploring artificial intelligence adoption in public organizations: a comparative case study", *Public Manage. Rev.*, vol. 26, no. 1, pp. 114-141, 2024. [http://dx.doi.org/10.1080/14719037.2022.2048685]

[32] J. Pan, S. Ding, D. Wu, S. Yang, and J. Yang, "Exploring behavioural intentions toward smart healthcare services among medical practitioners: a technology transfer perspective", *Int. J. Prod. Res.*, vol. 57, no. 18, pp. 5801-5820, 2019. [http://dx.doi.org/10.1080/00207543.2018.1550272]

[33] Parveen. "India's AI adoption surges, poised for explosive growth". Retrieved from: https://www.indiabusinesstrade.in/blogs/indias-ai-adoption-surges-poised-for-explosive-growth/

[34] L. Petersson, I. Larsson, J.M. Nygren, P. Nilsen, M. Neher, J.E. Reed, D. Tyskbo, and P. Svedberg, "Challenges to implementing artificial intelligence in healthcare: a qualitative interview study with healthcare leaders in Sweden", *BMC Health Serv. Res.*, vol. 22, no. 1, p. 850, 2022. [http://dx.doi.org/10.1186/s12913-022-08215-8] [PMID: 35778736]

[35] Roy. "AI adoption in key Indian sectors touches 48% in FY24". Retrieved from: https://economictimes.indiatimes.com/tech/technology/ai-adoption-in-key-in-ian-sectors-touches-48-in-fy24/articleshow/110060391.cms?from=mdr

[36] T.L. Saaty, "The analytic hierarchy process (AHP)", *J. Oper. Res. Soc.*, vol. 41, no. 11, pp. 1073-1076, 1980.

[37] M. Sharma, and R. Sehrawat, "A hybrid multi-criteria decision-making method for cloud adoption: Evidence from the healthcare sector", *Technol. Soc.*, vol. 61, p. 101258, 2020. [http://dx.doi.org/10.1016/j.techsoc.2020.101258]

[38] K. Sood, P. Pathak, J. Jain, and S. Gupta, "How does an investor prioritize ESG factors in India? An assessment based on fuzzy AHP", *Manag. Finance,* vol. 49, no. 1, pp. 66-87, 2023. [http://dx.doi.org/10.1108/MF-04-2022-0162]

[39] Steerling E, Siira E, Nilsen P, Svedberg P, Nygren J. Implementing AI in healthcare—the relevance of trust: a scoping review. Frontiers in health services. 2023 Aug 24;3:1211150.

[40] O. Strachna, and O. Asan, "Reengineering clinical decision support systems for artificial intelligence", *2020 IEEE International Conference on Healthcare Informatics (ICHI),* pp. 1-3, 2020. [http://dx.doi.org/10.1109/ICHI48887.2020.9374370]

[41] D. Ueda, T. Kakinuma, S. Fujita, K. Kamagata, Y. Fushimi, R. Ito, Y. Matsui, T. Nozaki, T. Nakaura, N. Fujima, F. Tatsugami, M. Yanagawa, K. Hirata, A. Yamada, T. Tsuboyama, M. Kawamura, T. Fujioka, and S. Naganawa, "Fairness of artificial intelligence in healthcare: review and recommendations", *Jpn. J. Radiol.,* vol. 42, no. 1, pp. 3-15, 2024. [http://dx.doi.org/10.1007/s11604-023-01474-3] [PMID: 37540463]

[42] N. Upadhyay, A. Kamble, and A. Navare, "Virtual healthcare in the new normal: Indian healthcare consumers adoption of electronic government telemedicine service", *Gov. Inf. Q.,* vol. 40, no. 2, p. 101800, 2023.

[http://dx.doi.org/10.1016/j.giq.2022.101800]

[43] V. Venkatesh, M.G. Morris, G.B. Davis, and F.D. Davis, "User acceptance of information technology: Toward a unified view", *Manage. Inf. Syst. Q.,* vol. 27, no. 3, pp. 425-478, 2003. [http://dx.doi.org/10.2307/30036540]

[44] V. Venkatesh, J.Y.L. Thong, and X. Xu, "Consumer acceptance and use of information technology: extending the unified theory of acceptance and use of technology", *Manage. Inf. Syst. Q.,* vol. 36, no. 1, pp. 157-178, 2012. [http://dx.doi.org/10.2307/41410412]

[45] P. Vichitkraivin, and T. Naenna, "Factors of healthcare robot adoption by medical staff in Thai government hospitals", *Health Technol. (Berl.),* vol. 11, no. 1, pp. 139-151, 2021. [http://dx.doi.org/10.1007/s12553-020-00489-4]

[46] J. Yang, B. Luo, C. Zhao, and H. Zhang, "Artificial intelligence healthcare service resources adoption by medical institutions based on TOE framework", *Digit. Health,* vol. 8, 2022. [http://dx.doi.org/10.1177/20552076221126034] [PMID: 36211801]

[47] T. Ye, J. Xue, M. He, J. Gu, H. Lin, B. Xu, and Y. Cheng, "Psychosocial factors affecting artificial intelligence adoption in health care in China: cross-sectional study", *J. Med. Internet Res.,* vol. 21, no. 10, p. e14316, 2019. [http://dx.doi.org/10.2196/14316] [PMID: 31625950]

[48] R. Yeoh, H.K. Kim, H. Kang, Y.A. Lin, A.D. Ho, and K.F. Ho, "What determines intentions to use mobile fitness apps? The independent and joint influence of social norms", *Int. J. Hum. Comput. Interact.,* vol. 40, no. 2, pp. 121-130, 2024. [http://dx.doi.org/10.1080/10447318.2022.2111040]

[49] Zadeh LA. Information and control. Fuzzy sets. 1965 Jun 3;8(3):338-53.

[50] A. Kapoor, R. Sindwani, M. Goel, and A. Shankar, "Mobile wallet adoption intention amid COVID-19 pandemic outbreak: A novel conceptual framework", *Comput. Ind. Eng.,* vol. 172, p. 108646, 2022. [http://dx.doi.org/10.1016/j.cie.2022.108646]

[51] A. Kapoor, and R. Sindwani, "Artificial Intelligence as a Catalyst for Advancing Contactless Payments: Unveiling Key Adoption Drivers", In: *AI Marketing and Ethical Considerations in Consumer Engagement.* IGI Global Scientific Publishing, 2025, pp. 321-338. [http://dx.doi.org/10.4018/979-8-3373-3476-9.ch016]

CHAPTER 9

Multidisciplinary Advances in Healthcare

Srinjoy Chatterjee[1,*] and **Shouvik Das**[2]

[1] *Department of Dentistry, The West Bengal University of Health Sciences, Kolkata, West Bengal, India*

[2] *Department of Animal Biology and Biotechnology, University of Hyderabad, Hyderabad, Telangana, India*

Abstract: In today's rapidly evolving healthcare landscape, collaboration across various disciplines has become essential to addressing complex health challenges. This chapter explores the importance of a multidisciplinary approach in healthcare, where the combined expertise of medical professionals, engineers, policymakers, and others leads to innovative solutions. It begins with a historical perspective, highlighting the evolution of healthcare through multidisciplinary collaboration and showcasing key milestones such as the integration of technology in surgery and the synergistic efforts of public health and epidemiology.

Key areas of multidisciplinary advances are examined, including biomedical engineering's role in diagnostics and treatments, and the impact of artificial intelligence in clinical decision-making. The chapter also delves into the pharmaceutical industry's collaboration with life sciences to advance personalized medicine, as well as the contributions of public health professionals in shaping global health policies. Special focus is placed on dentistry, showing how oral health is connected to overall well-being and its importance in multidisciplinary care teams.

The chapter emphasizes the role of interdisciplinary research and education in training future healthcare professionals, highlighting case studies of institutions fostering cross-disciplinary learning. Technological innovations such as telemedicine, robotics, and genomic medicine are explored as key drivers of multidisciplinary care, offering transformative possibilities in patient treatment and health monitoring. It concludes by addressing challenges such as communication barriers and ethical dilemmas in multidisciplinary teams, while envisioning future trends like precision medicine and wearable health technology that will shape global health initiatives and foster deeper collaboration across healthcare disciplines.

* **Corresponding author Srinjoy Chatterjee:** Department of Dentistry, The West Bengal University of Health Sciences, Kolkata, West Bengal, India; E-mail: dr.srinjoychatterjee@gmail.com

Arun Kumar Rana, Mandeep Kaur & Sumit Kumar Rana (Eds.)

Keywords: Artificial intelligence, Bioinformatics, Biomedical engineering, Dentistry, Drug discovery, Epidemiology, Genomic medicine, Healthcare advancements, Life sciences, Machine learning, Medical technology, Multidisciplinary collaboration, Oral health, Robotics surgery, Telemedicine.

INTRODUCTION

Multidisciplinary research offers a flexible strategy for tackling complex issues by combining insights and techniques from multiple fields. In today's world, marked by intricate and interconnected challenges, this approach has become vital, as single-discipline research often falls short [1]. By leveraging expertise from different areas, multidisciplinary research promotes a deeper understanding of problems and increases the likelihood of discovering innovative solutions [2].

In the past, research was typically confined to individual disciplines, resulting in specialized knowledge but minimal interaction between fields [3]. However, as global challenges like climate change, public health emergencies, and technological progress have become more intricate, the drawbacks of these traditional boundaries have become evident [4]. Multidisciplinary research aims to overcome these limitations by promoting collaboration among various disciplines, offering a more comprehensive approach to addressing these complex problems [5].

The current healthcare landscape faces a range of complex challenges, including the rise of chronic diseases, aging populations, mental health concerns, and emerging infectious diseases. These issues are often interconnected, requiring more than just a single discipline's expertise to address them effectively. Multidisciplinary approaches in healthcare have become essential for tackling these problems, as they combine knowledge from various fields such as medicine, public health, data science, psychology, and engineering. By fostering collaboration between experts in different areas, these approaches enable more comprehensive solutions that consider not only the medical aspects but also social, technological, and behavioral factors. This integrative strategy is critical for developing innovative treatments, improving patient outcomes, and addressing public health issues on a larger scale.

KEY AREAS OF MULTIDISCIPLINARY ADVANCES

Medical Technology and Engineering

Role of Biomedical Engineering in Diagnostics and Treatment

Biomedical engineering plays a critical role in both diagnostics and treatment by integrating principles of engineering with biological and medical sciences to enhance healthcare. In diagnostics, it has contributed to the development of advanced imaging technologies, such as MRI, CT scans, and ultrasound, which enable accurate detection and monitoring of diseases. Biomedical engineers also design diagnostic devices, such as biosensors and wearable health monitors, that provide real-time data on patients' conditions. In terms of treatment, biomedical engineering has led to innovations in medical devices like pacemakers, prosthetics, and surgical robots, improving the effectiveness and precision of medical procedures. Furthermore, it contributes to the development of drug delivery systems and regenerative medicine, which aid in faster recovery and personalized treatment. Through these innovations, biomedical engineering is transforming the way healthcare is delivered, leading to better patient outcomes and more efficient medical practices.

Integration of Artificial Intelligence and Machine Learning in Clinical Decision-making

Artificial Intelligence (AI), particularly methods like Machine Learning (ML), reinforcement learning, and deep learning, is highly effective in addressing the data and challenges in healthcare. AI can assist physicians in complex tasks such as risk stratification for interventions, identifying patients at high risk of rapid deterioration, and analyzing multiple smaller outcomes to improve overall patient care. The next major shift in medical education will involve integrating physicians into AI model development and educating them about these technologies. The complexity of AI methods varies, affecting how easily physicians can understand and interpret the results. For instance, while decision trees are commonly used and easy to interpret, they are limited by their static structure [6]. In contrast, deep learning models like convolutional neural networks are harder to interpret, making it difficult to establish causal links [7], and therefore require clinicians' active involvement [8]. Neural networks, often used to analyze patient images, also rely on radiologists to curate suitable data for training [9]. Collaboration between AI developers and knowledgeable physicians is essential to define the accuracy and interpretability needed in specific clinical settings.

Pharmaceutical and Life Sciences

Collaboration Between Pharmacists, Biochemists, and Healthcare Providers

Collaboration between pharmacists, biochemists, and healthcare providers is essential for delivering comprehensive patient care and improving health outcomes. Pharmacists, with their expertise in drug formulation and administration, play a key role in ensuring the safe and effective use of medications. Biochemists, on the other hand, contribute their understanding of biochemical processes, helping to identify molecular mechanisms of diseases and develop new therapies. Healthcare providers, including doctors and nurses, oversee patient diagnosis, treatment, and management. By working together, these professionals can optimize treatment plans, personalize therapies based on biochemical insights, and minimize the risk of adverse drug reactions. This interdisciplinary collaboration not only enhances the accuracy of diagnoses and the effectiveness of treatments but also fosters innovation in developing new diagnostic tools and therapeutic interventions, ultimately improving patient care.

Advances in Personalized Medicine and Drug Discovery

The blockbuster strategy, which focuses on developing drugs with sales exceeding USD 1 billion, has enabled pharmaceutical companies to generate sufficient resources to cover the high costs of Research and Development (R&D). However, this model is becoming less sustainable due to growing criticism regarding its therapeutic effectiveness. Research has shown that many blockbuster drugs are only effective for a small majority of patients. Additionally, the model lacks the predictability needed to develop innovative, safe, and effective treatments for patients with specific disease subtypes. Issues like suboptimal treatments, adverse drug reactions, and incomplete or inaccurate diagnoses are still common. As a result, the industry's goal of improving treatment outcomes while reducing costs remains a significant challenge. Unfortunately, many efforts to achieve these goals have been costly, complex, time-consuming, or ineffective. Moreover, regulatory authorities are increasingly demanding evidence-based therapeutics, pushing the industry toward a new, more suitable approach to drug discovery and development. This shift is closely linked to the growing interest in biomarkers. According to the National Institutes of Health (NIH), a biomarker is "a characteristic that is objectively measured and evaluated as an indicator of normal biological processes, pathogenic processes, or pharmacologic responses to a therapeutic intervention." In the future, an individual's genetic profile will play a crucial role in clinical decision-making, particularly in selecting the most appropriate treatments for each patient [10].

Biomarkers are key to understanding patient variability, allowing the drug discovery industry to shift from mass-marketed products to targeted therapies. The insights provided by biomarkers enhance the understanding of cellular and biological processes, creating new commercial opportunities in areas such as target identification, diagnostic development, clinical trial design, outcomes analysis, product launches, and market expansion.

Public Health and Policy

Influence of Epidemiologists, Social Workers, and Policymakers in Managing Global Health Crises

Epidemiologists, social workers, and policymakers play a crucial role in managing global health crises. Epidemiologists provide critical insights by studying the patterns, causes, and spread of diseases, enabling the identification of high-risk populations and guiding prevention and control measures. Their data-driven analysis helps shape effective public health strategies. Social workers, on the other hand, address the social and psychological impacts of health crises by supporting vulnerable communities, ensuring access to essential services, and promoting mental health and well-being. Policymakers are responsible for translating scientific data and social insights into actionable policies, allocating resources, and coordinating large-scale interventions to control the spread of disease. Together, these professionals work to ensure a comprehensive response, balancing scientific, social, and political aspects to mitigate the impact of health emergencies on global populations.

Impact of Multidisciplinary Teams in Health Policy Development

A multidisciplinary team (MDT) in oncology refers to the collaboration of various specialized professionals involved in cancer care, with the primary goal of enhancing treatment effectiveness and improving patient outcomes. Head and Neck Cancers (HNC) encompass a range of distinct diseases, each requiring different therapeutic approaches. Symptoms, treatment side effects, and the physical and psychological impacts vary depending on the cancer's location and treatment plan. Coordinating efforts among diverse specialists is seen as a significant improvement over the outdated model of a single physician managing all aspects of care [11].

The multidisciplinary approach gained traction in oncology in the mid-1980s, when the addition of chemotherapy to radiotherapy and surgery demonstrated increased survival rates. During this time, organ-preservation strategies for HNC began to emerge with new therapeutic techniques [12]. Initially, MDTs functioned as formal committees that reviewed new cancer cases, with medical and radiation oncologists and surgical specialists collaborating on treatment plans based on clinical expertise and current evidence.

As the benefits of this approach in improving patient care became evident, additional specialists focusing on supportive care were incorporated into MDTs. Their inclusion helped to mitigate treatment side effects, improving patient adherence and compliance with therapies [13]. This approach evolved further with the development of oncological functional units, which focus on specific cancer types and streamline the coordination of services for cancer patients [14]. These units integrate multidisciplinary committees from all departments involved in a patient's care, reducing delays in diagnosis and treatment initiation.

Dentistry, Oral Health, and General Medicine

Contributions of dentistry to oVerall Health (e.g., Systemic Diseases and Oral Health Connections)

Two key questions for dental practitioners are, "How will tissue engineering impact dentistry?" and "Which oral tissues can potentially be engineered?" While the full impact is still being determined, tissue engineering is expected to revolutionize the field of dentistry. As for the second question, nearly all types of oral tissues have the potential to be engineered. Tissue engineering's influence on dentistry comes from its broad application to various tissues related to the oral cavity, such as bone, cartilage, skin, oral mucosa, dentin, dental pulp, and salivary glands.

Bone

Tissue engineering is expected to have its greatest impact in dentistry through advancements in bone tissue engineering and regeneration. Bone defects caused by injury, disease, or congenital conditions pose a significant health challenge. Current methods to repair these defects involve using autografts, allografts, and synthetic biomaterials. While these approaches can restore stability and function to a reasonable extent, they have limitations. This has sparked interest in engineering bone through all three tissue engineering strategies. Both conductive and inductive methods can be applied to regenerate small bone defects. Guided Tissue Regeneration (GTR) following periodontal surgery is a conductive technique for bone regeneration. Bone Morphogenetic Proteins (BMPs) and related proteins, as well as the genes that encode them, enable inductive bone engineering in cases where GTR falls short. Additionally, cell transplantation offers the potential to create large bone structures, such as an entire mandible, which may not be achievable through other strategies. These structures can even be fully developed in the laboratory before being used in major reconstructive procedures [15] (Fig. **1**).

Cartilage

In the field of craniofacial reconstruction, the development of polymer scaffolds with specific mechanical and degradative characteristics has paved the way for advancements in cartilage repair. Cartilage damage, often caused by trauma or diseases such as degenerative joint conditions at the temporomandibular joint, is challenging due to the tissue's limited ability to regenerate and the absence of growth-promoting molecules. This has led researchers and manufacturers to focus on cell transplantation techniques for cartilage engineering. Clinically, cell transplantation without a carrier is already being used to treat small cartilage defects [17]. Additionally, studies in animal models have shown that new cartilage tissue, with accurately defined sizes and shapes for maxillofacial reconstruction (*e.g.*, nasal septum, temporomandibular joint), can be created using biodegradable scaffolds designed to support cell growth [18, 19].

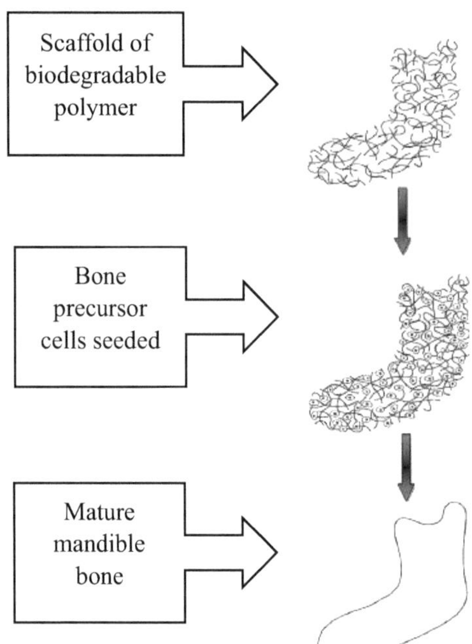

Fig. (1). A potential strategy for cell transplantation to reconstruct half of a mandible after extensive resective surgery (such as in cancer patients) involves designing a polymer scaffold shaped like half the mandible. Bone precursor cells are placed onto the scaffold and cultivated in a bioreactor. As the scaffold gradually degrades, it promotes the growth of new bone in the form of the mandible [16].

Skin and Oral Mucosa

The most successful achievement in tissue engineering so far is the creation of skin equivalents. Lab-grown skin, incorporating both dermal and epidermal layers, is produced using a combination of cells and various polymer carriers. This engineered skin is used in aesthetic treatments for individuals disfigured by severe burns, invasive cancer surgeries, and major trauma like shotgun wounds and knife lacerations. Engineered skin products were the first tissue-engineered products approved by the FDA for clinical use [20, 21]. A similar method has been developed for replacing oral mucosa, although it has not yet been commercially available [22, 23]. Engineering and transplanting oral mucosa and gingiva could become an important new approach for periodontal graft surgery and treating gingival recession.

Dentin and Dental Pulp

Tissue engineering strategies have also shown success in producing dentin and dental pulp in both animal and laboratory studies. These engineered tissues hold significant promise for treating tooth decay, one of the most widespread diseases among children and young adults. "Root canal" is often one of the most feared terms in dentistry, but new methods are emerging to regenerate lost dentin and dental pulp. Research suggests that even if odontoblasts (the cells responsible for producing dentin) are destroyed by cavities, it may be possible to generate new cells from pulp tissue using certain BMPs (Bone Morphogenetic Proteins) [24 - 26]. These newly formed odontoblasts can create new dentin. Additionally, it may be possible to engineer dental pulp tissue itself by utilizing cultured fibroblasts and synthetic polymer scaffolds [27]. If further developed, these approaches could transform the way we treat cavities, potentially revolutionizing dental care.

Salivary Gland

One of the most difficult challenges in tissue engineering is the replacement of entire organs, and notable advancements have been made in engineering salivary gland function. Loss of salivary gland tissue or function, whether as a result of radiation therapy for cancer or diseases like Sjogren's syndrome, can severely impact quality of life, particularly in medically vulnerable individuals. One treatment method for salivary gland dysfunction involves inductive gene therapy, which aims to convert existing non-secretory ductal epithelial cells, damaged by radiation, into secretory cells capable of fluid movement. This approach has shown success in animal models [28, 29]. Another method involves cell transplantation. Recently, Baum and colleagues have developed an artificial salivary gland substitute, consisting of a polymer tube lined with epithelial cells [30]. This simple device could be implanted into the buccal mucosa of patients with damaged or non-functional salivary glands and has the potential to deliver fluid to the mouth. These innovative approaches hold promise for treating conditions resulting from lost salivary gland function, such as difficulty swallowing, altered taste, severe tooth decay, and mucosal infections.

Role of Dental Professionals in Multidisciplinary Care Teams

A multidisciplinary approach involves social practices carried out by a team of professionals who work together to provide treatment from a comprehensive perspective, addressing the patient's needs in a holistic and compassionate manner [31]. Integrality aims to ensure that individuals are evaluated as a whole, fully meeting their needs through practices and knowledge focused on human beings, supporting, assisting, and valuing them in the process of health promotion [32]. Health care networks must ensure that there is coordinated action across various levels of care to positively impact people's health and quality of life. The integration process seeks to expand the scope of healthcare services by fostering collaboration among various healthcare professions and multidisciplinary teams [33]. This approach to comprehensive patient care creates a new dynamic, promoting the exchange of knowledge between different fields, encouraging mutual respect among healthcare professionals, and finding new ways to incorporate the unique contributions of each profession [34].

Effective treatment requires a multidisciplinary approach, as every dental procedure depends on the patient's overall health, which is managed by other healthcare professionals. This comprehensive care considers the patient's physical, nutritional, emotional, spiritual, and physiological well-being, which influences the type of dental treatment recommended and whether it can be applied [35]. Another study emphasized the vital role of dental professionals in the care of patients with heart disease, underscoring the value of a multidisciplinary team approach. It highlighted the importance of collaboration among different healthcare specialties to improve patient outcomes. This aligns with one of the key principles of the Universal Health System, which advocates for a comprehensive, integrated approach to healthcare delivery [36].

In hospitalized patients, oral changes are common due to infrequent proper oral hygiene, highlighting the essential role of the dental team within the multidisciplinary care group [37]. Their involvement is crucial for assessing this patient population, linking oral health to clinical factors, addressing necessary cases, and promoting the importance of maintaining good oral hygiene [38]. In this context, a study assessed the prevalence of oral toxicities caused by cancer treatment in children and adolescents at Hospital Estadual da Criança, finding that nearly 50% experienced oral issues. Some patients even had to pause their antineoplastic therapy due to these complications. This highlights the critical role of dental surgeons within the oncology multidisciplinary team. The study also emphasized the importance of addressing clinical variables, attending to necessary cases, and promoting good oral health to support treatment continuity [39, 40].

A study conducted within the Interdisciplinary Home Hospitalization Program (PIDI), which supports cancer patients in palliative care at the Federal University's Teaching Hospital, highlighted the high prevalence of oral manifestations in this population. This underscores the vital role of dental surgeons within the multidisciplinary palliative care team [41, 42]. "Hospital centers often have dental services that collaborate with the broader team, offering tools and education. Dentists are responsible for evaluating clinical situations and guiding the prevention and treatment of oral pathologies. It is crucial that Intensive Care Units (ICUs) recognize the importance of dental surgeons, as their involvement can help reduce risks in hospitalized patients, particularly those on prolonged ventilation, through proper oral hygiene management and care for related injuries" [43].

A study on the inclusion of oral health in the Street Office Program (PCR) in Curitiba-PR highlighted the crucial role of oral health professionals in the program's multidisciplinary team. Their involvement has fostered a stronger bond with the homeless population, leading to better treatment adherence. The experience in Curitiba-PR demonstrated that integrating oral health into care for the homeless plays a key role in boosting self-esteem and supporting social reintegration [44]. In relation to comprehensive care for children, another study evaluating the collaboration between a Multiprofessional Residency Program and a Family Health Strategy (ESF) unit showed that professional interaction, with each contributing their expertise, can enhance prevention and promotion of oral health. This collaboration strengthens the field of dentistry and promotes interprofessional teamwork [45]. A summary of the previously analyzed works of other authors is shown in Table **1**.

Table 1. Summary table of the analyzed publications.

Refs.	Aim
36	To describe a clinical case of dental care os a child patient with tetralogy of Fallot in a hospital
38	To evaluate the prevalence of oral toxicities resulting from cancer treatment in children
39	To highlight the performance of the dental surgeon in different stages of treatment, highlighting the importance of maintaining oral health
40	To report a sign of cases of patients assisted at the dental service of the oncology centre of the Oswaldo Cruz University Hospital

(Table 1) cont.....

Refs.	Aim
41	To report the experience of in-service training in dentistry in a multiprofessional residency program in the oral health care network
42	To evaluate the prevalence of the main oral manifestation in patients with cancer in CP admitted to PIDI of HE/UFPel.

FHS professionals encounter various challenges in fostering teamwork, particularly in interpersonal relationships. These difficulties are compounded by changes in Primary Health Care, such as the integration of the oral health team. While ESF professionals generally recognize the importance of teamwork in the current primary care model, the oral health team often feels excluded and underappreciated by the rest of the team. Given this, it is crucial for managers and team members to prioritize the inclusion of oral health within the ESF and develop strategies to promote engagement and collaboration among all members [46].

The Function of Primary Dental Care Services

Dentists provide services at subdistrict hospitals, particularly where there are no full-time dentists, handling procedures beyond the scope of dental hygienists, such as complex tooth extractions or fitting dentures for the elderly. The frequency of dentist visits varies, with some areas seeing a dentist once a week, while others only once a month. Dental hygienists focus on delivering primary dental care, preventing oral diseases, and promoting oral health in the community. These tasks were already part of the dental team's routine before the implementation of the Family Care Team Policy, making them familiar responsibilities [47].

The Role of Identifying Risks and Providing Services Accordingly

Most dentists have conducted screenings for denture needs, oral cancer, and oral health assessments related to diabetes and kidney disease in elderly patients, in line with the policy of the Dental Public Health Bureau, Ministry of Public Health. This policy directs dentists to focus on risk screenings and service provision, with a particular emphasis on older adults, as they are the primary target group during this period [47].

The Importance of Promoting Health and Preventing Oral Diseases

Most respondents indicated that the role of dental personnel is already integrated into their workload, in line with the policies of the Dental Public Health Bureau, Ministry of Public Health. These policies focus on providing preventive oral health services for different age groups, including preschool children, school-aged children, working adults, and the elderly. Key performance indicators set by the Ministry include ensuring children aged 0–12 are cavity-free, increasing the percentage of 12-year-olds without tooth decay, and ensuring elderly individuals have at least 20 teeth and 4 pairs of functional teeth. "The role of promoting health and preventing oral diseases is already part of our responsibilities and aligns with the policy of the Dental Public Health Bureau, which mandates age-specific preventive services [47]."

TECHNOLOGICAL INNOVATIONS DRIVING MULTIDISCIPLINARY CARE

Telemedicine and Remote Care

According to the World Health Organization (2010), telemedicine is defined as "the delivery of health care services where distance is a crucial factor, utilizing information and communication technologies for the exchange of valid information for diagnosis, treatment, and prevention of diseases and injuries." Telemedicine offers numerous benefits, such as reducing hospital stays and rehospitalization rates, minimizing unnecessary travel for patients and healthcare professionals, fostering educational opportunities among healthcare workers, delivering faster and more targeted care, improving access to care in rural areas, and enhancing medical follow-up [48 - 51]. Additionally, during the COVID-19 pandemic, telemedicine has provided a safe way to deliver care without physical contact, particularly for chronic conditions and early diagnosis of COVID-19 [52].

The benefits for one group may lead to dissatisfaction for others [53], so a holistic view considering all stakeholders is essential. Finally, telemedicine implementation is highly context-dependent, and outcomes may differ by location and other aspects [54]. To fully grasp the challenges of implementing telemedicine, several factors must be considered. First, telemedicine is not a simple, ready-to-use technology; it involves both technological and sociotechnical components. Its adoption necessitates changes not only in infrastructure but also in work organization [55], potentially impacting organizational perspectives and business models. Therefore, it's important to address both technical and strategic aspects. Second, telemedicine is a complex innovation [56] introduced into an already intricate context. Its implementation requires interdisciplinary approaches that account for the dynamic interactions within the system and the human factors involved [57]. Different medical practices of telemedicine are shown in Table **2**.

Table 2. The five main acts of telemedicine [55].

Medical Practice	Definition	Nature
Teleconsultation	Diagnosing and consulting with a patient remotely	Synchronous
Tele-expertise	Consultation with one or more healthcare professionals from a distance	Synchronous/ Asynchronous
Telemonitoring	Monitoring a patient's health remotely	Asynchronous
Tele-assistance	Providing remote support to another healthcare professional during a medical or surgical procedure	Synchronous
Tele-emergency	A preliminary assessment to initiate the most appropriate response in emergency situations	Synchronous

Telemedicine is more than just a technology; it is a sociotechnical practice, meaning that the obstacles to its implementation go beyond the technology itself [58, 59]. These challenges arise from the interaction between the technology and the broader ecosystem surrounding it. This ecosystem is made up of various elements, including healthcare professionals, patients, technology providers, healthcare organizations, and the National Health System (NHS). As shown in Fig. (**2**), the advantages of telemedicine extend to patients, the healthcare system, and healthcare professionals.

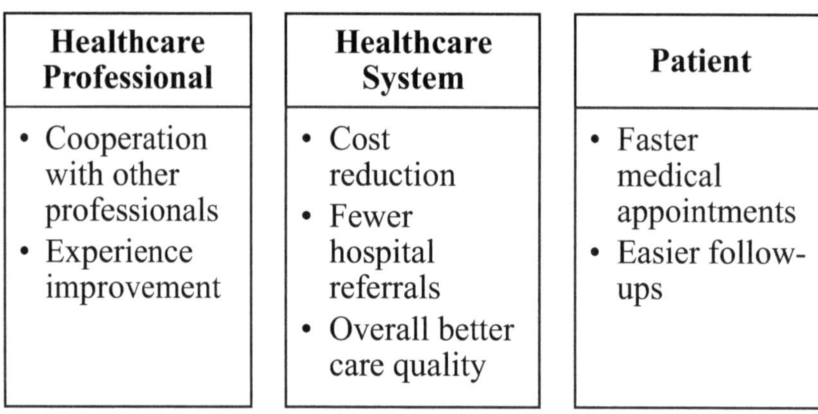

Fig. (2). The advantages of telemedicine extend to patients, the healthcare system, and healthcare professionals [55].

Robotics and Minimally Invasive Surgery

In an era of mechanical automation and computerization, where devices and software can either replace or augment human abilities, what defines a skilled surgeon and a successful surgery? A good surgery, from the patient's perspective, leads to an enhanced quality of life. The surgeon's skilled hands and trained eyes are essential for performing effective operations, as surgery traditionally involved manual cutting and stitching with tools like scalpels and knives. Surgeons need dexterous hands to engage with the surgical site, utilizing tactile feedback, along with sharp vision and sound judgment [60]. However, the human eye and hand have limitations when it comes to accessing the body's interior, which is why medical devices have been introduced into the operating room to increase surgical precision and accuracy [61]. Surgical robotics represents a multidisciplinary field that integrates engineering for system design, computer science for control and intelligence, and surgery for clinical application, while also drawing upon medical imaging, human factors, and biomedical sciences to ensure safe, precise, and effective healthcare solutions. To overcome these human limitations, automated and computerized machines have been integrated into hospital care. Modern technologies, whether surgical or biomedical, are designed to extend human abilities and reduce errors, thereby improving overall performance [62, 63]. The underlying belief is that mechanizing surgical procedures enhances both human dexterity and the quality of surgery [64, 65].

As new surgical innovations are developed, they are introduced into operating rooms not solely due to their novelty. Instead, their adoption depends on various factors, including social, economic, interpersonal, and administrative contexts [66], along with marketing efforts [67]. When these innovations reach the operating room, they are often promoted through media and commercial channels, emphasizing their ability to reduce pain and invasiveness, with a focus on technical and scientific features. This tech-centric portrayal appeals to patients, surgeons, and hospital administrators, suggesting that these advanced procedures will improve the quality of care by supplementing or replacing human hands and vision. This belief in technological determinism has contributed to the gradual replacement of direct human interaction with patients in the operating room. Consequently, hospital administrators, surgeons, and patients may feel compelled to adopt these technologies due to their perceived benefits, significance, and utility [68].

Genomic Medicine and Bioinformatics

Bioinformatics, an interdisciplinary field combining biology, computer science, and information technology, plays a pivotal role in genomics and personalized healthcare. It extends beyond traditional boundaries, influencing various medical fields, including dentistry, as noted by Natarajan (2022) [69]. For instance, its application in dentistry impacts diagnostic, therapeutic, and prognostic practices, showcasing the broad utility of bioinformatics in addressing diverse healthcare challenges. At its core, bioinformatics in personalized healthcare involves managing and analyzing vast amounts of genomic data, which is essential for developing personalized medicine. This approach focuses on tailoring medical treatments to individual patient characteristics, enhancing treatment efficacy and safety. Bioinformatics facilitates this by interpreting complex genomic data, which is crucial for identifying disease risks and customizing therapies.

However, integrating genomics into healthcare presents numerous challenges. Al Kawam *et al.* (2018) [70] highlight obstacles such as data generation, storage, representation, and the integration of genomic data with clinical information. To address these issues, bioinformatics must manage not only large volumes of data but also ensure that it is meaningfully interpreted in clinical settings. One of the major challenges involves ethical and legal concerns surrounding genomic data. Ensuring patient privacy and data security is critical, requiring stringent protections for sensitive information. Additionally, issues of consent and data ownership necessitate clear legal frameworks to guide the use of genomic data in healthcare. Education is another challenge, as healthcare professionals need to be trained to interpret and apply genomic data in clinical practice, emphasizing the importance of incorporating bioinformatics and genomics into medical curricula.

Economic considerations also play a role, as building and maintaining bioinformatics infrastructure requires substantial investment. The cost-effectiveness of personalized medicine must be evaluated to ensure its sustainability within healthcare systems. Despite these challenges, the benefits of integrating bioinformatics and genomics into healthcare are substantial. Personalized medicine offers the potential for more accurate diagnoses, more effective treatments, and the ability to prevent diseases before they arise. Bioinformatics is crucial in unlocking this potential by translating genomic data into actionable insights for patient care [71].

CHALLENGES IN MULTIDISCIPLINARY HEALTHCARE

Multidisciplinary healthcare, while offering comprehensive patient care through collaboration among various specialists, faces several challenges. One of the primary issues is effective communication and coordination among team members from different disciplines, which can lead to fragmented care or misaligned treatment plans. Another challenge is the varying approaches and priorities of different specialists, which may result in conflicting opinions regarding patient management. Additionally, time constraints in busy healthcare environments make it difficult to organize regular multidisciplinary meetings, limiting the opportunity for thorough case discussions. Resource allocation and funding for maintaining such teams can also be a hurdle, particularly in systems where budgets are stretched. Furthermore, patients may feel overwhelmed by interacting with multiple healthcare providers, making it harder for them to follow complex treatment plans. Overcoming challenges in healthcare requires strategies that combine innovation, collaboration, and adaptability. Digital health tools such as electronic health records, telemedicine, and wearable devices improve access and monitoring. Artificial intelligence and data analytics support faster diagnosis and personalized treatment. Robotics and automation enhance surgical precision and reduce workload. Interdisciplinary collaboration among clinicians, engineers, and data scientists fosters holistic solutions, while continuous training ensures professionals adapt to evolving technologies. Patient-centered approaches, strong regulatory frameworks, and investment in infrastructure further strengthen healthcare systems. Together, these strategies and tools improve efficiency, safety, and equity in delivering quality care. Despite these challenges, multidisciplinary healthcare remains crucial for delivering holistic and personalized care, but addressing these issues is vital for its success.

FUTURE TRENDS

The potential of tissue engineering in dentistry is immense, but significant challenges must be addressed over the next 15 to 20 years for it to realize its full potential. Many of these challenges are not scientific but relate to the practical application of the technology. Once we gain a comprehensive understanding of how to create functional, viable tissues in the lab, the question remains: how will this knowledge be translated to widespread clinical use? A key issue will be the cost of these therapies. Can the industry produce tissue-engineered products at a cost that makes them affordable for patients? Additionally, for these innovations to be accessible to the general public, healthcare centers equipped to apply these products will be necessary, alongside professionals trained to utilize these therapies. This will require new training programs for scientists, clinicians, and support staff. Ethical concerns also present significant challenges, particularly regarding the source and type of cells used in tissue engineering (*e.g.*, patient-derived *vs.* donated cells, adult *vs.* fetal cells). Questions surrounding who should receive these therapies—whether based on need, financial capability, or other factors—remain unresolved. Moreover, the stance of third-party payers on covering these new treatments is unclear, adding another layer of complexity. Diverse perspectives on these issues, influenced by individual, cultural, and scientific values, will undoubtedly shape the future of tissue engineering in dentistry.

This is an exciting period for dentistry and the broader biomedical community. In the next 20 to 25 years, dentistry will likely undergo significant changes, much as it has over the past few decades. Dental schools and postgraduate programs are already reassessing their curricula to meet public oral health needs, taking into account advances in genetics, cell and molecular biology, and materials science. At the undergraduate level, tissue engineering offers an excellent opportunity for students to engage in multidisciplinary learning that integrates cell biology, molecular biology, bioengineering, and biomaterials with clinical practices in oral surgery, periodontics, restorative dentistry, and oral medicine. This will allow students to observe firsthand the connection between scientific principles and clinical application. Such training will also promote collaboration between biomedical scientists, dentists, and physicians—something that is often lacking in dental education. At the postgraduate level, there is a growing need for D.D.S./Ph.D.-trained professionals who are experts in tissue engineering to serve as practitioners, researchers, and educators. Continuing education programs for practicing dentists can also raise awareness of tissue engineering as a treatment option for various oral health issues and foster connections between community dentists and academic health centers specializing in tissue engineering. As the public becomes more aware of these advanced treatments, they will demand nothing less than the best options. Clinicians who can integrate tissue engineering into their practice will continue to thrive in the evolving landscape of dentistry [15].

Global health initiatives increasingly rely on multidisciplinary approaches to tackle pandemics and address health inequities. By integrating expertise from fields, such as epidemiology, public health, social work, economics, and policy-making, these initiatives create more comprehensive strategies to combat global health crises. This collaboration enables a more holistic response to pandemics, ensuring that not only the medical aspects are addressed, but also the social determinants of health that contribute to disparities. Multidisciplinary efforts foster innovation, improve healthcare access, and promote equitable outcomes by addressing the unique needs of diverse populations, particularly those most vulnerable to health inequities.

CONCLUSION

Multidisciplinary approaches in healthcare and research are becoming increasingly essential in addressing the complexities of modern challenges. These approaches allow for a more integrated, comprehensive perspective that traditional single-discipline methods often lack. In today's world, where issues like climate change, public health crises, and technological advancements are interconnected, leveraging expertise from various fields offers a more robust framework for problem-solving and innovation. Multidisciplinary research promotes deeper insights, which are crucial in developing innovative solutions that meet the nuanced needs of global challenges.

The rise of biomedical engineering exemplifies how merging different disciplines can revolutionize both diagnostics and treatment. By integrating engineering principles with medical sciences, biomedical engineering has significantly advanced healthcare, particularly in diagnostic imaging technologies like MRI, CT scans, and ultrasound. These innovations have dramatically improved the accuracy of disease detection and monitoring, leading to better patient outcomes. Furthermore, the incorporation of Artificial Intelligence (AI) into healthcare is another major step forward, particularly in machine learning and deep learning applications. AI helps physicians by analyzing vast amounts of data to predict patient outcomes, stratify risk, and optimize interventions. The integration of AI into clinical practice is poised to become a key aspect of medical education, with physicians needing to understand and contribute to AI model development for improved healthcare delivery. The role of biomarkers in drug discovery and personalized medicine further highlights the importance of multidisciplinary collaboration. Biomarkers, which provide critical insights into patient variability, are shifting the pharmaceutical industry from mass-marketed products to more targeted, individualized therapies. This approach not only enhances treatment efficacy but also opens up new commercial opportunities, such as diagnostics development, clinical trial design, and market expansion. The ability to better understand cellular and biological processes through biomarkers is transforming the drug development landscape, making treatments more precise and tailored to specific patient needs.

Multidisciplinary teams (MDTs) in oncology provide a practical example of how collaboration among diverse specialists can significantly improve patient care. Head and Neck Cancer (HNC) treatment has benefited greatly from this approach, where oncologists, radiologists, surgeons, and other healthcare professionals work together to formulate and execute more effective treatment plans. This multidisciplinary strategy, which emerged in the 1980s, has not only increased survival rates but also improved the quality of life for cancer patients by addressing treatment side effects and psychological well-being. The development of functional oncological units, focusing on disease-specific care, further streamlines this process by integrating all departments involved in patient care, ensuring timely diagnosis and treatment. In dentistry, tissue engineering represents a revolutionary shift, enabling the regeneration of oral tissues like bone, cartilage, skin, and dental pulp. This technology has the potential to transform dental care, providing solutions to complex problems such as craniofacial reconstruction and treating tooth decay. The advancements in tissue engineering highlight how multidisciplinary collaboration between dental practitioners, biologists, and engineers can lead to groundbreaking improvements in patient care. The broader integration of bioinformatics into personalized healthcare is yet another area where multidisciplinary efforts are crucial. By managing and analyzing vast genomic datasets, bioinformatics plays a pivotal role in the development of personalized medicine, which tailors treatments to individual genetic profiles. This approach has the potential to revolutionize healthcare by making it more predictive, preventive, and participatory. However, the integration of genomics into clinical practice presents numerous challenges, including data management, ethical concerns, and the need for healthcare professionals to be trained in genomic interpretation. Addressing these challenges will require collaboration across disciplines, including bioinformatics, clinical medicine, law, and education.

Despite the numerous challenges—such as communication gaps, coordination difficulties, and resource constraints—multidisciplinary healthcare remains vital for delivering holistic, patient-centered care. The complexities of modern medicine demand a collaborative approach, as no single discipline can fully address the intricate needs of today's patients. Overcoming these challenges will be key to ensuring that multidisciplinary strategies continue to enhance healthcare outcomes and drive innovation in the field. Hence, multidisciplinary collaboration is essential across healthcare and research, offering flexible, innovative solutions to some of the world's most complex problems. As the fields of biomedical engineering, drug discovery, oncology, dentistry, and bioinformatics continue to evolve, the importance of interdisciplinary teamwork will only grow, shaping the future of personalized, effective, and compassionate healthcare.

DECLARATION

The English language of the article was improved with ChatGPT.

ACKNOWLEDGEMENTS

The authors are thankful to the Department of Animal Biology and Biotechnology, University of Hyderabad, India, for providing the necessary facilities and support.

REFERENCES

[1] J.T. Klein, *Discourses of interdisciplinarity.* Routledge, 2017.

[2] M. Borrego, L.K. Newswander, and S.Y. Yoon, "Characteristics of interdisciplinary research in engineering education", *J. Eng. Educ.,* vol. 102, no. 3, pp. 280-301, 2013.

[3] B. Tress, G. Tress, G. Fry, and P. Opdam, "Clarifying integrative research concepts in land and water management", *Environ. Sci. Policy,* vol. 8, no. 3, pp. 203-217, 2005.

[4] A.F. Repko, and R. Szostak, *Interdisciplinary research: Process and theory.* Sage Publications, 2017.

[5] National Academy of Sciences, *Facilitating interdisciplinary research.* National Academies Press, 2005.

[6] C. Giordano, M. Brennan, B. Mohamed, P. Rashidi, F. Modave, and P. Tighe, "Accessing Artificial Intelligence for Clinical Decision-Making", *Front. Digit. Health,* vol. 3, p. 645232, 2021. [http://dx.doi.org/10.3389/fdgth.2021.645232] [PMID: 34713115]

[7] M. Prosperi, Y. Guo, M. Sperrin, J.S. Koopman, J.S. Min, X. He, S. Rich, M. Wang, i.e. Buchan, and J. Bian, "Causal inference and counterfactual prediction in machine learning for actionable healthcare", *Nat. Mach. Intell.,* vol. 2, no. 7, pp. 369-375, 2020. [http://dx.doi.org/10.1038/s42256-020-0197-y]

[8] F. Wang, R. Kaushal, and D. Khullar, "Should health care demand interpretable artificial intelligence or accept “black box” medicine?", *Ann. Intern. Med.,* vol. 172, no. 1, pp. 59-60, 2020. [http://dx.doi.org/10.7326/M19-2548] [PMID: 31842204]

[9] Martín Noguerol T, Paulano-Godino F, Martín-Valdivia MT, Menias CO, Luna A. Strengths, weaknesses, opportunities, and threats analysis of artificial intelligence and machine learning applications in radiology. J Am Coll Radiol. (2019) 16(Pt. B):1239–47. [http://dx.doi.org/10.1016/j.jacr.2019.05.047]

[10] A. Amir-Aslani, and V. Mangematin, "The future of drug discovery and development: Shifting emphasis towards personalized medicine", *Technol. Forecast. Soc. Change,* vol. 77, no. 2, pp. 203-217, 2010. [http://dx.doi.org/10.1016/j.techfore.2009.09.005]

[11] M. Taberna, F. Gil Moncayo, E. Jané-Salas, M. Antonio, L. Arribas, E. Vilajosana, E. Peralvez Torres, and R. Mesía, "The Multidisciplinary Team (MDT) Approach and Quality of Care", *Front. Oncol.,* vol. 10, p. 85, 2020. [http://dx.doi.org/10.3389/fonc.2020.00085] [PMID: 32266126]

[12] T. Ruhstaller, H. Roe, B. Thürlimann, and J.J. Nicoll, "The multidisciplinary meeting: An indispensable aid to communication between different specialities", *Eur. J. Cancer,* vol. 42, no. 15, pp. 2459-2462, 2006. [http://dx.doi.org/10.1016/j.ejca.2006.03.034] [PMID: 16934974]

[13] S. Maslin-Prothero, "The role of the multidisciplinary team in recruiting to cancer clinical trials", *Eur. J. Cancer Care (Engl.),* vol. 15, no. 2, pp. 146-154, 2006. [http://dx.doi.org/10.1111/j.1365-2354.2005.00625.x] [PMID: 16643262]

[14] F.C. Wright, C. De Vito, B. Langer, and A. Hunter, "Multidisciplinary cancer conferences: A systematic review and development of practice standards", *Eur. J. Cancer,* vol. 43, no. 6, pp. 1002-1010, 2007. [http://dx.doi.org/10.1016/j.ejca.2007.01.025] [PMID: 17329094]

[15] Kaigler, D. and Mooney, D., (2001). Tissue Engineering’s Impact on Dentistry, Transfer of Advances in Sciences into Dental Education.

[16] E. Alsberg, E.E. Hill, and D.J. Mooney, "Craniofacial tissue engineering", *Crit. Rev. Oral Biol. Med.,* vol. 12, no. 1, pp. 64-75, 2001. [http://dx.doi.org/10.1177/10454411010120010501] [PMID: 11349963]

[17] M. Brittberg, A. Lindahl, A. Nilsson, C. Ohlsson, O. Isaksson, and L. Peterson, "Treatment of deep cartilage defects in the knee with autologous chondrocyte transplantation", *N. Engl. J. Med.,* vol. 331, no. 14, pp. 889-895, 1994. [http://dx.doi.org/10.1056/NEJM199410063311401] [PMID: 8078550]

[18] W.C. Puelacher, D. Mooney, R. Langer, J. Upton, J.P. Vacanti, and C.A. Vacanti, "Design of nasoseptal cartilage replacements synthesized from biodegradable polymers and chondrocytes", *Biomaterials,* vol. 15, no. 10, pp. 774-778, 1994. [http://dx.doi.org/10.1016/0142-9612(94)90031-0]

[19] W.C. Puelacher, J. Wisser, C.A. Vacanti, N.F. Ferraro, D. Jaramillo, and J.P. Vacanti, "Temporomandibular joint disc replacement made by tissue-engineered growth of cartilage", *J. Oral Maxillofac. Surg.,* vol. 52, no. 11, pp. 1172-1177, 1994. [http://dx.doi.org/10.1016/0278-2391(94)90538-X] [PMID: 7965312]

[20] N. Parenteau, "The organogenesis story", *Sci. Am.,* vol. 280, pp. 83-84, 1999.

[PMID: 10232963]

[21] G. Naughton, "The advanced tissue sciences story", *Sci. Am.,* vol. 280, no. 4, pp. 84-85, 1999. [PMID: 10232964]

[22] H. Mizuno, N. Emi, A. Abe, I. Takahashi, T. Kojima, H. Saito, Y. Sumi, K.I. Hata, and M. Ueda, "Successful culture and sustainability *in vivo* of gene-modified human oral mucosal epithelium", *Hum. Gene Ther.,* vol. 10, no. 5, pp. 825-830, 1999. [http://dx.doi.org/10.1089/10430349950018571] [PMID: 10210149]

[23] J.A. Garlick, and E.S. Fenjves, "Keratinocyte gene transfer and gene therapy", *Crit. Rev. Oral Biol. Med.,* vol. 7, no. 3, pp. 204-221, 1996. [http://dx.doi.org/10.1177/10454411960070030101] [PMID: 8909878]

[24] M. Nakashima, "The induction of reparative dentine in the amputated dental pulp of the dog by bone morphogenetic protein", *Arch. Oral Biol.,* vol. 35, no. 7, pp. 493-497, 1990. [http://dx.doi.org/10.1016/0003-9969(90)90078-O] [PMID: 2222252]

[25] Y. Lianjia, G. Yuhao, and F.H. White, "Bovine bone morphogenetic protein-induced dentinogenesis", *Clin. Orthop. Relat. Res.,* no. 295, pp. 305-312, 1993. [PMID: 8403667]

[26] R.B. Rutherford, J. Wahle, M. Tucker, D. Rueger, and M. Charette, "Induction of reparative dentine formation in monkeys by recombinant human osteogenic Protein-1", *Arch. Oral Biol.,* vol. 38, no. 7, pp. 571-576, 1993. [http://dx.doi.org/10.1016/0003-9969(93)90121-2] [PMID: 8368953]

[27] D.J. Mooney, C. Powell, J. Piana, and B. Rutherford, "Engineering dental pulp-like tissue in vitro", *Biotechnol. Prog.,* vol. 12, no. 6, pp. 865-868, 1996. [http://dx.doi.org/10.1021/bp960073f] [PMID: 8983211]

[28] B.J. Baum, and B.C. O'Connell, "*In vivo* gene transfer to salivary glands", *Crit. Rev. Oral Biol. Med.,* vol. 10, no. 3, pp. 276-283, 1999. [http://dx.doi.org/10.1177/10454411990100030201] [PMID: 10759409]

[29] C. Delporte, B.C. O'Connell, X. He, H.E. Lancaster, A.C. O'Connell, P. Agre, and B.J. Baum, "Increased fluid secretion after adenoviral-mediated transfer of the aquaporin-1 cDNA to irradiated rat salivary glands", *Proc. Natl. Acad. Sci. USA,* vol. 94, no. 7, pp. 3268-3273, 1997. [http://dx.doi.org/10.1073/pnas.94.7.3268] [PMID: 9096382]

[30] B.J. Baum, S. Wang, E. Cukierman, C. Delporte, H. Kagami, Y. Marmary, P.C. Fox, D.J. Mooney, and K.M. Yamada, "Re-engineering the functions of a terminally differentiated epithelial cell *in vivo*", *Ann. N. Y. Acad. Sci.,* vol. 875, no. 1, pp. 294-300, 1999. [http://dx.doi.org/10.1111/j.1749-6632.1999.tb08512.x] [PMID: 10415576]

[31] M.S. Clemente, *Oral rehabilitation of patient in home care service: case report.* UFU, Institutional Repository, 2019, pp. 1-20.

[32] P.H.D.A. Rodrigues, "[Political challenges facing the consolidation of the Sistema Único de Saúde: a historical approach]", *Hist. Cienc. Saude Manguinhos,* vol. 21, no. 1, pp. 37-59, 2014. [http://dx.doi.org/10.1590/S0104-59702014000100003] [PMID: 24789485]

[33] M.V.S. Silva, G.B.N. Miranda, and M.A. Andrade, "Diverse meanings of comprehensiveness: between the presupposed and the experienced in a multi-disciplinary team", *Interface Comum Saúde Educ.,* vol. 21, no. 62, pp. 589-599, 2017.

[34] L. Horiguchi, L.L. Carvalho, E. Umeda, and M. Borba, "Harmonic performance of multidisciplinary health teams: Humanized hospital discharge", *Rev. Bioet.,* vol. 30, pp. 564-574, 2022.

[35] M.Z. Marini, I. Arrieira, and C. Jacotec, "Experience report of the dental team in home care at a teaching hospital in the city of Pelotas, RS, Brazil", *Journal of the Faculty of Dentistry-UPF.,* vol. 22, no. 2, 2017.

[36] C.L. Chandler, and M.F. Silva-Junior, "Dental care of hospitalized pediatric patient with tetralogy of Fallot: a case report", *RGO Rev. Gaúch. Odontol.,* vol. 70, p. e20220004, 2022. [http://dx.doi.org/10.1590/1981-86372022000420200049]

[37] K.M. Lima, K.A.A. Calado, C.F.S. Menezes, and F.F. Lopes, "Analysis of the case series of the oral condition of patients in the surgical clinic of a university hospital", *CES Dentistry.,* vol. 34, no. 1, pp. 4-13, 2021.

[38] L.D.B. Alves, I.S. Cerqueira, F. Arsati, A.L.P. Valente Pires, and V.S. Freitas, "Oral toxicities of cancer therapy in children and adolescents: A descriptive study", *CES Dentistry,* vol. 34, no. 2, pp. 30-45, 2021.

[39] I.S. Oliveira, N.M. Nascimento, M.G.A.M. Chaves, T.C. Esteves, L.C. Lenz e Silva, and G.M.C. Fabri, "Dental intervention prior to and subsequent to the diagnosis of acute myeloid leukemia: case report", *RGO Rev. Gaúch. Odontol.,* vol. 70, p. e20220017, 2022. [http://dx.doi.org/10.1590/1981-86372022001720190157]

[40] T.S. Macêdo, M.C.F. Melo, and A.K.L. Vidal, "Hospital and oncological dental care: a series of cases", *RGO Rev. Gaúch. Odontol.,* vol. 67, p. e20190036, 2019. [http://dx.doi.org/10.1590/1981-86372019000363610]

[41] S.F. Mestriner, W.M. Junior, L.D. de Macedo, and L.P. de Mesquita Lago, "Dentistry in the multiprofessional health residency: Experience of training in the oral health care network", *Revista da ABENO,* vol. 22, no. 2, pp. 674-1674, 2022.

[42] Da Fonseca Orcina B, Jaccottet CMG & Savian MCB. Prevalence of Oral Manifestations in Cancer Patients Assisted in a Home Care Program in the City of Pelotas-RS. Brazilian Cancerology. 2021;67(2).

[43] C. Humeres-Sigala, A. Márquez, P. González Ritchie, R. Valenzuela-Ramos, M. Rivera Saavedra, P. Vásquez, and C. Araya-Salas, "Multidisciplinary management of the oral cavity in COVID-19 patients under invasive mechanical ventilation. List of dental equipment", *Int. J. Odontostomatol.,* vol. 14, no. 4, pp. 701-704, 2020. [http://dx.doi.org/10.4067/S0718-381X2020000400701]

[44] De Albuquerque RAL, da Silva Nascimento AC, Freitas RS, Wollmann A, da Silva ROC & Ditterich RG. "The implementation of oral health in the street clinic program in Curitiba-PR", *Tempus–Actas de Saúde Coletiva.* 2019; 13(3): ág-191.

[45] De Araújo DC, de Souza Lucena EE, Tavares TRP, de Araújo TB, de Araújo CM, da Costa BMB & de Araújo Medeiros Filho JS. Promotion of oral health in growth and development consultations in primary care: A report collaboration. of interprofessional Revista Ciência Plural. 2018;4(2):87-101.

[46] H.E. Peruzzo, A.G. Bega, A.P.A.T. Lopes, M.D.C.F.L. Haddad, A.M. Peres, and S.S. Marcon, *The challenges of teamwork in the family health strategy.* Anna Nery School, 2018, p. 22.

[47] S. Sangouam, "The Roles of Dental Professionals Team among the Family Care Team Policy in Lower-Northern Region, Thailand", *Journal of Dentistry Indonesia,* vol. 25, no. 3, pp. 148-152, 2018. [http://dx.doi.org/10.14693/jdi.v25i3.1257]

[48] A. Lockamy, and D.L. Smith, "Telemedicine: a process enabler for enhanced healthcare delivery systems", In: *Business Process Management Journal* vol. 15. , 2009, no. 1, pp. 5-19. [http://dx.doi.org/10.1108/14637150910931433]

[49] F. Mold, J. Hendy, Y.L. Lai, and S. de Lusignan, "Electronic consultation in primary care between providers and patients: systematic review", *JMIR Med. Inform.,* vol. 7, no. 4, p. e13042, 2019. [http://dx.doi.org/10.2196/13042] [PMID: 31793888]

[50] T. Cravo Oliveira, J. Barlow, and S. Bayer, "The association between general practitioner participation in joint teleconsultations and rates of referral: a discrete choice experiment", *BMC Fam. Pract.,* vol. 16, no. 1, p. 50, 2015. [http://dx.doi.org/10.1186/s12875-015-0261-6] [PMID: 25896515]

[51] R. Speyer, D. Denman, S. Wilkes-Gillan, Y. Chen, H. Bogaardt, J. Kim, D. Heckathorn, and R. Cordier, "Effects of telehealth by allied health professionals and nurses in rural and remote areas: A systematic review and meta-analysis", *J. Rehabil. Med.,* vol. 50, no. 3, pp. 225-235, 2018. [http://dx.doi.org/10.2340/16501977-2297] [PMID: 29257195]

[52] W.R. Smith, A.J. Atala, R.P. Terlecki, E.E. Kelly, and C.A. Matthews, "Implementation guide for rapid integration of an outpatient telemedicine program during the COVID-19 pandemic", *J. Am. Coll. Surg.,* vol. 231, no. 2, pp. 216-222e2, 2020. [http://dx.doi.org/10.1016/j.jamcollsurg.2020.04.030] [PMID: 32360960]

[53] J. Barlow, D. Singh, S. Bayer, and R. Curry, "A systematic review of the benefits of home telecare for frail elderly people and those with long-term conditions", *J. Telemed. Telecare,* vol. 13, no. 4, pp. 172-179, 2007. [http://dx.doi.org/10.1258/135763307780908058]

[54] J. Barlow, S. Bayer, and R. Curry, "Implementing complex innovations in fluid multi-stakeholder environments: Experiences of 'telecare'", *Technovation,* vol. 26, no. 3, pp. 396-406, 2006. [http://dx.doi.org/10.1016/j.technovation.2005.06.010]

[55] A. Khodadad-Saryazdi, "Exploring the telemedicine implementation challenges through the process innovation approach: A case study research in the French healthcare sector", *Technovation,* vol. 107, p. 102273, 2021. [http://dx.doi.org/10.1016/j.technovation.2021.102273]

[56] T. Greenhalgh, S. Shaw, J. Wherton, G. Hughes, J. Lynch, C. A'Court, S. Hinder, N. Fahy, E. Byrne, A. Finlayson, T. Sorell, R. Procter, and R. Stones, "SCALS: a fourth-generation study of assisted living technologies in their organisational, social, political and policy context", *BMJ Open,* vol. 6, no. 2, p. e010208, 2016. [http://dx.doi.org/10.1136/bmjopen-2015-010208] [PMID: 26880671]

[57] T. Greenhalgh, J. Wherton, C. Papoutsi, J. Lynch, G. Hughes, C. A'Court, S. Hinder, N. Fahy, R. Procter, and S. Shaw, "Beyond adoption: a new framework for theorizing and evaluating nonadoption, abandonment, and challenges to the scale-up, spread, and sustainability of health and care technologies", *J. Med. Internet Res.,* vol. 19, no. 11, p. e367, 2017. a [http://dx.doi.org/10.2196/jmir.8775] [PMID: 29092808]

[58] Papoutsi, C., Wherton, J., Shaw, S., Morrison, C., Greenhalgh, T., 2020. Putting the social back into sociotechnical: case studies of co-design in digital health. J. Am. Med. Inf. Assoc. [http://dx.doi.org/10.1093/jamia/ocaa197]

[59] J. Wherton, S. Shaw, C. Papoutsi, L. Seuren, and T. Greenhalgh, "Guidance on the introduction and use of video consultations during COVID-19: important lessons from qualitative research", *BMJ Leader,* vol. 4, no. 3, pp. 120-123, 2020. [http://dx.doi.org/10.1136/leader-2020-000262]

[60] M.J. Mack, "Minimally invasive and robotic surgery", *JAMA,* vol. 285, no. 5, pp. 568-572, 2001. [http://dx.doi.org/10.1001/jama.285.5.568] [PMID: 11176860]

[61] Kim Leland, "Google Glass Delivers New Insight During Surgery," USCF News Center (California), Oct. 30, 2013, Available from: https://www.ucsf.edu/news/2013/10/109526/surgeon-improves-safe-y-eiciency-operating-room-google

[62] L.F. Hogle, "Enhancement Technologies and the Body", *Annu. Rev. Anthropol.,* vol. 34, no. 1, pp. 695-716, 2005. [http://dx.doi.org/10.1146/annurev.anthro.33.070203.144020]

[63] M. Eunjeong, "Body and Enhancement Technology: An Introduction", *East Asian Sci. Technol. Soc.,* vol. 10, no. 1, pp. 1-4, 2016.

[64] K. Moorthy, Y. Munz, A. Dosis, J. Hernandez, S. Martin, F. Bello, T. Rockall, and A. Darzi, "Dexterity enhancement with robotic surgery", *Surg. Endosc.,* vol. 18, no. 5, pp. 790-795, 2004.

[http://dx.doi.org/10.1007/s00464-003-8922-2] [PMID: 15216862]

[65] T. Schlich, *Surgery, Science and Industry: A Revolution in Fracture Care.* Palgrave Macmillam: Houndmills, 2002.
[http://dx.doi.org/10.1057/9780230513280]

[66] D. Howell, *Joel, Technology in the Hospital: Transforming Patient Care in the Early Twentieth Century.* The Johns Hopkins University Press: Baltimore, 1996.
[http://dx.doi.org/10.56021/9780801850202]

[67] C. Van den Bulte, and G.L. Lilien, "Medical Innovation Revisited: Social Contagion versus Marketing Effort", *Am. J. Sociol.,* vol. 106, no. 5, pp. 1409-1435, 2001.
[http://dx.doi.org/10.1086/320819]

[68] P. Abrishami, A. Boer, and K. Horstman, "Understanding the adoption dynamics of medical innovations: Affordances of the da Vinci robot in the Netherlands", *Soc. Sci. Med.,* vol. 117, pp. 125-133, 2014.
[http://dx.doi.org/10.1016/j.socscimed.2014.07.046] [PMID: 25063968]

[69] P. Manickam Natarajan, "Dental Bioinformatics – Current Scope and Future perspectives", *Research Journal of Pharmacy and Technology,* vol. 15, no. 6, pp. 2351-2356, 2022.
[http://dx.doi.org/10.52711/0974-360X.2022.00391]

[70] Al Kawam, A., Sen, A., Datta, A., & Dickey, N. (2018). Understanding the Bioinformatics Challenges of Integrating Genomics into Healthcare," in IEEE Journal of Biomedical and Health Informatics, 22(5), 1672-1683.
[http://dx.doi.org/10.1109/JBHI.2017.2778263]

[71] Oluwatoyin Ayo-Farai, Oluwatosin Ogundairo, Chinyere Onwumere, O. Ogundairo, C.P. Maduka, C.C. Okongwu, and C. Onwumere, "Bioinformatics and personalized medicine in the U.S.: A comprehensive review: Scrutinizing the advancements in genomics and their potential to revolutionize healthcare delivery", *World Journal of Advanced Research and Reviews,* vol. 21, no. 1, pp. 335-351, 2024.
[http://dx.doi.org/10.30574/wjarr.2024.21.1.0016]

CHAPTER 10

Mobile Health Apps: Improving Healthcare Delivery and Patient Outcomes

Sanjay Kumar[1,*], **Vivek Agrawal**[2] and **Kuldeep Singh Kaswan**[2]

[1] *Department of Electronics and Communication Engineering, Galgotias College of Engineering and Technology, Greater Noida, Uttar Pradesh, India*

[2] *School of Computer Science & Engineering, Galgotias University, Greater Noida, Uttar Pradesh, India*

Abstract: The mobile technology landscape has dramatically evolved from simple communication devices to highly sophisticated tools that serve critical functions across all aspects of daily life, especially in the health sector. Initially limited to texting and calling, mobile phones have transformed into powerful computing platforms with the advent of smartphones and advancements in wireless technology. These devices now support a wide range of applications capable of executing complex tasks, including health management. Among the most significant developments in mobile technology is the emergence of health applications. These advanced apps deliver healthcare solutions by leveraging smartphone features such as sensors, GPS, and internet connectivity. Mobile health applications have revolutionized healthcare delivery—from tracking calories and exercise routines to managing chronic conditions and enabling remote consultations. With ongoing advancements in mobile technology and the integration of cloud computing, big data analytics, and artificial intelligence, health applications are poised to become an integral component of the modern healthcare system.

Keywords: Artificial intelligence, Chronic condition management, Healthcare, Mobile technology, mHealth applications, Smartphones.

INTRODUCTION

Background

Overview of Mobile Technology Evolution

There is not much we can argue against in the statement that the world around us has changed largely due to mobile technology over the years, with mobile devices transitioning from simple tools used solely for messaging to advanced instru-

* **Corresponding author Sanjay Kumar:** Department of Electronics and Communication Engineering, Galgotias College of Engineering and Technology, Greater Noida, Uttar Pradesh, India; E-mail: skakhil@gmail.com

Arun Kumar Rana, Mandeep Kaur & Sumit Kumar Rana (Eds.)

ments. Over time, who would have imagined that mobile telephones in the 90s would evolve to encompass different dimensions today, enabling us to interact with our surroundings? Yes, to begin with, and with the introduction of the first incarnations, mobile phones were mostly utilized for communicating voice and text messages [1]. Conclusively, within the realm of hand-held devices, mobile networked phones are rapidly evolving into multicore processor devices due to the growth of smartphones and technological shifts in wireless systems. Among them are numerous enhanced functionalities, including health organization-related activities.

MHealth, or mobile mental health, is gaining prominence as the next big breakthrough in mobile technology innovation. With application usage and the GPS capabilities of hand-held devices and phones, many different tasks can now be performed—including internet access—where health innovations show great promise [2]. The latest usage metrics for these apps speak volumes. By simply monitoring physical activity and nutrition, managing chronic diseases, or enabling telehealth sessions, mobile health apps have reshaped the delivery and consumption of healthcare services. Moreover, due to the fast-paced growth of mobile technologies—embracing further complements, such as artificial intelligence, deep analytics, and cloud systems—the scope of mobile health has become truly magnificent.

Importance of Health Management in the Modern Era

With chronic diseases becoming more common, the population aging, and individuals desiring personalization, health management has gained significant importance in the present day. Health management is necessary because it can impact patient recovery, contain healthcare expenditure, and, overall, improve quality of life. As healthcare systems grow more complicated, the need for various tools and technologies that help individuals manage their health and coordinate with care providers effectively is clearly evident [3].

Mobile technology—in this case, mobile health applications—can be considered at the forefront of addressing such issues. These applications encourage patients to be active participants in their health management by providing convenient access to health information and resources. They support patients in tracking health parameters, identifying suitable treatment regimens, and taking appropriate steps regarding their health [4]. Such applications also enable communication between patients and care providers at every stage of health management, helping to prevent disease and perform other managerial functions, such as care coordination.

In times when healthcare systems are burdened with the mandate to deliver operational efficiency and effectiveness, mobile technology appears to be a promising solution for achieving these goals in healthcare.

Scope and Objectives

Purpose of the Chapter

The aim of this chapter is to explore the impact of mobile health applications, or apps, in transforming the domain of health management. With enhanced technological advancement, the use of mobile devices has broadened in the health sector, and new ways have emerged to increase patient engagement and interaction, improve communication between patients and healthcare providers, and ultimately enhance health outcomes. This chapter provides a detailed evaluation of self-health practices among patients through mobile health applications and how these practices are influencing the provision of health services. The chapter also examines the emerging challenges to the widespread adoption of these technologies and the future trends of mobile health in the rapidly evolving healthcare environment.

The focus of the chapter is to investigate the benefits and barriers of mobile health applications and to appraise their future development trends. The details and content of this chapter will assist researchers, technology developers, policymakers, and healthcare practitioners who are committed to enhancing healthcare through the use of mobile technology.

Key Questions the Chapter Will Address

This chapter will address several key questions to provide a deeper understanding of the impact of mobile health apps on health management:

1. **How do mobile health apps empower patients in managing their health?**
   - Bankruptcy is looking at advances in how these apps allow patients to disclose their health information, control treatment plans, and make informed choices, and empower them to manage chronic conditions on their own.
2. **What role do mobile health apps play in enhancing communication between patients and healthcare providers?**
   - Bankruptcy looks at how these apps help coordinate interventions, virtual counseling, and remote monitoring to improve affected individuals' attendance and care planning.
3. **What are the challenges associated with the use of mobile health apps in healthcare?**

   - The chapter will cover technical, ethical, and social issues, such as protecting data security and privacy, inequalities in access across generations, and consumer barriers to accepting them, from eliminating the source
4. **What are the potential future directions for mobile health apps in health management?**
   - This chapter will consider trends and technologies advancing through artificial intelligence and big data, which will likewise improve the efficiency of mobile health apps, as well as how the study had to find long-term impact in the 19th century

HISTORICAL PERSPECTIVE OF MOBILE TECHNOLOGY IN HEALTH

Early Applications of Mobile Technology in Healthcare

Mobile devices have been embedded in healthcare since the early days of telecommunications. Mobile phones were originally just basic devices for sending texts and talking on the phone, but as they evolved, their potential in the medical field was explored. Mobile devices have been embedded in healthcare since the early days of telecommunications [5]. Mobile phones were originally just basic devices for sending texts and talking on the phone, but as they evolved, their potential in the medical field was explored.

Initial Uses of Mobile Devices in Health Management

By current standards, the early application of mobile technology towards health management was pretty straightforward. By the late 1990s and the early 2000s, doctors were texting people to remind them of their appointments. These reminders mainly dealt with appointment setting, medication, and visits. The ease of use made it an easily accessible strategy in promoting patient adherence to treatment regimens, while available health care was very limited within such low-resource settings.

Mobile phones were even used in early public health interventions to disseminate information on health promotion and disease prevention. For instance, during infectious disease outbreaks caused by HIV/AIDS and tuberculosis, mobile phones were utilized to transmit instructional messages to at-risk groups [6]. Such an early application of mobile technology in public health showed just how efficiently, immediately, and widely these devices can reach mass populations.

Case Studies of Early Implementations

The adoption of mobile technology in health care is very well documented in many case studies from the early 2000s. A good example is a UK "Text2Remind" campaign that used cell phones. It was one of the earliest programs to use text messages to remind patients to take prescriptions and appear for follow-up appointments. As a result of such programs, participants' drug adherence rates substantially increased, which could be seen to pave the way for mobile health interventions to be adopted broadly. Another example of early adoption would have been the use of mobile phones in maternal and child health programs in sub-Saharan Africa. For instance, "Mobile for Mothers" leveraged mobile technology in reminding pregnant women about prenatal care visits as well as making available crucial health information [7]. These interventions increased the health status of mothers and children in areas where access to health services had been limited.

Another case of chronic illness management engaged the use of mobile technology with remote monitoring systems. By utilizing mobile phones, early experimental programs in the US and Europe were possible; health information, like blood pressure or glucose levels, was transferred from the patient to the doctor. Such systems made possible the monitoring of happenings in real-time and immediate interventions, which are always very crucial for chronic conditions such as diabetes and hypertension [8]. These early usages of mobile technology created all the groundwork for more advanced applications of mobile health (mHealth). The history of the development of mobile health (mHealth) is characterized by a slow progression in sophistication and technology that changed simple handheld devices from pure communication machines into real health management devices. MHealth started as a simple application a few decades ago, but it has evolved into a very complex system that has proven to be necessary to ensure contemporary health care is delivered.

Evolution of Mobile Health (mHealth)

Mobile health (mHealth) is a case of growing technological advances and sophistication, transforming mobile devices from simple communication tools into effective health care delivery systems. From simple applications to the most sophisticated systems required for modern healthcare, mHealth has evolved over the last few decades.

Development from Basic Mobile Tools to Advanced Applications

The first phase of mHealth development focused on the use of simple features of early mobile phones. The most common mHealth applications in the late 1990s and early 2000s were simple text messaging services that delivered patients' health information and reminders; although these early applications were not very functional, they demonstrated how mobile technology could enhance patient compliance and impact health behaviors.

As mobile technology advanced, so did the scope of mHealth applications. The launch of the smartphone became a revolutionary moment that led to much more complex and interactive health applications. This was why the inclusion of sensors, GPS, and internet connectivity within the smartphone was necessary for it to become a fully functional tool for health management [9]. The developers have created applications that started monitoring a wide variety of health metrics: exercise, food intake, sleep patterns, and drug adherence. Such apps give individuals instant feedback and personalized recommendations, making them much more enthusiastic about their health.

While advancement in the capabilities of mHealth applications goes in tandem with an advance in mobile technology, perhaps a great watershed moment came when the arrival of smartphones enabled the development of ever more complex and interactive health applications. The inclusion of sensors, GPS, and internet connectivity moved the smartphones toward becoming effective health management tools. Many developers went on to develop health-related applications, including apps that could track medication compliance, sleep habits, food, and activity levels [10]. In this way, these apps can provide users with individualized advice, real-time feedback, and encourage an active role on the part of the users in managing their health and well-being.

The Role of Mobile Networks in Health Management Growth

Healthcare Providers embrace mHealth growth largely based on mobile network development. Due to mobile technology, data collection, monitoring, and analysis can now be done on an enormous scale. Development in mobile health or mHealth solutions has also risen. They offer numerous benefits in the health and wellness sphere. They ensure patient engagement as well as make healthcare more accessible. They also give providers a way of monitoring health and giving care that has never been experienced [11]. Despite the exponential growth of mHealth, there Are Still some key challenges. Integration of mHealth into health systems is one of the most significant challenges. mHealth needs to be integrated into existing workflows. This is to ensure the effectiveness and efficiency of care delivery. It should also be applied in a way that is accepted and trusted by the patients.

Another major challenge is the security and confidentiality of health information. The use of mHealth solutions will also depend on the transfer and storage of patient health information. This makes Data Security Measures an imperative. Medical data Privacy Policies are also essential. They safeguard Patient Privacy as well as Confidentiality. There is a need for a strong framework to protect data. It is designed to ensure compliance with the law and regulations regarding data protection. It also assures the sensitive health data, keeping it safe. Accessibility and Equity in mHealth adoption are also some of the issues. Technological access barriers exist in some populations [12]. It can be worse for the Existing health disparities. Healthy solutions have to be designed for all users. In some places, internet access and smartphone ownership are still limited; therefore, solutions must reach everyone.

Limited evidence of the effectiveness of Healthy solutions and regulatory ambiguity are the other challenges. The NIH has acknowledged that there is little evidence for mHealth-related solutions. It is an area that needs rigorous evaluations of mHealth solutions. This way, they can be sure to have some measurable health benefits. Besides, the complexities of mHealth regulation have also come under notice. Implementing mHealth solutions must not put the Patient at risk. The potential for Harm and Misuse requires the regulation.

Ensuring a clear regulatory framework on the development and use of mHealth solutions is fundamental. Although many of these challenges present significant hurdles, the potential to transform healthcare offered by mHealth is colossal. The potential for revolutionizing health care delivery in ways never imaginable before is enormous. mHealth is a very rapidly advancing practice. Its full potential has yet to be realized. It will, however, mark the beginning of a much more patient-centered, accessible, and efficient health care era. This is a very short account of how mHealth has grown with the mobile network. When the origin of mobile technologies was first formulated, they were largely restricted to 2G networks [13]. They had limited bandwidth and coverage. This imposed constraints on mHealth applications. However, the development of mobile networks was not stagnant. There was 3G and then 4 G. Now there is 5G. This significantly increased the mHealth potential. In fact, the move from 2G to 3 G networks improved the data speed, which had more reliability with the connections. This opened up a wide range of health applications. It made the applications relatively more interactive. More data-intensive applications were possible.

Patients could make use of devices. They enjoyed improved access to a broader array of health resources. These included video consultations with health care givers, live health care data transmission. The rollout of 4G networks also further fueled mHealth deployment. They provided the much-needed infrastructure for seamless high-definition video streaming. Moreover, high-speed data exchange was also beneficial. This technology allowed health care providers to provide for remote consultation. They could offer Telemedicine services with quality and speed [14]. The above were impossible before. Patients in remote areas benefited greatly from such programs. They have been prevented from reaching healthcare facilities. The advent of recent 5G networks is going to revolutionize mHealth with ultra-low latency and increased bandwidth, which can support a huge number of connected devices. 5G will be enabled with high-order applications such as remote surgeries. Real-time health monitoring through wearable devices is also feasible. AI-driven diagnostics can easily be integrated. All the enhancements in connectivity that 5G is going to provide will also support the growth of IoMT. Connected devices and sensors are used here to collect and transmit health data. This, in turn, strengthens our understanding of patient health.

MOBILE HEALTH TECHNOLOGIES

Types of Mobile Health Applications

The biggest advancement in healthcare is the use of mobile health technology, which takes advantage of the growing popularity of mobile devices to improve treatment and treatment delivery. So this technology has many uses, from telemedicine and remote counseling methods to fitness tracking and health monitoring. Below is an in-depth analysis of the types of mobile health apps that are transforming healthcare today:

Health Monitoring Apps

Health-monitoring applications are devised to track a variety of health parameters. It provides immediate answers to both patients and service delivery personnel in healthcare. The apps use sensors packed in smartphones and wristwatch-like devices. These sensors have the capability of keeping Track of vital signs. They can track heart rate, blood pressure, glucose levels, and sleep patterns. The data obtained through the apps becomes A subject of scrutiny [15]. It can identify early warning signs of health disorders. On this count, the Apps permit interventions on time.

Consider diabetes Management apps. Very useful for those who have to monitor their blood glucose levels. These apps also track diet. They remind people to take medication. On similar lines, there are apps for people suffering from hypertension. They track the blood pressure readings. This enables the handling of the situation more effectively. Apps like these can share health data with healthcare providers. Sharing is the most important feature of it. It better coordinates care. It also helps in formulating plans of treatment for patients.

They confer power to the users. They take charge of their health. Users have the power to adopt a proactive role. They actively manage their State of health. These apps furnish users with continuous responses [16]. Alerts are given continuously. Users are aided in adhering to treatment strategies. Healthy behaviors are both promoted and sustained. Complications are also prevented. Technology is advancing rapidly. This is likely to result in the further sophistication of health monitoring apps. They will integrate with other health systems. Artificial intelligence will be used for predictive insights.

These insights will be at the Forefront of healthcare management. They will be useful for personalized patient care. The future looks bright. Technology will certainly play a major Role in healthcare.

Telemedicine and Remote Consultation Platforms

Telemedicine applications, through which people can take the advice of doctors from anywhere, are now a very popular application used in the present day, especially due to the prevalence of the COVID-19 pandemic. They prevent patients from visiting hospitals in person to get opinions, diagnoses, or treatments from doctors. Video conferencing, chat-based consultation, and the sharing of medical records with healthcare providers are common components of the telemedicine apps [17].

How telemedicine can be of greater advantage includes increased access by people living in disadvantaged or rural areas. Telemedicine allows consultation with experts, a second opinion, and mental health services for patients from their comfort at home. The patients are seen in time, decongesting medical facilities.

Text Telemedicine systems often include the integration of remote monitoring devices. With connected devices, a patient suffering from chronic diseases can forward his or her clinical data to their healthcare provider for adjustment of treatment programs [18]. Since it leads to continuous monitoring, reduced hospital admissions, and improvements in quality of services are experienced.

Fitness and Wellness Tracking Apps

- Fitness and wellness tracking applications have helped facilitate a healthier way of living by tracking wellness-related indicators, such as diet and physical activity. Many use these applications to keep fit, lose weight, or gain a fitness level. Other elements that are tracked by these applications include heart rate, steps, calories burned, and even sleep patterns through sensors in smartphones or wearable technology [19].

- Well-known fitness apps, which provide guided regimes to count daily steps, encourage users to achieve the desired fitness goals. Nutrition-oriented applications guide users to log their food intakes, hydration levels, macronutrient ratios, and calorie levels. Some other applications provide personalized workout programs and nutrition plans to the likes and health goals of users.
- Wellness tracking applications have functionalities like stress management, mindfulness exercises, and meditation guides. Such applications tend to be holistic, integrating mental wellness with physical wellness to embrace overall well-being fully.

Mobile Health Devices

Mobile health devices have greatly revolutionized the management of health care. Some of the devices include wearable technologies and sensors that are connected to the Internet of Things devices. These functions will empower patients as well as healthcare practitioners in monitoring real-time health, early detection of problems, and better chronic disease management. In this paper, two considerable categories of mobile health devices are discussed below: wearable technology and sensors connected to Internet of Things devices.

Wearable Technology

The core of mobile health is wearable technology that gives personal insights and continuous health monitoring [20]. Body-worn gadgets monitor a host of physiological parameters, thus making it possible for individuals to have mastery over health.

Fitbits and Garmins are many fitness watches that track daily activities, with heart rate taking a snapshot of calories burned and steps taken. Setting and pursuing healthy beauty goals simplifies the motivation for the wearer when it comes to pursuing an active lifestyle.

- Smart watches: Apart from fitness, smart watches like Samsung Galaxy Watch and Apple Watch have also gained momentum, for health monitoring functions like blood oxygen level, ECG reading, and fall detection, which will be particularly useful for them, seniors who may need daily care or become ill.
- Medical Variables: Such devices can provide real-time analysis, with high levels of disease management information. Examples include wearable blood pressure monitors or continuous glucose monitors (CGMs) for people with diabetes [21]. For example, CGMs allow diabetics to monitor their blood sugar levels without having to tap their fingers repeatedly, making diabetes care easier.

- Improved healthcare: Enforced technology for remote quality monitoring and early detection of health problems; as a result, healthcare improves. Information between the patient and the health care provider can lead to better treatment planning and more informed treatment decisions.

Sensors and IoT Devices in Health Management

The integration of sensors and IoT (Internet of Things) devices in healthcare represents the next wave of innovation. This technology can easily collect, transmit, and analyze health data, providing a comprehensive view of a patient's health status.

Key Aspects of IoT in Health Management

- **Distant tracking**: Sensors, internal smart watches, health bands, or maybe medical wearables would collect several fitness metrics constantly. These encompass heart rate, blood pressure, and glucose levels. IoT networks can use these statistics to permit healthcare companies to receive records that would allow faraway tracking and timely intervention with reference to a patient. For example, in the case of heart arrhythmia, the patient has to be constantly monitored for the doctor to detect an abnormal heart rhythm.
- **Smart Home Health Devices:** For asthma patients, IoT-enabled sleep monitoring, connected scales, and smart inhalers provide critical information about a patient's schedule and how that patient could manage their treatment, because it is flexible, real-time, and treatment planning based on collected data
- **Smarter hospital:** An IoT-enabled smart hospital will utilize numerous IoT devices to provide patient care with optimum operational efficiency. The IoT device tracks their location and usage; in addition, it monitors patients' status in real-time and provides prescriptions accurately due to sensors, which eventually results in minimizing errors, quicker responses, and a better patient experience.
- **Challenges and Considerations:** IoT devices and wearable technologies have several advantages. However, it includes shortcomings in protecting privacy and data security. Users must be assured that their information is handled securely because the devices possess vast amounts of sensitive health information that needs to be safeguarded from attack. Most importantly, these must remain usable.

Integration with Other Technologies

Integration with AI, IoT, and Big Data

- Incorporation of big data, the Internet of Things (IoT), and artificial intelligence (AI) has enabled better capabilities in mobile health programs. Artificial intelligence improves the price of mobile fitness apps by means of providing choice assistance gear and offering insights via predictive analytics and personalization [22]. For instance, AI can have a look at tendencies in a consumer's clinical records, become aware of possible dangers, and offer customized remedies. With those talents, one can have a proactive method to health management, for instance, by predicting the outbreak of sicknesses and suggesting preventive remedies.

- The Internet of Things extends the possibility of cellular health control as it connects disparate fitness devices and sensors right into a community. Examples of IoT-enabled gadgets encompass wearables and clever domestic healthcare home equipment that are constantly collecting statistics and forwarding them to healthcare providers for timely movements and far-flung monitoring [23]. For instance, if blood sugar leaves the regular range, an Internet of Things-enabled glucose monitor can be configured to give a notification to the affected person and the healthcare provider so that instant action may be taken.
- The terrific volume of facts that AI and IoT devices generate calls for big data to process them. Healthcare specialists can perceive styles, point out population fitness problems, and make advanced choices with the aid of analyzing large datasets [24]. For instance, big data analytics may be used to track sickness outbreaks in real-time, thereby assisting public health employees to act more skillfully. Big data also permits the design of custom-designed medicinal drugs, as it makes it feasible to deliver remedy styles alongside strains of a patient's genetic makeup and scientific records.
- In addition to enhanced patient care, the adoption of AI, IoT, and big data in mobile healthcare has enabled a shift to value-based, focused healthcare more on outcomes than on costs.

Cloud Computing in Mobile Health Management

Another important technology that has spurred the development of mobile healthcare is cloud computing. With cloud services, mobile health applications can store and process large amounts of data without any restrictions on how it is stored on individual devices. It enables better coordination between patient providers, real-time data integration, and electronic access to medical records.

Cloud computing enables efficient storage of health information and enables on-demand access without loss of privacy. It also leverages scalability, where an entire healthcare application can scale up to handle a large number of users and critical data types [25]. For example, cloud-based healthcare services can scale up in times of public health crisis, and everyone who needs their services needs to continue to have access to them.

Cloud computing makes it easier to connect multiple healthcare apps and systems, thus achieving a more integrated healthcare environment. For example, a healthcare professional on behalf of a patient will analyze data obtained from their wearable device transferred to the cloud. Based on the EHR, the workflow with this kind of integration is streamlined, effectively reduces operational workflow, and improves the accuracy of health information.

IMPACT OF MOBILE TECHNOLOGY ON HEALTH MANAGEMENT

Enhancing Patient Engagement

Mobile technologies are central to patient engagement for better health outcomes. Patient engagement can be defined as people who are actively involved in decisions related to their health care, self-care, and overall health care. Especially, mobile technology in the form of smartphone apps has enabled this participation to evolve and become more involved with a more knowledgeable and capable patient base, of patient-provider contact. Contributions have been made.

Improved Communication between Patients and Healthcare Providers

One of the influences of cell technology on patient engagement is improved communication between the patient and healthcare providers. In the beyond, conversation mainly happened during face-to-face appointments or cell phone calls, which then caused neglected opportunities for data sharing or lengthy wait instances for provider transport. Mobile generation has closed this gap through non-stop real-time communication.

With cell health programs and structures, users can talk with their fitness care experts via video conferencing, via messaging systems, or through secured portals. No longer must a patient anticipate a visit to a clinical facility to record symptoms or ask questions because this line of communication is open and allows for spontaneous help [26]. Examples consist of sufferers who are managing long-term sicknesses, including diabetes or high blood pressure, and can forward their day-by-day measurements to their clinician for remote help or a change in treatment plans.

The mobile era also permits for extra personalized and tailored conversation. A clinician can remind a patient of ongoing follow-up care, appointments, or adherence to medication prescriptions through cellular generation for continuous involvement with the patient in the course of the path of care. These tactics in verbal exchange build an ongoing relationship with the patient and the clinician, thereby fostering belief and improving the person's pride [27].

Enhanced coordination in care has additionally been facilitated through the progress conversation that has been made feasible via mobile technologies. Where care involves a couple of companies, mobile applications make certain that all are on the same page and informed; consequently, any mistakes or false impressions, the possibility of which is lower, are minimized.

Role of Mobile Apps in Patient Education

Patient communication and education about mobile apps can be improved. More educated patients are more likely to actively manage their health, adhere to their treatment plans, and make intelligent decisions about their care.

Mobile apps can make health information and educational information more understandable to patients. Issues range from understanding medical issues and available treatments to preventative care and healthy lifestyles. Information that is often interesting and approachable is easier for the patient to understand and use.

Mobile health apps also include other media such as movies, quizzes, and personalized presentations, which are often included to enhance the learning process. For example, a person with asthma can use the application on their smartphone to learn interactive lessons about triggers, medications, and breathing techniques so patients can manage their disease better while avoiding complications [23].

Another valuable aspect of patient education is the ability of mobile apps to provide immediate support and trigger feedback. The typical smoker may be a quit smoker who tracks behavior through a smartphone application over time, receives encouragement, and is then reminded of the tools he or she can use to overcome the craving. Such continued support will ensure that the patient remains committed to health goals and behaviors.

The advent of mobile technology has made it easier than ever to educate patients. Information will be available to patients whenever they feel it would be most convenient for them—whether at home, at work, or on the go—and the continuous flow ensures that education becomes part of the patient's daily life and not at the bottom.

Data Collection and Analysis

Because of mobile technology, the series and analysis of health facts have been totally converted in the healthcare enterprise. It is because of the very high availability and sophisticated capabilities that cellular gadgets have emerged as an important tool for collecting large volumes of data about health. By processing and analyzing this record, healthcare could be made much more effective and tailored to the needs of each patient.

How Mobile Devices Facilitate Health Data Collection

A strong simplification of health data collection is the use of mobiles such as smartphones, tablets, and wearable devices. This enables constant real-time data collection and provides a much better view of a person's health status than previous methods that once relied on manual record-keeping or infrequent visits to health facilities Perhaps the greatest way mobile devices facilitate data collection are health apps that can track all kinds of metrics: blood pressure, heart rate, activity level, sleep patterns and this capability continues to improve with technology a worn such as smart watches and fitness trackers It can synchronize data with mobile health apps by tracking key features regularly [24]. This reduces the possibility of errors or omissions in the system because they can continue to collect data without user intervention. Another way mobile devices collect data is through self-report measures in which users record symptoms, medication adherence, or other health information. A good example is how a person with diabetes can use an application on a smartphone to see their blood sugar levels during the day. She can then take this information to her doctor for review. This type of input can lead to faster treatment when needed because it provides insightful information about the patient's condition.

Additionally, mobile technology helps collect data from multiple sources, such as medical devices, lab results, and EHRs. As a result, both the patient and the healthcare professional make better decisions because they have a more complete understanding of the patient's health status.

Use of Analytics in Personalizing Healthcare

Advanced analytics can signify large volumes of records created by cellular devices that could also be used to customize healthcare. Personalized healthcare refers to the variation of scientific interventions and remedies according to each affected person's particular desires, options, and traits. Such a level of personalization requires mobile technologies and data analytics.

Analytics software can process and analyze the data coming from the mobiles to identify correlations or patterns that might otherwise not have been noticed by analyzing the data manually. For instance, analytics can point out certain patterns in a patient's heart rate, blood sugar, and activity levels and correlate them with other variables such as stress, food, or medicines [25]. Such patterns could be used by health care providers to understand and thus change the treatment regimens for patients.

According to previous data, some algorithms of machine learning, based on advanced analytics, can further predict health outcomes. For example, predictive analytics, given by data patterns, predict how likely a patient is to experience relapse or complications, and then doctors can take it and change their treatment pattern according to the condition to avoid undesirable results.

Analytics can also be used in personalizing patient interventions and health recommendations. Mobile health apps can evaluate data in real-time, based on the individual's health profile, and offer tailored feedback such as nutrition recommendations or reminders for prescriptions. Since patients tend to be more apt to follow recommendations tailored to their individual needs, this level of customization also improves patient engagement and adherence to the treatment plans [26].

Mobile technology and analytics enable population health management, which aggregates and analyzes data from thousands of patients at the community/population level to identify trends or risk factors. Used to allow for effective resource allocation and the creation of focused interventions, this will improve general public health outcomes.

Reducing Healthcare Costs

In addition to improving patient care, mobile devices have dramatically reduced healthcare costs and revolutionized healthcare. Analysis of the total cost of mobile technology in healthcare and the benefits derived from mobile healthcare are two factors contributing to this cost reduction.

Efficiency Gains from Mobile Health Management

- Helps to raise awareness of health-related best practices to achieve higher efficiency of the health system. The benefits here come from mobile device capabilities, which enable real-time data sharing, improved communication between patient and provider, and remote monitoring. MHealth applications reduce the burden on medical staff and locations because they do not require frequent personal visits, thus saving resources for emergencies.
- The most obvious areas of need for improvement in clinical practice are chronic diseases. Without much medical help, patients can easily use mobile apps to monitor symptoms, track disease progress, and track their treatment. This proactive positioning makes them less likely to have complications and easier to treat, which will result in fewer ER visits and hospital stays, thus improving coordination of care between different health care providers [27].
- Another aspect of mobile health technology is telemedicine. Thanks to these tools, remote counseling has greatly improved productivity. Aside from reducing

administrative costs and requiring physical resources, this feature enables healthcare professionals to treat more patients in less time. Mobile health apps can be common features, such as scheduling appointments, medication refills, and follow-up reminders, which work to further reduce the administrative burden on health systems.

Cost-Benefit Analysis of Mobile Technology in Healthcare

The value-advantage analysis is a very good tool for helping the implementation of cellular technology in healthcare. Even though there may be an up-front fee in growing and deploying cell health solutions, precise long-term savings transpire. Hospital costs, fees for operations, and patient care prices are all reduced through cell technology.

Since the packages no longer require patients to go to the medical doctor as regularly, health programs offer patients a reasonably-priced way of looking after their fitness. It is through this that it is less difficult to get access to healthcare offerings from home, resulting in better fitness outcomes at much less cost. An instance of the sort of health issues that can be reduced by way of remote monitoring of chronic conditions is medical institution readmission, which is often very costly to patients and the healthcare system [20].

From an issuer's perspective, the cell era saves on value in terms of personnel and physical infrastructure. Some operations are streamlined through cellular health programs, thereby lightening the workload of an administrative assist team; more importantly, telemedicine systems allow providers to look at extra patients without adding to the workplace space. Reduced running charges and more earnings have been reported as a result of these developments.

Furthermore, providing purchasers with custom-designed health recommendations and reminding them is a key component of preventive care via mobile health technology. The long-term financial savings of healthcare systems result from this because the fee of preventive therapy commonly outweighs the cost of advanced infection treatment. Simply placed, the cell era lets healthcare shift from reactive to proactive, which is the more monetary and sustainable technique.

CHALLENGES IN MOBILE HEALTH MANAGEMENT

Technical Challenges

Though there are lots of advantages on the side of mobile healthcare, the major technical problems that should be solved to implement the technology successfully are: there are two major and more technical issues: compatibility and connectivity problems of the device, as well as data security and privacy.

Data Security and Privacy Concerns

The largest technical difficulty in mobile health control is that of the protection and privacy of sensitive health information. The safety issues with cell devices are hacking, unauthorized access, and data breaches, among others [21]. The stakes in making sure that healthcare records are safe are very high as they hold as much economic information as clinical records and private records.

Violations concerning fitness records can cause very dire implications like identity robbery, monetary fraud, and inappropriate access to people's clinical data. Thus, healthcare providers and mobile health app builders need to first have in place strong security measures consisting of encryption, stable authentication procedures, and common security updates [22]. However, due to the huge variety and frequency of differing security settings among cell gadgets and operating systems, the realistic implementation of those measures is exceptionally difficult.

More stringent information protection controls are mandated, as in the case of HIPAA within the US. It can be looking to realize such norms for small or man or woman app developers. One of the most demanding situations in cellular fitness management packages is reaching the right balance between the need for stringent safety features and the requirements of consumer-friendly designs.

Device Compatibility and Connectivity Issues

One of the technological challenges in telehealth is the compatibility of contact information and devices. Issues with compatibility of health apps often arise due to different hardware, operating systems, or software versions for mobile devices, so more development and testing are needed to ensure mobile health software is wearable, and it works well on tablets, smartphones, *etc*. platforms.

Connectivity issues, along with device compatibility issues, are the major barriers to mobile health monitoring. Most mobile healthcare systems rely on a continuous Internet connection to provide telemedicine services, remote monitoring, and real-time data connectivity. Poor connectivity can affect such services, making them less effective where network charging is inconsistent or poor, such as in remote or isolated locations [23]. The consequences of this poor connectivity are subject to delays in data transfer, interruptions during remote assessment, and, generally, health care failures.

Moreover, trust in mobile networks is associated with reliability issues related to data transfer. Even in an area with high-speed internet, network outages are possible. This can result in inadequate or very slow exchange of information between patients and healthcare professionals. This impacts the standard of care, especially in complex cases where information needs to be available immediately.

Ethical and Legal Issues

Although telehealth is transforming healthcare, it also raises ethical and legal concerns. Many of these issues are complex and multifaceted and include patient access, data availability, and regulatory constraints that are critical to the use of mobile health devices, as well as the theory.

Patient Consent and Data Ownership

The most important ethical issues in mobile health monitoring relate to appropriate patient consent and data ownership definition. Data ownership is one of the most important questions in digital health because patients' medical and personal information is frequently collected, saved, and distributed through such mobile applications.

Patient consent is perhaps the simplest ethical principle that requires individuals to decide for informed and voluntary consent to the collection, use, and sharing of personal information. Providing informed consent implementation is difficult, especially in mobile healthcare settings. Often, when a user downloads and uses an app, they do not fully understand the terms they agree to [24]. Consent may be more implied than indicated, mainly because privacy policies are broad and the wording can sometimes be vague or overly general. Data ownership is a controversial issue affecting consent in mobile health contexts. While patients used to own their health information, ownership is slowly eroding as the number of mobile health apps grows. Potential conflicts of interest may arise from claims by app developers, claims by healthcare providers, or other groups. The most important ethical issue to be addressed is that it remains within the ownership and control of patients, who can access, view, or delete their data.

Regulatory Challenges in mHealth Applications

The ever-changing regulatory landscape for mobile health applications, or mHealth, presents significant regulatory challenges. Consistent implementation of existing requirements can be challenging as telehealth applications often fall at the intersection of infrastructure and health services. Such ambiguity creates accountability and compliance problems.

Of particular legal and regulatory concern are the rules and regulations governing specific mHealth services. Not all mobile health apps are considered medical devices in the United States, although some are regulated by the FDA. When the line between wellness and medical or health care starts to blur, determining whether an app needs FDA approval or other types of regulatory oversight becomes a bit of a challenge.

Another challenge is the use of mobile healthcare systems, due to their global reach. Patients from other countries may use apps developed in one country, and potential multilateral conflicts over jurisdiction [25]. Application developers and service providers also face the daunting task of negotiating these complex national and international laws and regulations.

Ensuring compliance with data protection requirements, for example, the EU General Data Protection Regulation, adds a level of complexity. These laws are very strict when it comes to the processing of personal data, and the terms are very strict if they are not followed. So, they have to comply with all those regulations in developing mobile health apps, which is challenging because different countries have different regulatory requirements.

User Adoption Barriers

In mobile healthcare, such systems are highly dependent on user adoption, but there are several barriers to widespread adoption. Such barriers stem from usability problems, hence digital literacy, patient confidence, and other problems. These barriers need to be overcome to ensure the effectiveness of mobile health technologies to improve health outcomes.

Accessibility and Usability Challenges

Indeed, the problems of mobile healthcare are more problems of accessibility and usability than any other question, which is critical for marginalized or technologically underserved communities. As soon as the devices were launched, it became clear that not every citizen has access to the latest smartphone or reliable internet; The digital exclusion causes these apps to spread unevenly in low-income or rural communities.

Technology is not a trouble; however, the use of cell fitness structures can be. Many apps have complicated person interfaces that are too complex to effortlessly understand for most customers, in particular, older or less familiar ones. Applications could be hard to use, specifically because of those necessities: brief textual content, complex navigation, or multiple steps involved in working through a task [26]. These packages must be designed with an ergonomic user-targeted design approach, while considering the need for exceptional groups of customers to triumph over those challenges.

Language is any other usability and likely layout. As a maximum of the mobile fitness apps are available in some languages, those who do not understand English or whose mother tongue is one of the different, less regularly spoken languages will no longer be able to make use of Multilingual help while developing cellular fitness apps. Taking into account cultural differences in cellular health, there are also available apps that can be used.

Digital Literacy and Patient Trust

Digital literacy constitutes any other vital venture towards the implementation of cellular health management systems. Digital literacy may be defined as the ability to efficiently use digital equipment and technologies. Not all sufferers experience the use of an app-based fitness management application or being conversation-friendly with cell technologies. This is especially so with people with a whole lot less exposure to virtual platforms, older humans, and people who are less conversant [27].

It is not clean for patients to download apps, generate money owed, use functions, or access the fitness records that are sent to them. In some respects, the difficulty can be as essential as understanding how to link the tool to the internet. Improved virtual literacy via instruction and assistance will therefore help ensure that all patients can benefit from mobile fitness gadgets.

The second factor that affects the adoption of cellular health programs is the affected person's trust. Hesitation on the part of sufferers to adopt these technologies might be due to their worries about the protection and confidentiality of their scientific information. If they accept as true that their records will no longer be handled correctly or morally, then they are even less unwilling to apply the cellular fitness systems. There needs to be an open conversation about the use, storage, and safety of statistics to make certain that they agree with what is built. Moreover, mobile health applications need to comply with all relevant laws and regulations.

CASE STUDIES AND REAL-WORLD APPLICATIONS

Successful Implementations

Many of its programs in various healthcare settings show that the new mHealth era has promise in reworking the management of health.

Case Study 1: Management of Diabetes via Mobile Apps

One of the greatest success stories may be the management of diabetes through mobile apps on smartphones. Apps like Miser and Glooko, among others, allow patients to monitor their blood glucose levels, track their food intake, and receive customized feedback. According to a leading healthcare provider, individuals who used these apps had significantly lower HbA1c levels compared to those receiving standard care. Improved adherence to treatment plans and overall health outcomes were observed due to the convenience of the apps and the instant feedback they provide.

Case Study 2: Remote Monitoring of Patients with Heart Failure

The ability to monitor patients with heart failure through mobile technology has been effectively implemented. An American hospital launched a program to track patients' blood pressure, heart rate, and other vital signs using wearable devices and smartphone applications. The data was communicated in real time to healthcare providers, who responded accordingly. Hospital readmissions among these patients dropped by 30%, and both patient outcomes and healthcare costs improved significantly.

Case Study 3: Mobile Apps for Treating Mental Health Conditions

In this context, mobile apps such as Headspace and Calm have become valuable tools in mental health care, helping patients manage stress, anxiety, and even sexual health concerns. A study conducted in the UK found that frequent users of these applications experienced a 45% reduction in anxiety and depression. Through mobile technology portals, attending therapy or accessing caregiver support has become much easier, leading to improved mental health outcomes for patients.

Comparative Studies

Comparative Study 1: Health vs. mHealth – Traditional Care for Chronic Diseases

A comparative study conducted in 2022 evaluated the effectiveness of mHealth treatments versus conventional medications in managing chronic conditions such as diabetes, hypertension, and asthma. The findings revealed that patients using mobile health apps had better disease control compared to those receiving traditional care. The study also found that fewer patients visited the emergency room, and medication adherence among mHealth users was 20% higher. It supported the argument that mobile health can enhance patient self-management and reduce the burden on healthcare systems.

Comparative Study 2: Telemedicine vs. In-person Consultation

To examine the effectiveness of telemedicine compared to in-person visits for managing non-emergency cases, a study included more than 5,000 patients from various medical centers. Results showed that telemedicine specialists were as effective as in-person consultations for most conditions, with patient satisfaction rates exceeding 90%. Additionally, telemedicine emerged as a strong alternative to traditional care, significantly reducing the time and cost of healthcare visits.

Comparative Study 3: Patient Education through Mobile Applications

Compared to traditional methods, patient education through mobile applications has proven to be more effective than books and personal meetings. The use of apps such as Ada, WebMD, and others has increased treatment adherence by 25%, as patients have become more aware of diseases and treatment options. One of the most important factors contributing to this success is that mobile apps are personalized and interactive, allowing patients to learn and engage more effectively.

Comparative Study 4: mHealth in Urban vs. Rural Settings

A comparative study examining the effectiveness of mHealth interventions in urban and rural settings found that while mHealth was beneficial in both contexts, it had a greater impact on patients in rural areas who had limited access to traditional healthcare providers. Health outcomes improved by 40% in rural environments and by 25% in urban environments due to mHealth activities. These findings underscore the importance of mHealth as a tool to bridge healthcare disparities among marginalized populations.

FUTURE TRENDS IN MOBILE HEALTH MANAGEMENT

Emerging Technologies

The incorporation of new technologies into healthcare systems signals major breakthroughs ahead for the field of mobile health, or mHealth. It is set to transform health management in unimaginable ways, expanding the possibilities of mHealth solutions.

Artificial Intelligence and Machine Learning

Machine learning and artificial intelligence are reshaping the mHealth landscape. These technologies can analyze large volumes of health data to improve diagnosis, forecast health outcomes, and recommend individualized treatments. The complexity of AI-powered virtual health assistants and chatbots is increasing, providing patients with real-time support and guidance. With improved machine learning algorithms, predictive analytics will become more effective, enhancing proactivity in managing chronic illnesses and enabling earlier detection of potential health issues.

Health Parameter Measurement

Health parameter measurement is rapidly advancing through devices such as fitness trackers and smartwatches within wearable technology. The Internet of Medical Things (IoMT) refers to connected medical devices that collect, share, and analyze health data for clinical decision-making. These technologies allow continuous monitoring of vital signs, medication adherence, and lifestyle factors, giving healthcare professionals deeper insights into a patient's health status. Future developments in IoMT are expected to include more advanced sensors and greater integration with electronic health records.

Blockchain for Secure Health Data

Blockchain technology offers the potential to enhance the security and privacy of health data. It enables secure patient data exchange between providers by preventing unauthorized access and maintaining an immutable record of health information. This technology can address many of the current data security challenges in mHealth, creating a more reliable and safe system for health information exchange.

AR and VR Applications

Health education is increasingly using AR and VR technologies to engage patients. For example, VR can deliver immersive experiences in patient education and therapy, while AR can create interactive visualizations of medical conditions and treatment plans. These features are likely to improve health outcomes by enhancing patient understanding and engagement.

International Perspectives

Regional differences in healthcare infrastructure, legal frameworks, and cultural perspectives influence the uptake and impact of mobile health technologies.

Developed Countries

Mobile health technologies are increasingly being integrated into the conventional healthcare systems of developed countries to promote patient participation, cost-effective treatment delivery, and improved care provision. These countries have highly advanced healthcare systems that utilize mHealth for telemedicine, personalized health recommendations, and chronic disease management. Key considerations include interoperability across different health systems and concerns regarding data protection.

Developing Nations

Mobile health technologies are addressing major gaps in healthcare delivery and access in developing nations. In regions with limited healthcare infrastructure, mobile health programs are primarily used to enhance disease management, provide virtual consultations, and facilitate the transmission of vital health information. Examples of mHealth applications improving health outcomes include mobile clinics and SMS-based health education programs. Despite its potential, challenges such as connectivity, infrastructure limitations, and digital literacy must be addressed to realize the full benefits of mHealth.

Global Health Initiatives

International organizations and global health initiatives are increasingly recognizing the potential of mobile health technologies to address global health challenges. Cooperative efforts focus on using mHealth for health education, vaccination and immunization campaigns, and epidemic monitoring. International collaborations are essential for sharing best practices, establishing uniform standards, and ensuring equitable access to mobile health solutions across diverse geographical regions.

Driven by technological breakthroughs and changing healthcare needs, mobile health management is expected to undergo substantial changes and advancements in the future.

- Integration and Interoperability: To properly exploit mHealth technologies, they would need to be integrated into existing electronic health records and healthcare systems. Interoperability of the various systems and devices will enhance coordination of care, reduce duplication in healthcare procedures, and facilitate smooth interchange of data.
- Personalization and Precision: The advanced mHealth technologies to be developed in the near future will take the role of precision medicine and

personalization further. Using personal data and lifestyle factors combined with genetic information, treatment and therapy then become even more efficient and focused in themselves. Patients will have a motive to manage their health with greater self-care and increased proactivity as they utilize evidence-based mHealth personalized solutions.

- **Ethical and Legal Advancement:** Developments For mHealth technologies to gain wide acceptance, ethical as well as legal issues need to be addressed. Patient's consent, safety of data, and their privacy shall remain most vital. The regulatory agencies shall have to develop and update the guidelines in pace with new technology development so that mHealth solutions are safe, efficient, and compliant with the relevant standards.
- **Health Equity:** The main goals for the near future are to use mobile health technologies to promote the elements of health equity. The dependability, of course, shall lie in making mHealth solutions useful and accessible to a range of groups, and most especially to the marginalized and underprivileged groups, to build an effort aimed at bridging digital divides and removing the enablers of barrier technology adoption regarding sharing the advantages of mHealth fairly.

CONCLUSION

The chapter on mobile health management provides a critical study of the advantages and disadvantages of mobile technology's impact on healthcare. Mobile technology has promoted patient involvement in various ways—from personal educational needs and real-time feedback to enhanced communication networks between patients and healthcare providers. Patients are now actively and wisely participating in health management more than ever before. Constant and real-time collection of health data through mobile technologies enhances the accuracy and completeness of health monitoring. Advanced analytics, including AI and machine learning, provide predictive insights and personalized healthcare.

Mobile health technologies reduce costs through efficiency improvements, reduced reliance on physical infrastructure, and support for preventive care. The shift toward proactive healthcare lowers operational and overall patient care costs. Technical challenges include connectivity issues, device compatibility, and concerns about data privacy and security. Ethical and legal issues involve patient consent, data ownership, and compliance with laws and regulations. These concerns also relate to barriers in user adoption, including digital literacy, usability, accessibility, and trust.

Future mHealth technologies expected to reshape the landscape include blockchain, AI, IoMT, and AR/VR. Upcoming developments will focus on inclusion, individualization, ethical considerations, and health equity, as global perspectives influence adoption levels and barriers. As one of the major advancements in healthcare administration, mobile health technology offers significant benefits in patient participation, data precision, and cost efficiency. However, overcoming its inherent challenges is essential to realize the potential of these technologies fully. As mobile health solutions continue to advance, they hold the promise of improving healthcare outcomes and delivery worldwide.

ACKNOWLEDGEMENTS

The author would like to express their sincere gratitude to all those who contributed to the successful completion of this work on mobile health technologies. They extend their appreciation to the academic and healthcare professionals whose insights and research have shaped the understanding of mHealth's transformative role in modern healthcare systems.

Special thanks to the author's colleagues for their continuous support, constructive feedback, and encouragement throughout this endeavour. Their guidance has been invaluable in refining the content and ensuring its relevance to both academic and practical contexts.

REFERENCES

[1] C. Free, G. Phillips, L. Galli, L. Watson, L. Felix, P. Edwards, V. Patel, and A. Haines, "The effectiveness of mobile-health technology-based health behaviour change or disease management interventions for health care consumers: a systematic review", *PLoS Med.,* vol. 10, no. 1, p. e1001362, 2013.
[http://dx.doi.org/10.1371/journal.pmed.1001362] [PMID: 23349621]

[2] J.C. Sieverdes, F. Treiber, C. Jenkins, and K. Hermayer, "Improving diabetes management with mobile health technology", *Am. J. Med. Sci.,* vol. 345, no. 4, pp. 289-295, 2013.
[http://dx.doi.org/10.1097/MAJ.0b013e3182896cee] [PMID: 23531961]

[3] M.C. Hung, and W.Y. Jen, "The adoption of mobile health management services: an empirical study", *J. Med. Syst.,* vol. 36, no. 3, pp. 1381-1388, 2012.
[http://dx.doi.org/10.1007/s10916-010-9600-2] [PMID: 20878452]

[4] G. Kalem, and Ç. Turhan, "Mobile technology applications in the healthcare industry for disease management and wellness", *Procedia Soc. Behav. Sci.,* vol. 195, pp. 2014-2018, 2015.
[http://dx.doi.org/10.1016/j.sbspro.2015.06.216]

[5] K. Fan, and Y. Zhao, "Mobile health technology: a novel tool in chronic disease management", *Intelligent Medicine,* vol. 2, no. 1, pp. 41-47, 2022.
[http://dx.doi.org/10.1016/j.imed.2021.06.003]

[6] R.S.H. Istepanian, D. Casiglia, and J.W. Gregory, "Mobile health (m-Health) for diabetes management", *British Journal of Healthcare Management,* vol. 23, no. 3, pp. 102-108, 2017.
[http://dx.doi.org/10.12968/bjhc.2017.23.3.102]

[7] V. Mohan, S. Muralidharan, H. Ranjani, R.M. Anjana, and S. Allender, "Mobile health technology in the prevention and management of Type 2 diabetes", *Indian J. Endocrinol. Metab.,* vol. 21, no. 2, pp. 334-340, 2017.
[http://dx.doi.org/10.4103/ijem.IJEM_407_16] [PMID: 28459035]

[8] A.A. Dinakrisma, P.W. Laksmi, T. Abdiel, J.P. Fernandez, N. Indahwati, A.P. Susanto, A.A. Indrajaya Lukmana, and P.A. Yusuf, "The role of digital mobile technology in elderly health management among health care workers in Indonesia: Analysis of knowledge, attitudes, and practice", *Digit. Health,* vol. 8, 2022.
[http://dx.doi.org/10.1177/20552076221102771] [PMID: 35646377]

[9] S. Sharma, B. Kumari, A. Ali, R.K. Yadav, A.K. Sharma, K.K. Sharma, K. Hajela, and G.K. Singh, "Mobile technology", *J. Family Med. Prim. Care,* vol. 11, no. 1, pp. 37-43, 2022.
[http://dx.doi.org/10.4103/jfmpc.jfmpc_1114_21] [PMID: 35309626]

[10] C. Free, G. Phillips, L. Watson, L. Galli, L. Felix, P. Edwards, V. Patel, and A. Haines, "The effectiveness of mobile-health technologies to improve health care service delivery processes: a systematic review and meta-analysis", *PLoS Med.,* vol. 10, no. 1, p. e1001363, 2013.
[http://dx.doi.org/10.1371/journal.pmed.1001363] [PMID: 23458994]

[11] A. Garavand, F. Ameri, F. Salehi, A.H. Talebi, Z. Karbasi, and A. Sabahi, "A Systematic Review of Health Management Mobile Applications in COVID-19 Pandemic: Features, Advantages, and Disadvantages", *BioMed Res. Int.,* vol. 2024, no. 1, pp. 1-11, 2024.
[http://dx.doi.org/10.1155/2024/8814869] [PMID: 38230030]

[12] K.V. Kreitmair, "Mobile health technology and empowerment", *Bioethics,* vol. 38, no. 6, pp. 481-490, 2024.
[http://dx.doi.org/10.1111/bioe.13157] [PMID: 36950727]

[13] J.L.H. Shi, and R.W.S. Sit, "Impact of 25 Years of Mobile Health Tools for Pain Management in Patients With Chronic Musculoskeletal Pain: Systematic Review", *J. Med. Internet Res.,* vol. 26, p. e59358, 2024.
[http://dx.doi.org/10.2196/59358] [PMID: 39150748]

[14] P. Galetsi, K. Katsaliaki, and S. Kumar, "Exploring benefits and ethical challenges in the rise of mHealth (mobile healthcare) technology for the common good: An analysis of mobile applications for health specialists", *Technovation,* vol. 121, p. 102598, 2023.
[http://dx.doi.org/10.1016/j.technovation.2022.102598]

[15] Oloruntoba Babawarun, Rawlings Chidi, J.O. Arowoogun, A.O. Adeniyi, and R. Chidi, "The role of mobile health applications in improving patient engagement and health outcomes: A critical review", *International Journal of Science and Research Archive,* vol. 11, no. 1, pp. 2566-2574, 2024.
[http://dx.doi.org/10.30574/ijsra.2024.11.1.0334]

[16] Y. Zheng, B. Campbell Rice, G.D.E. Melkus, M. Sun, S. Zweig, W. Jia, N. Parekh, H. He, Y. Zhang, and J. Wylie-Rosett, "Dietary Self-Management Using Mobile Health Technology for Adults With Type 2 Diabetes: A Scoping Review", *J. Diabetes Sci. Technol.,* vol. 17, no. 5, pp. 1212-1225, 2023.
[http://dx.doi.org/10.1177/19322968231174038] [PMID: 37162011]

[17] W. Fan, and G. Liu, "The power of collaboration in facilitating mobile technology adoption in health care", *J. Med. Internet Res.,* vol. 26, p. e60350, 2024.
[http://dx.doi.org/10.2196/60350] [PMID: 38976864]

[18] V. Sapouna, P. Kitixis, E. Petrou, T. Michailidou, P. Dalamarinis, and E. Kortianou, "Mobile health applications designed for self-management of chronic pulmonary diseases in children and adolescents: a systematic mapping review", *J. Bras. Pneumol.,* vol. 49, no. 5, p. e20230201, 2023.
[http://dx.doi.org/10.36416/1806-3756/e20230201] [PMID: 37909552]

[19] M. Guo, F. Meng, Q. Guo, T. Bai, Y. Hong, F. Song, and Y. Ma, "Effectiveness of mHealth management with an implantable glucose sensor and a mobile application among Chinese adults with type 2 diabetes", *J. Telemed. Telecare,* vol. 29, no. 8, pp. 632-640, 2023.
[http://dx.doi.org/10.1177/1357633X211020261] [PMID: 34152238]

[20] K. Sleurs, S.F. Seys, J. Bousquet, W.J. Fokkens, S. Gorris, B. Pugin, and P.W. Hellings, "Mobile health tools for the management of chronic respiratory diseases", *Allergy.,* vol. 74, no. 7, pp. 1292-1306, 2019.

[21] E. Rochmawati, F. Kamilah, and A. C. Iskandar, "Acceptance of e-health technology among older people: a qualitative study", *Nurs. Health Sci.,* vol. 24, no. 2, pp. 437-446, 2022. [PMID: 35646377]

[22] S. Dhawan, A. K. Rana, S. K. Rana, and K. Nisar, "Internet of medical things devices: A review", *Converg. Deep Learn. Artif. Intell. Internet Things,* pp. 135-148, 2022.

[23] S. Vyas, D. Bhargava, J. Bhola, J.A. Ujjan, S. Eswaran, and A.W. Rahmani, "Critical Retrospection of Performance of Emerging Mobile Technologies in Health Data Management", *J. Healthc. Eng.,* vol. 2022, no. 1, pp. 1-12, 2022. [http://dx.doi.org/10.1155/2022/8903604] [PMID: 35345655]

[24] A. Scarry, J. Rice, E.M. O'Connor, and A.C. Tierney, "Usage of mobile applications or mobile health technology to improve diet quality in adults", *Nutrients,* vol. 14, no. 12, p. 2437, 2022. [http://dx.doi.org/10.3390/nu14122437] [PMID: 35745167]

[25] K. Moon, M. Sobolev, and J.M. Kane, "Digital and mobile health technology in collaborative behavioral health care: scoping review", *JMIR Ment. Health,* vol. 9, no. 2, p. e30810, 2022. [http://dx.doi.org/10.2196/30810] [PMID: 35171105]

[26] N. Bonini, M. Vitolo, J.F. Imberti, M. Proietti, G.F. Romiti, G. Boriani, S. Paaske Johnsen, Y. Guo, and G.Y.H. Lip, "Mobile health technology in atrial fibrillation", *Expert Rev. Med. Devices,* vol. 19, no. 4, pp. 327-340, 2022. [http://dx.doi.org/10.1080/17434440.2022.2070005] [PMID: 35451347]

[27] T. Liu, and M. Liu, "Effect of Mobile Internet Technology in Health Management of Heart Failure Patients Guiding Cardiac Rehabilitation", *J. Healthc. Eng.,* vol. 2022, no. 1, pp. 1-5, 2022. [http://dx.doi.org/10.1155/2022/7118919] [PMID: 35251573]

CHAPTER 11

A Phase-Based Health Recommendation and Prediction System for Women

Gurjot Kaur[1], **Kushagra Agrawal**[2,*] and **Shaveta Jain**[2]

[1] *Apex Institute of Technology (CSE), Chandigarh University, Mohali, Punjab, India*

[2] *Department of Computer Science and Engineering, Manav Rachna International Institute of Research and Studies, Faridabad, Haryana, India*

Abstract: Numerous women's health apps worldwide monitor menstrual cycles and forecast related outcomes. However, the majority of these apps focus primarily on symptom tracking and cycle prediction. There are relatively few solutions designed to enhance women's physical health and immunity during menstruation. Additionally, there is a lack of comprehensive frameworks offering personalized exercise and dietary recommendations tailored to the user's menstrual phase. Even fewer systems provide individualized lifestyle guidance and raise awareness about menstrual health by leveraging Generative AI. To address these gaps, we have developed a Phase-Based Women's Health Recommendation and Prediction System that leverages optimization algorithms to deliver personalized exercise, dietary, and lifestyle recommendations based on the user's current menstrual phase. The system integrates a prediction model to forecast both the menstrual cycle date and phase, along with a large language model to raise awareness by answering common user queries, empowering women to improve their overall health. The predictive model predicted the length of menses with 97% accuracy. The system emphasizes the importance of integrating menstrual phase-based health recommendations to foster improved cycle health and well-being.

Keywords: Large language model, Machine learning, Menstruation, Menstrual prediction, Menstrual phases, Nutrition, Recommendation system, Women's health.

INTRODUCTION

Technology is transforming women's healthcare by enabling more personalized wellness. User and healthcare provider feedback are both crucial for developing effective healthcare applications [1].

[*] **Corresponding author Kushagra Agrawal:** Department of Computer Science and Engineering, Manav Rachna International Institute of Research and Studies, Faridabad, Haryana, India; E-mail: agrawal_kushagra@rediffmail.com

Arun Kumar Rana, Mandeep Kaur & Sumit Kumar Rana (Eds.)

There are numerous menstrual tracking, prediction, and health tracking systems for women. However, they primarily concentrate on identifying the symptoms andestimating the next menstrual cycle date. There are relatively few applications that concentrate on enhancing women's physical well-being and health [1].

Women's energy metabolism levels have been reported to be impacted by changes in ovarian hormones depending on the menstrual phase of the cycle [2]. In a study to report differences in muscle fatigue levels demonstrated by males and females, it was observed that females during the follicular and luteal phases showed higher fatigue levels [3]. As a result, energy intake must also vary throughout the menstrual cycle. Women experience higher energy intake during the luteal phase than during the follicular phase, suggesting that tailoring nutritional intake to match the specific needs of each phase could be beneficial [4]. Apart from hormonal changes, factors like energy imbalance, intensity of physical activity, and food habits can also affect menstrual regularity, particularly in female athletes. In cases where women engage in intense or high-frequency exercise without relevant nutrition intake, they may experience disturbances in their menstrual cycle. Such disruptions can lead to menstrual dysfunctions like amenorrhea, which is characterized by the absence of menstruation, and can negatively affect bone health, cardiovascular function, and overall well-being [5]. Therefore, a healthy diet and active lifestyle play a pivotal role in the prevention of such hormonal disorders.

The menstrual cycle consists of four phases: menstrual, follicular, ovulatory, and luteal, and each requires specific dietary and exercise considerations. During the menstrual phase, iron-rich foods and gentle exercise, such as yoga, are recommended to address menstrual loss and discomfort. The follicular phase benefits from a diet rich in protein and healthy fats, coupled with strength training to maximize energy. The ovulatory phase sees an optimal time for antioxidants and vigorous exercise, while the luteal phase requires magnesium-rich foods and moderate workouts to manage premenstrual symptoms (PMS). These recommendations are supported by research in nutrition and exercise physiology, highlighting the importance of phase-specific interventions [6].

Monitoring menstrual health awareness in girls before menarche is also a crucial indicator of their readiness for the onset of menstruation. Being informed about menstrual health and understanding how the process works directly contributes to their confidence, reducing anxiety and misconceptions [7]. Early education in this area empowers girls to approach menstruation with a positive mindset. To support this educational goal, a variety of digital solutions have been developed, providing engaging platforms for Menstrual Health Education (MHE) by utilizing interactive tools such as comic arts and question-and-answer forums. These platforms offer engaging and accessible ways for young girls to learn about menstruation, providing vital information in a user-friendly format that fosters both understanding and comfort with the subject [8].

Designing a phase-based women's health recommendation and prediction system should consider diverse health needs, accurately predict menstrual cycle phases, and offer tailored health recommendations using machine learning and optimisation algorithms and user-centered design. Using a large language model and machine learning, our proposed system can provide recommendations based on menstrual phases, empowering users with valuable insights into their health. Through continuous refinement based on user feedback, the accuracy and relevance of the recommendation system can be enhanced, and user empowerment and engagement can be fostered.

Additionally, our initiative mainly focuses on lifestyle changes and holistic methods as potential preventive measures against polycystic ovarian syndrome (PCOS) and polycystic ovarian disease (PCOD). PCOS is a common cause of anovulation and a leading cause of infertility. As it is a chronic illness, there is no known cure. However, medication, lifestyle modifications, and fertility treatments can all help with some symptoms [9]. The proposed solution will equip users with lifestyle suggestions that can help prevent such disorders and promote healthy well-being.

In summary, a solution is required that aims to not only track the health status of a woman during each phase of the menstrual cycle but also helps them regulate their overall physical and mental health.

Existing Menstrual Tracking Applications and Methodologies

Menstrual tracking apps are emerging as essential tools for people looking to track their menstrual cycles and manage their reproductive health. With increasing awareness of the importance of menstrual health, these apps allow users to track cycles, manage symptoms, and receive insights into their general well-being. To systematically examine the landscape of these applications, we ran a comprehensive search on the Google Play Store using keywords: "menstrual tracking," "period tracking," "ovulation tracking," "family planning," and "fertility tracker." Our selection criteria included applications with a user rating of more than 4.5, availability in the English language, and at least one million user downloads. These criteria guaranteed a focus on widely used applications that reflect a wide range of user experiences and needs.

Following this process, we identified various applications for further analysis. Each of these apps offers unique capabilities to help users track their menstrual cycles and manage their reproductive health. However, they did show limitations that can affect user engagement and satisfaction, as explained in Table 1.

Table 1. Key features and limitations in various identified menstrual apps.

Application Name	Ratings (out of 5) and Downloads on the Play Store as of 2024	Key Features	Limitations
My Calendar - Period Tracker	4.9 10M	Three modes available: cycle tracking, try to conceive, and track pregnancy. Self-care articles section, partner mode is available. A public chat forum is available where users can post questions on various topics, including menstrual health, fashion, sleep, and more. Animal-based themes to increase user interaction	The application fails to provide users with detailed health insight forecast reports. Lack of food and exercise recommendations based on the forecast, no menopause or menarche guidance provided
Flo Period & Pregnancy Tracker	4.8 100M	Symptom tracking with detailed insights, self-assessments for PCOS, endometriosis, and uterine fibroids are available. A public chat room under specialists' guidance, pregnancy mode, and the option to add a partner are available.	Health or exercise recommendation insights are not present in detail; there is a risk of personal information leakage in a public chat room, and no menopause guidance.
Femometer - Fertility Tracker	4.8 1M	Three modes are available: period tracking, trying to conceive, and pregnancy. App offers integration with hardware devices like the femometer ring, IV, Fitbit, and Apple Watch. Users can earn app points by adding symptoms and checking in to increase user interaction, and a public chat forum.	Detailed BBT insights and detailed health reports for symptom forecast and analysis are paid features; partnering accounts are also a paid feature.
Ovulation & Period Tracker	4.8 10M	Two modes available: cycle tracking and pregnancy tracking. Self-care articles available, app security pin available, animal-based themes with soundscapes to increase user interaction	No detailed symptom analysis feature for free. No menopause guidance or public chat room is available. Most educational articles require the user to upgrade.
Period Calendar, Cycle Tracker	4.9 10M	Three modes: cycle tracking, trying to conceive, and tracking pregnancy. Provides meditation and breathing exercises. Security pin for security	Previous cycle reviews and detailed analysis are premium features.

(Table 1) cont.....

Application Name	Ratings (out of 5) and Downloads on the Play Store as of 2024	Key Features	Limitations
MeetYou - Period Tracker	4.7 10M	Four modes available: period mode, pregnancy preparation mode, pregnancy mode, and parenting mode. Health summaries are available for each mode. The parenting mode has baby feed tracking and insights features, and articles explaining postpartum changes.	No public chat forum available to answer user queries, and limited health recommendations
Maya - Period | Pregnancy	4.7 5M	Four modes available: track cycle and health, avoid pregnancy, try to conceive, and track pregnancy. Friendly user interface. Provides tips based on research journals, public chat forums with featured articles, and expert opinions	Limited health improvement recommendations
Period Tracker Ovulation Cycle	4.6 5M	Two modes: cycle tracking and tracking pregnancy. An Artificial Intelligence (AI) chatbot to address user queries. App lock option for security. The app also provides contraception and pregnancy surveys.	Fails to address users going through menopause and menarche.
Clue Period and Cycle Tracker	4.4 50M	Four modes are made available: period tracking, trying to conceive, tracking pregnancy, and perimenopause. Provides detailed health analysis reports with customized tracking options.	Blogs, detailed tracking analysis, and detailed symptom insights are all paid features. Only period tracking and pregnancy tracking modes are available for free, with limited functionality.
Clover - Period Tracker	4.4, 5M	Helps maintain a detailed record of body health, promoting self-care. Detailed health analysis report	Most features require user plan upgrades for access. No public chat forums
Ovia - Period Tracker	4.3, 1M	Three modes are available: cycle tracking, conceive, and menopause. The health guidance section, named Ovia Health, provides articles and information for 15+ programs if opted for.	Community page with limited interactive functionality for users. The application mostly focuses on conceiving and fertility and fails to give detailed health insights.

For example, while some applications thrive at providing community support and educational materials, they may struggle with privacy issues or sophisticated user interfaces. Others may charge a monthly price for premium features, discouraging consumers looking for low-cost alternatives.

One of the existing menstrual tracking methodologies is MC-tracking that utilizes an inertial measurement unit (IMU) signals to monitor the menstrual cycle. It is a robust method that can predict cycle onset, seven days in advance, with an average error of 0.56 days. The system is robust to emotions, age, and biological clock [10]. Another approach is BeReady, which provides recommendation system capabilities against diagnosed PCOS/PCOD users, menstrual prediction, and chatbot features [11]. Another work highlights the importance of menstrual health education in women and implements machine learning to help answer the most common queries related to gynecological problems and suggests visiting a doctor when any problem is identified [12]. Another fem-tech solution, MonAmie, focuses on cycle tracking, PCOD detection, menstrual product awareness, and doctor consultation [13].

This section not only summarizes the current state of menstrual health apps but also indicates potential gaps and opportunities for innovation in this critical field of fem-health technology.

Major Drawbacks in Existing Menstrual Tracking Applications

After conducting a thorough analysis of various widely used menstrual tracking applications, the following limitations were identified, as mentioned in Fig. (**1**) as well.

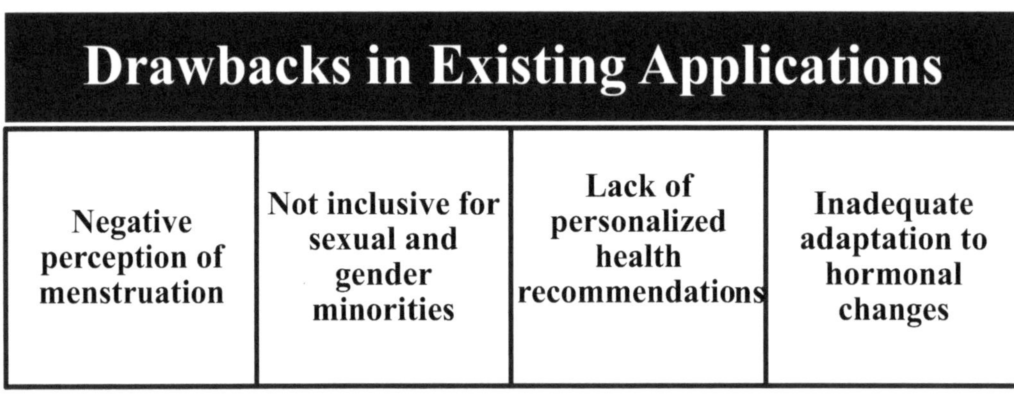

Fig. (1). discusses the drawbacks of existing menstrual tracking applications.

Inadequate Adaptation to Hormonal Fluctuations: Many menstruation tracking applications in the market do not account for the complex hormonal changes that occur during different life stages like menarche, menopause, and hormonal disorders [14]. This inaccuracy leads to erroneous dates being forecast, compromising the reliability of tracking systems. In addition, they disregard hormonal imbalances that could impact the menstrual cycle.

Lack of Personalised Phase-based Health Recommendations: Positive lifestyle interventions are often hindered by the lack of proactive health suggestions in menstrual tracking applications, leaving users without guidance on cycle-specific best practices. Most apps do not recommend which diet to follow or which exercises are appropriate for each phase of the menstrual cycle, limiting their ability to support comprehensive health management. Additionally, there is a shortage of personalized health recommendations tailored to meet the specific needs of individual users.

Negative Perception of Menstruation: Many existing applications inadvertently perpetuate a negative perception of menstruation among users [15]. Due to their inability to promote positive awareness of menstrual health, these applications contribute to the stigma surrounding menstruation, a natural biological occurrence.

Not Inclusive for Sexual and Gender Minorities: Use of gendered language in applications like she/her, with assumptions about sexuality, neglects diverse reproductive and sexual health needs of lesbian, gay, bisexual, transgender, and questioning or queer (LGBTQ) individuals [16].

Proposed Solution

The proposed Phase-Based Women's Health Recommendation and Prediction System offers a comprehensive and user-centric approach to tracking menstruation and encouraging physical well-being by bridging the health recommendation gaps mentioned in the previous section. Our system combines machine learning algorithms with innovative features to deliver precise phase and cycle forecasts, promote a positive menstruation narrative, and provide personalized advice on healthy behaviors.

Phase-based Diet Recommendations: Hormonal fluctuations during each menstrual phase affect energy levels and nutrient needs of individuals [16]. Planned diet plans can help alleviate symptoms like fatigue, bloating, and cramps, while supporting hormonal balance and overall health. It includes utilising sophisticated language models to provide personalised food and lifestyle advice that coincides with menstrual cycle stages.

Phase-based Exercise Recommendations: Recommending workout schedules for each phase can help maintain energy levels throughout the menstrual cycle, promoting reduced PMS, easy recovery for the next cycle, better hormonal balance, and improved mental health.

Accurate Menstrual Cycle Tracking: Creating predictive analytics using machine learning for reliable menstrual cycle monitoring and phase prediction that adjusts to hormonal swings throughout life.

Positive Menstrual Health Promotion: Central to our solution is the promotion of a positive and empowering narrative surrounding menstruation. Through educational resources, supportive content, and community engagement features, we aim to dismantle stigma and foster a culture of informed menstrual health management. This includes leveraging Large Language Models (LLMs) for addressing menstruation-related user queries.

Our solution employs user-centric design principles to provide accurate tracking, promote a positive narrative surrounding menstruation, and deliver personalized health recommendations tailored to individual needs, as shown in Fig. (**2**). By empowering women with comprehensive insights and actionable strategies, we aim to foster a culture of informed menstrual health management and holistic wellness.

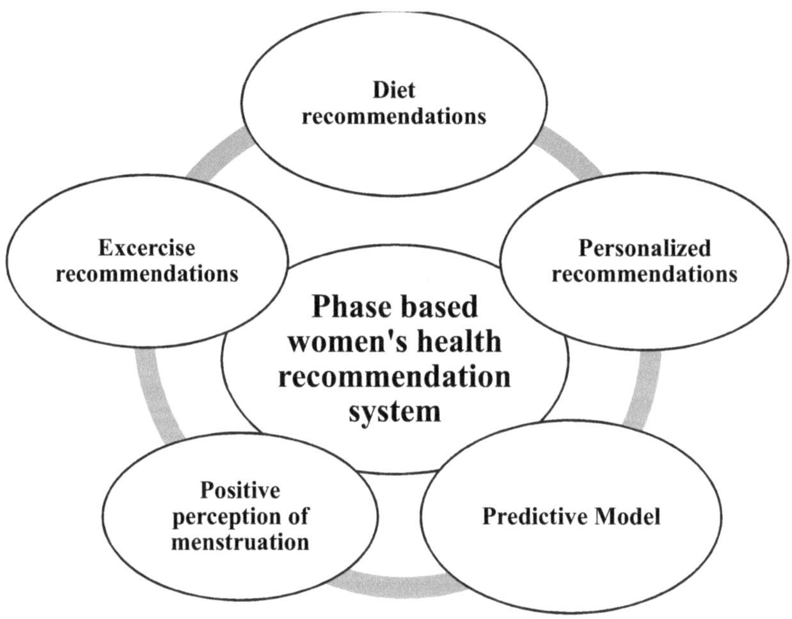

Fig. (2). Explains the various aspects of our proposed solution.

Feedback Optimisation Algorithms for Personalised Recommendations: Establish mechanisms for users to submit ratings and feedback on recommendations, enabling a continuous improvement of the recommendation system and generating personalised diet and exercise plans over time.

LITERATURE REVIEW

The study examines menstrual cycle data collected through the Natural Cycles app to describe cycle characteristics and explore relations between cycle length, age, and Body Mass Index (BMI). 612, 613 ovulatory cycles from 124,648 users were analyzed, revealing a mean cycle length of 29.3 days. The follicular phase averaged 16.9 days, while the luteal phase averaged 12.4 days, which is different from theoretical estimations. Variations in cycle characteristics caused by BMI and age were also analysed. These findings highlight lesser-known variations in menstrual cycle characteristics with implications for health and well-being [17].

This paper explores the Chi-squared mechanism for feature selection and Gaussian naive Bayes to predict PCOS with a 100% accuracy and time computations of 0.002 seconds using a dataset with clinical and physical parameters of women. Prolactin, blood pressure systolic and diastolic, thyroid-stimulating hormone, relative risk (RR-breaths), and pregnancy were revealed to be the prominent factors for PCOS prediction [18].

When it comes to accurately capturing biological states and predicting cycle lengths, hierarchical HIDDEN MARKOV MODELS (HMMs) outperform Single Hidden Semi-Markov Models (HSMMs) (75%) and hierarchical HMMs (61%) with a much greater accuracy of 93%. The model's capacity to adjust to long-term shifts in tracking behavior improves its long-term accuracy in labeling self-tracked health records. The method anticipates cycle lengths of ongoing cycles with substantially lower error rates (2.88 times lower on average) than baseline methods, especially for users with irregular cycles. The inability of the framework to express within-state dependencies between variables at the time of model initialization may have an impact on its capacity to represent intricate relationships found in the data [19].

The study analyzes menstrual tracking in English and Chinese menstrual tracking apps for adolescents, focusing on literacy, cross-cultural differences, and symptom framing. It involved content analysis of 15 popular apps (8 English, 7 Chinese) sampled from December 2022 to January 2023. Both English and Chinese apps lacked information on symptom management, and English apps had more emotional symptoms than physical ones, contrasting with Chinese apps. Chinese apps also tended to frame symptoms more negatively compared to the English ones. The study underscores the importance of evidence-informed communication about symptoms in menstrual tracking apps, highlighting historical taboos and negative perceptions around menstruation. It notes socio-cultural differences in attitudes and experiences, emphasizing the need for improvement to benefit adolescent sexual and reproductive health [15].

In this case study, a new data donation strategy is proposed where menstrual datasets from 35 donors were received, out of which 13 donors participated in the recontextualization of their data. The donors were actively involved in reconstructing the data *via* offline and online meetings. This study explores a unique approach of actively involving the donors in the process of data analysis obtained from the menstrual health tracking app. This covers the importance of effectively involving user feedback in a more intimate way for the improvement of the recommendation apps [20].

This case study explores all existing traditional as well as Machine Learning approaches for the detection of polycystic ovary syndrome. A comparative study is done of different methods as well as algorithms used in detection. The algorithm performance is compared, and possible solutions are mentioned for the challenges faced by those studies. It is observed that the available datasets for PCOD detection are not standardized, are small in size, and are greatly imbalanced. In addition, the suggestion is made for the usage of more clustering and object detection algorithms for detection [21].

An evaluative study is done where 34 menstrual tracking applications are evaluated on the parameters of non-duplicacy, reviews greater than 10,000, last updated less than 180 days ago, written in Korean or English, available free of charge, and currently operational. It is found that the Mobile Application Rating Scale (MARS) and user version of mobile application rating scale (uMARS) scores have no correlation, and the applications that show high MARS scores generally have low uMARS scores. It is observed that the feedback of consumers and health care providers is necessary for a menstrual recommendation system that incorporates all beneficial aspects [1].

This review highlights the lack of specific research on female athletes and the consequences of inadequate nutrition. It recommends female athletes aim for approximately 45 kcal per kg, FFM per day, and pay attention to menstrual cycles for signs of deficiency. Micronutrient intake, hydration, and consulting sports dietitians are emphasized. Additionally, it underscores the need for more research to address the complexities of female physiology and advocate for equal investment in female athletes' success. Female athletes should monitor changes in their menstrual cycle that may signify nutritional deficiency, as missing cycles is unhealthy for an athlete [22].

Exercise-induced menstrual dysfunction, including amenorrhea and irregular menstruation, is common among female athletes and impacts health and performance. Factors like energy imbalance, exercise intensity, and disordered eating contribute to this dysfunction, with individual variations in susceptibility.

Poor energy intake and food selection lead to inadequate intake of essential nutrients, notably calcium, B vitamins, iron, and zinc. Improving energy balance can reverse menstrual dysfunction, safeguarding reproductive health and bone density. Athletes may require supplementation to meet nutrient needs and prevent deficiencies, particularly in bone-building nutrients like calcium and vitamin D [7].

Menstrupedia, an Indian digital platform, addresses the taboo of menstruation by providing menstrual health education (MHE) *via* its website and comic. Through qualitative research and a feminist lens, Menstrupedia's effectiveness and user perceptions were analyzed. While its Q&A forum is underutilized, the platform garners over 4 million views. Menstrupedia's diverse engagement methods, including comics in multiple languages, cater to varied audiences. Menstrupedia provided important information on vaginal discharge, dietary habits, different colors of blood, PMS, and more. Interviews reveal their friendly format and valuable information, yet challenges persist, highlighting the need for nuanced technology-based MHE dissemination strategies and understanding of user dynamics [8].

Obesity and high body mass index (BMI) pose risks for anovulation and infertility, impacting menstrual cycle parameters. A study with 244 women aged 20-54, over 2,035 cycles, found differences in luteal phase and menses length among normal, overweight, and obese BMI groups. Overweight and obese women were 34% less likely to have a positive urinary Luteinizing Hormone (LH) surge, indicating reduced ovulation probability. Anovulation rates were higher in overweight and obese women, suggesting a link between obesity, anovulation, and infertility. Further research is necessary to explore obesity's full impact on menstrual cycle parameters and functions, addressing infertility concerns [23].

Heavy Menstrual Bleeding (HMB) has a prominent impact on one's life and can correlate to underlying health issues, yet measuring it accurately remains challenging. We investigated the accuracy of self-reported menstrual data compared to the data tracked from Clue, which is a menstrual health app. Among 6,546 users, the reported period heaviness was associated with app-tracked cycle duration and heavy flow days, influencing the quality of life and daily activities. While 44% accurately recalled period length, overestimation was common. Users with longer tracked periods tended to underestimate length, potentially leading to underdiagnosis of HMB. The study highlights the complexity of period heaviness and suggests real-time app tracking could enhance understanding of menstrual bleeding patterns and inform treatment. Limitations include the study's age demographics and the lack of validation for app-reported flow volume levels, necessitating further research, especially among younger users [24].

A generative machine learning based model that gives probabilistic outputs based on Poisson regression to make informed predictions of cycle lengths based on a dataset of 186108 users. The model follows a novel approach of countering the irregularity of users in menstrual tracking and takes into account any potential cycle length skips. The model can generate daily predictions as well as get the probability of the user skipping tracking her cycle. This is achieved by computing data log-likelihood using the Monte Carlo approach. The model's predictive performance is found to be superior and has much lower Root Mean Square Error (RMSE) than other baselines in prediction, like mean, median, and neural-network-based methods [25].

The study aims to take variability in the statistics of the cycle length of users to differentiate between symptoms for users on opposite sides of the spectrum. A threshold of a median Cycle Length Difference (CLD) is taken to split the menstrual experience and symptoms reported in the dataset of 378,694 users worldwide, between 21 and 33 years of age. This leads to two separate groups with differing cycle durations, variations, and symptom tracking behaviours- the majority of 92.32% and 7.68%. The latter group is constantly very variable and has severe fluctuations in cycle length. The method used for calculation is the Kolmogorov-Smirnov test. The median cycle length of 29 resulted from the dataset aligning with the previous study of cycle length, which had higher values and wider ranges than what was stereotyped [26].

This suggested model uses sequential Bayesian filtering techniques to calculate the log likelihood for forecasting menstrual cycle stages and the next menstruation day using daily Basal Body Temperature data. Data was acquired from 29 continuous cycles of 20 Ran' tale website visitors, which is QQL Corporation. This study uses the calendar calculation approach as a baseline for comparison, providing more precise results for the later parts of the cycle [27].

A research that considers both regular and irregular menstrual cycles and produces findings for both groups using 305 qualifying cycles with ovulation from 89 women with normal and 77 qualified cycles with ovulation from 25 irregular women. The data is collected using an ear thermometer for BBT and a Huawei Band 5 for Heart Rate. The algorithm correctly forecasted the fertile window for regular cycles with an accuracy of 87.46% and 75.51% for inconsistent cycles and menses with an accuracy of 89.60%, sensitivity of 70.70%, specificity of 94.30%, and area under the curve (AUC) of 0.7849 for regular cycles. For irregular cycles, accuracy, sensitivity, specificity, and AUC were 75.90%, 36.30%, 84.40%, and 0.6759, respectively, for menses prediction. The results obtained from using both wearable devices outperformed algorithms that used only BBT as a parameter to predict fertile windows and menstruation in both regular and irregular cycles [28].

The proposed work focuses on food nutrition recommendations during menstrual cycles. It implemented melia dubia liquid and fermented rice water to identify issues like back pains, stomachache during menstruation, using collaborative filtering and content-based filtering techniques. The study suggested using the proposed liquid results in improved menstrual health when used over three cycles. The research got 97% recognition accuracy [29].

Table **2** lists the key findings and limitations of some of the previous works of other authors.

Table 2. Literature review.

Authors	Key Findings	Limitations
Ko S *et al.* [1]	It is observed that the Mobile Application Rating Scale (MARS) and user version of mobile application scale (uMARS) show no correlation. The feedback of both consumers and healthcare providers is necessary for menstrual tracking systems.	A small number of apps were evaluated and were not inclusive of all cultures.
Anupriya Tuli *et al.* [8]	Digital platform named Menstrupedia that addresses the taboo of menstruation and provides menstrual health education (MHE) in the form of comics in multiple languages and a Q&A forum.	Tailored technology-driven strategies and a deeper understanding of user needs are essential to effectively overcome challenges in disseminating mental health education.
Peng *et al.* [15]	Both English and Chinese apps lacked comprehensive information on symptom management or treatment, and English apps had more emotional symptoms than physical ones, contrasting with Chinese apps.	The causes of inherent taboo and any proposed methods to overcome them were not clearly defined.
Bull *et al.* [17]	Large and diverse data analyzed. Lesser-known variations in the menstrual cycle were realized.	Data can be further used to implement highly accurate prediction systems.
L. Symul *et al.* [19]	Hidden Markov Models (HMMs) outperform single Hidden Semi-Markov Models (HSMMs) (75%) and hierarchical HMMs (61%) with a much greater accuracy of 93%. The method forecasts cycle lengths of ongoing cycles with 2.88 times lower error rates than baseline methods.	The framework is unable to express the within-state dependencies between variables at the time of model initialization.
Alejandra Gomez Ortega *et al.* [20]	Proposes an inclusion of donors of datasets in a more intimate way, where they actively participate in the reconstruction of the context of the dataset.	Not many donors willingly donated their data, thus there was a lack of samples.

(Table 2) cont.....

Authors	Key Findings	Limitations
Kathy Li *et al.* [25]	The model is a novel approach that predicts the cycle date and the probability of a user skipping tracking the cycle. Data log-likelihood is computed using the Monte Carlo approach. The model shows superior performance to other baselines.	The study does not include data with inaccurate/nonstandard cycles.
Li *et al.* [26]	It takes variability in the statistics of cycle length as a threshold to differentiate between symptoms for users on opposite ends of the menstrual cycle length spectrum. It uses the Kolmogorov-Smirnov test for cycle length calculation.	Symptom tracking behavior is taken as a proxy for the true physiological behavior of the user.
Yu JL *et al.* [28]	For regular cycles, the fertile window was predicted with an accuracy of 87.46% menses and an accuracy of 89.60%. For irregular cycles, the fertile window was predicted with an accuracy of 75.51%, and menses 75.90%.	A lengthy approach, as users may fail to test or record their temperature measurements. The study can include more parameters.
L. E *et al.* [29]	The study worked on improving food nutrition recommendations during menstrual cycles. It implemented melia dubia liquid and fermented rice water for improved menstrual health. It got 97% recognition accuracy.	Calorie details can be included to plan a more thorough nutrition plan.

METHODOLOGY

Datasets

The predictive model's dataset, gathered in 2012 by Richard J. Fehring at Marquette University [30], includes a wide range of variables related to the menstrual cycle as well as several demographic, health, and lifestyle factors. The dataset includes information such as cycle number, study group, peak fertility indicators, cycle length, menstrual intensity, reproductive history, age, marital status, education, ethnicity, medical history, contraceptive use, and fertility intentions amongst 80 attributes. It records 1665 cycles of 159 individuals over a period of time. The data is thoroughly cleaned and pre-processed before applying predictive strategies. The data has been used to predict the phase of the menstrual cycle that a person is undergoing at a given time and their next cycle.

Websites offering complete, phase-specific diet plans and recipes from licensed female dietitians and health practitioners were scraped in order to compile the dataset for the recommendation system. To ensure the best possible model performance, the data was carefully cleaned, pre-processed, and sorted by nutrient content and menstrual phase once it was collected. Similarly, web scraping was used to collect the exercise suggestion dataset, which included suitable exercise intensities for each of the four menstrual stages. The data is pre-processed according to intensity level. The exercise plans include yoga, meditation, cardio, and gym workouts tailored to each phase.

For training a Retrieval-Augmented Generation (RAG) based chatbot aimed at providing menstrual health guidance, a curated dataset of over 50 key topics related to menstruation and menstrual health was assembled. Covering areas such as menstrual hygiene management, menopause, menarche, cultural and technological perspectives, menstrual health education, environmental impacts, treatments, taboos and stigma, menstrual products, health and fitness, nutrition, sanitation, hormonal phases, and related disorders, this dataset ensures the chatbot can respond effectively to a wide range of user queries on menstrual health and ensure an informed menstrual health management.

Recommendation System Architecture

Nutrient-Label-based Filtering: This includes making dietary and exercise recommendations based on user preferences, data that is currently available, and the nutrient requirements of each menstrual phase. For example, the system will advise recipes with more protein during the luteal phase and more carbohydrates during the follicular phase. Furthermore, foods high in iron and magnesium will be recommended during menstruation. With respect to exercise recommendations, lower-intensity pursuits like yoga and strolling are advised throughout the cycle, while high-intensity practices like weightlifting are advised during the follicular phase.

Modeling and Prediction: Based on user input, a K-Nearest Neighbors (KNN) algorithm is used to suggest customized diet and exercise schedules. The system generates vector representations of user data, ensuring that appropriate profiles are matched with relevant diet and workout plans to enhance recommendation accuracy.

The use case diagram shown in Fig. (**3**) discusses the flow of the Phase-Based Women's Health Recommendation and Prediction System, highlighting the predictive model, recommendation process, feedback mechanism, and querybot.

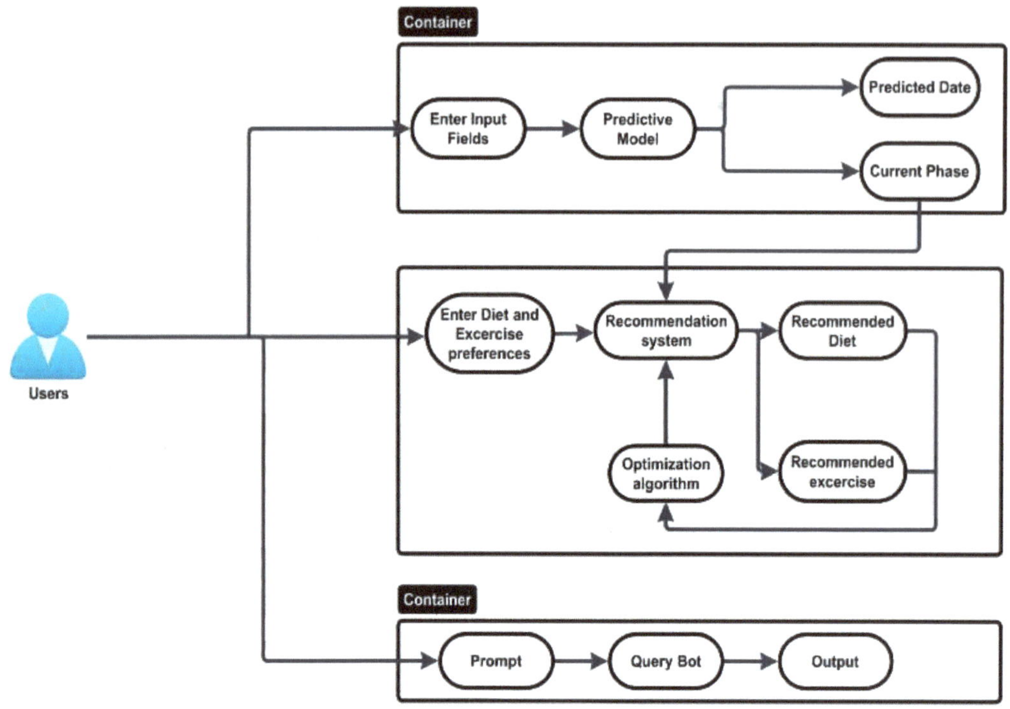

Fig. (3). Flow of the Phase-Based Women's Health Recommendation and Prediction System, highlighting the predictive model, recommendation process, feedback mechanism, and querybot.

User Profiling: Based on feedback on previously suggested recipes and workout schedules, customized user profiles are generated. This guarantees that recommendations in the future are more in line with personal tastes and objectives and helps to refine them.

Personalisation and Feedback Loop: To improve the system and update user profiles, feedback is gathered on each suggestion made. Over time, this ongoing feedback loop makes recommendations that are more precise and tailored to the individual.

Crowdsourcing: If the user is not satisfied with the provided recommendations, they will have an option to submit their own regional recipes. These submissions must include details such as nutrient balance, calorie count, preparation steps, and associated benefits. This will be used to further refine and personalize future recommendations, ensuring a more tailored experience for the user and providing similar recommendations for profiles from similar regions.

RESULTS

We examined the finer details of menstrual cycle patterns and found that there is a significant standard deviation of 3.92 days in when ovulation occurs in individuals. In order to successfully address this variability, we leveraged the predictive power of a random forest regressor model. The random forest regressor is a machine learning technique that creates different decision trees during training and provides their average prediction for regression problems. Impressively, as shown in Table **3**, our model exhibited a remarkable accuracy rate of 97% in forecasting the length of menstruation, showcasing its proficiency in this aspect. Using the menstrual cycle length, phases of menstruation were calculated and fed to the recommendation system. However, when it came to estimating the day of ovulation, our model demonstrated a comparatively lower accuracy rate of 56%. The system predicted the current menstrual phase, the recommendation system suggested relevant diet and exercise recommendations, and the chatbot answered any menstruation-related query.

Table 3. shows the model performance in forecasting the length of menses.

-	Accuracy	Precision	Recall
Logistic Regression	0.894231	0.909346	0.894231
Support Vector Machines	0.974359	0.982372	0.974359
Decision Trees	0.961538	0.962133	0.961538
Random Forest	0.977564	0.985687	0.977564
Naïve Bayes	0.958333	0.968850	0.958333
K-Nearest Neighbor	0.493590	0.524755	0.493590

Demonstration of the diet and yoga recommendations made by the recommendation model for the predicted Ovulation Phase is shown in Fig. (**4a,b**).

DISCUSSION

It was observed that the predictive model predicted the length of menses successfully with 97% accuracy. Further, it was found that while our dataset provided useful insights, its capacity to properly forecast ovulation dates was restricted due to the inherent variability in menstrual cycles between people. However, we saw chances for development and expansion in numerous critical areas. To begin with, there is a scarcity of open access to standardized menstrual datasets. This might be due to a variety of causes, including privacy concerns, cultural taboos, and the sensitive nature of the subject. To overcome data scarcity, we can collaborate with existing menstrual tracking applications for data access by complying with relevant data protection regulations and institutional guidelines. Additionally, expanding our large language model with more comprehensive and diverse training data could further enhance its ability to deliver more nuanced, personalized responses, ultimately improving user experience. Although predicting ovulation dates accurately remains challenging, these advancements hold promise for deepening our understanding of menstrual health and optimizing the effectiveness of our system.

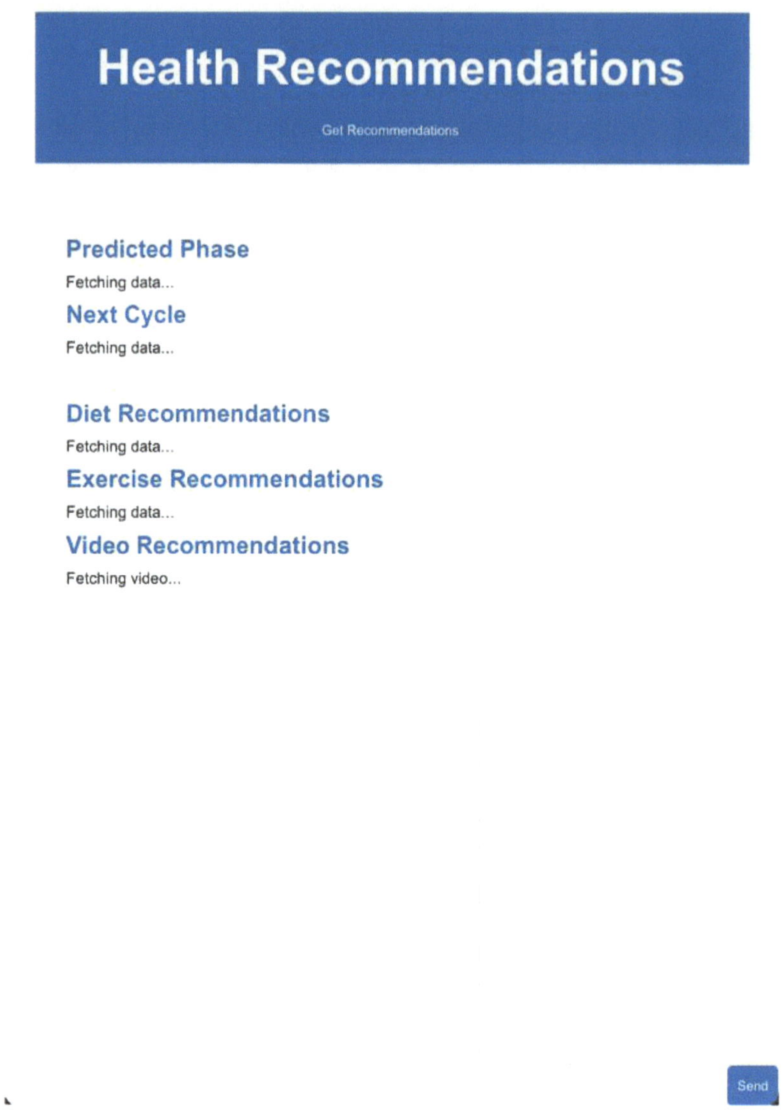

(Fig. 4) contd.....

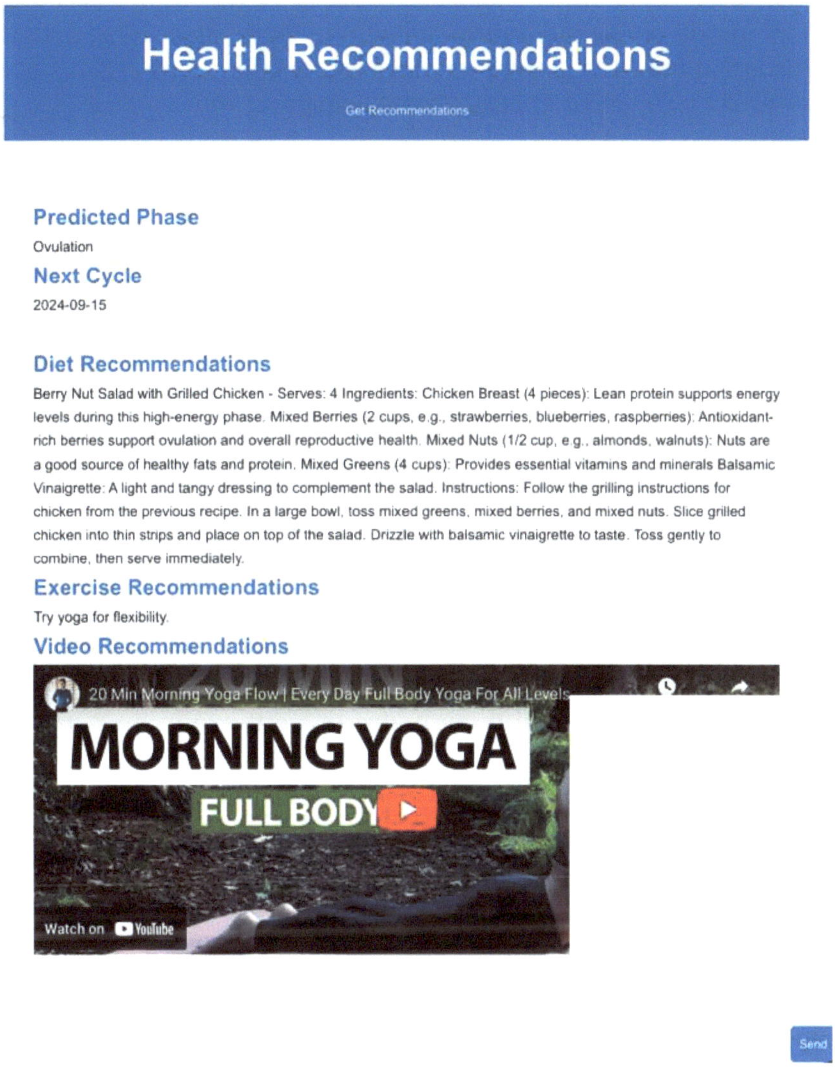

Fig. (4a & b). Show the demonstration of the diet and yoga recommendations made by the recommendation model for the predicted Ovulation Phase.

FUTURE WORK

While our dataset provided useful insights, reliably predicting ovulation dates and menses length is inherently challenging due to menstrual cycle variability. Therefore, expanding the dataset to include more real-world data points and integrating electrocardiogram (ECG) and basal body temperature data can also improve the predictive capabilities of the model [16, 31]. Furthermore, by increasing and enhancing exercise and diet recommendations to incorporate regional recipes, possibly through crowdsourcing by the users, we can further enhance the recommendation system. The solution can be further scaled up to include community pages that promote open dialogue among users to dismantle menstrual stigma, thus spreading more awareness about menstrual education and creating an informed menstrual health management.

CONCLUSION

The Phase-Based Women's Health Recommendation and Prediction System takes a novel approach to tackling significant flaws in existing period-tracking software while encouraging overall well-being for its users. Unlike standard cycle tracking apps, our solution provides a holistic, tailored experience by addressing specific health requirements associated with every menstrual phase. By recognizing and responding to these phase-specific expectations, the system promotes physical well-being and cycle regularity, laying the groundwork for holistic, proactive health management. Our technology transforms the menstruation-tracking experience by adding advanced machine learning algorithms that offer personalized health recommendations based on the user's current menstrual phase. Users receive nutrition, exercise, and lifestyle recommendations that are tailored to the individual demands of each phase, promoting physical and mental resilience. This strategy not only empowers women to take responsibility for their health but also fosters a positive narrative around menstrual health, inspiring users to prioritize their well-being with confidence. Additionally, personalized health recommendations based on user feedback allow users to make more educated decisions, promoting proactive health management as well as positive lifestyle changes.

To summarize, the Women's Health Recommendation and Prediction System tackles challenging women's health issues by bringing together menstrual phase-based health recommendations with large language models and modern machine learning methods. This collaboration of technology, data-driven insights, and user-centered design principles aims to empower women worldwide to live healthier, more fulfilling lives. By modifying the way women understand and manage their menstrual health, our approach promotes positive attitudes regarding menstruation, health, and well-being, fostering a society where women feel empowered and supported on their health journey.

REFERENCES

[1] S. Ko, J. Lee, D. An, and H. Woo, "Menstrual tracking mobile app review by consumers and health care providers: quality evaluations study", *JMIR Mhealth Uhealth,* vol. 11, no. 1, p. e40921, 2023. [http://dx.doi.org/10.2196/40921] [PMID: 36857125]

[2] A.C. Hackney, "Menstrual cycle hormonal changes and energy substrate metabolism in exercising women: a perspective", *Int. J. Environ. Res. Public Health,* vol. 18, no. 19, p. 10024, 2021. [http://dx.doi.org/10.3390/ijerph181910024] [PMID: 34639326]

[3] Salomoni S, Soares FA, de Oliveira Nascimento FA, da Rocha AF. Gender differences in muscle fatigue of the biceps brachii and influences of female menstrual cycle in electromyography variables. In2008 30th Annual international conference of the IEEE Engineering in Medicine and Biology Society 2008 Aug 20 (pp. 2598-2601).
[http://dx.doi.org/10.1109/IEMBS.2008.4649732]

[4] J.A. Tucker, S.F. McCarthy, D.P. Bornath, J.S. Khoja, and T.J. Hazell, "The effect of the menstrual cycle on energy intake: A systematic review and meta-analysis", *Nutr. Rev.*, p. nuae093, 2024.
[PMID: 39008822]

[5] M.M. Manore, "Dietary recommendations and athletic menstrual dysfunction", *Sports Med.,* vol. 32, no. 14, pp. 887-901, 2002.
[http://dx.doi.org/10.2165/00007256-200232140-00002] [PMID: 12427050]

[6] S. Rocha-Rodrigues, M. Sousa, P. Lourenço Reis, C. Leão, B. Cardoso-Marinho, M. Massada, and J. Afonso, "Bidirectional interactions between the menstrual cycle, exercise training, and macronutrient intake in women: a review", *Nutrients,* vol. 13, no. 2, p. 438, 2021.
[http://dx.doi.org/10.3390/nu13020438] [PMID: 33572821]

[7] J. Hennegan, Z.Y. Swe, K.K. Than, C. Smith, L. Sol, H. Alberda, J.N. Bukenya, S.P.S. Kibira, F.E. Makumbi, K.J. Schwab, and P.S. Azzopardi, "Monitoring menstrual health knowledge: awareness of menstruation at menarche as an indicator", *Front. Glob. Womens Health,* vol. 3, p. 832549, 2022.
[http://dx.doi.org/10.3389/fgwh.2022.832549] [PMID: 35400130]

[8] A. Tuli, S. Chopra, N. Kumar, and P. Singh, "Learning from and with menstrupedia: Towards menstrual health education in India", *Proceedings of the ACM on Human-Computer Interaction,* pp. 1-20, 2018.
[http://dx.doi.org/10.1145/3274443]

[9] World Health Organisation.(28 June 2023). Polycystic ovary syndrome. Available from: https://www.who.int/news-room/fact-sheets/detail/polycystic-ovary-syndrome

[10] Y. Wu, J. Zhang, Y. Chen, W. Shi, and H. Tan, "MC-Tracking: Towards Ubiquitous Menstrual Cycle Tracking Using the Smartphone", *IEEE Trans. Mobile Comput.,* 2023.

[11] A. Karia, A. Poojary, A. Tiwari, L. Sequeira, and M.K. Sokhi, "Beredy (period tracker & pcos diagnosis)", *2023 International Conference on Communication System, Computing and IT Applications (CSCITA),* pp. 142-147, 2023.
[http://dx.doi.org/10.1109/CSCITA55725.2023.10104755]

[12] Arunkumar P, Abarna K, Nagamithra N, Suweatha G, Varssha P. Application using machine learning to promote women's personal health. In2023 5th International Conference on Smart Systems and Inventive Technology (ICSSIT) 2023 Jan 23 (pp. 908-914).
[http://dx.doi.org/10.1109/ICSSIT55814.2023.10061126]

[13] N. Jeswani, N. Jain, A. Sharma, and S. Roychowdhury, "Comprehensive FemTech Solution for Feminine Health", *2023 International Conference on Signal Processing, Computation, Electronics, Power and Telecommunication (IConSCEPT),* pp. 1-6, 2023.

[14] Epstein DA, Lee NB, Kang JH, Agapie E, Schroeder J, Pina LR, Fogarty J, Kientz JA, Munson S. Examining menstrual tracking to inform the design of personal informatics tools. InProceedings of the 2017 CHI conference on human factors in computing systems 2017 May 2 (pp. 6876-6888).
[http://dx.doi.org/10.1145/3025453.3025635]

[15] S. Peng, Y. Yang, and M.G. Haselton, "Menstrual Symptoms: Insights from Mobile Menstrual Tracking Applications for English and Chinese Teenagers", *Adolescents,* vol. 3, no. 3, pp. 394-403, 2023.
[http://dx.doi.org/10.3390/adolescents3030027]

[16] G. Anuradha, and M. Mirza, "Study of Variations in Heart Rate., QT and QTc During Different Phases of Menstrual Cycle", *Int. J. Physiol.,* vol. 8, no. 02, p. 51, 2020.

[17] J.R. Bull, S.P. Rowland, E.B. Scherwitzl, R. Scherwitzl, K.G. Danielsson, and J. Harper, "Real-world menstrual cycle characteristics of more than 600,000 menstrual cycles", *NPJ Digit. Med.,* vol. 2, no. 1, p. 83, 2019.
[http://dx.doi.org/10.1038/s41746-019-0152-7] [PMID: 31482137]

[18] S. Nasim, M.S. Almutairi, K. Munir, A. Raza, and F. Younas, "A novel approach for polycystic ovary syndrome prediction using machine learning in bioinformatics", *IEEE Access,* vol. 10, pp. 97610-97624, 2022.
[http://dx.doi.org/10.1109/ACCESS.2022.3205587]

[19] L. Symul, and S. Holmes, "Labeling self-tracked menstrual health records with hidden semi-Markov models", *IEEE J. Biomed. Health Inform.,* vol. 26, no. 3, pp. 1297-1308, 2022.
[http://dx.doi.org/10.1109/JBHI.2021.3110716] [PMID: 34495854]

[20] Gomez Ortega A, Bourgeois J, Kortuem G. Reconstructing intimate contexts through data donation: a case study in menstrual tracking technologies. InNordic Human-Computer Interaction Conference 2022 Oct 8 (pp. 1-12).
[http://dx.doi.org/10.1145/3546155.3546646]

[21] S. Ahmed, M.S. Rahman, I. Jahan, M.S. Kaiser, A.S.M.S. Hosen, D. Ghimire, and S.H. Kim, "A review on the detection techniques of polycystic ovary syndrome using machine learning", *IEEE Access,* vol. 11, pp. 86522-86543, 2023.
[http://dx.doi.org/10.1109/ACCESS.2023.3304536]

[22] B. Holtzman, and K.E. Ackerman, "Recommendations and nutritional considerations for female athletes: health and performance", *Sports Med.,* vol. 51, no. S1, suppl. Suppl. 1, pp. 43-57, 2021.
[http://dx.doi.org/10.1007/s40279-021-01508-8] [PMID: 34515972]

[23] M.G. Lasquety, D. Rodriguez, and R.J. Fehring, "The influence of BMI levels on phases of the menstrual cycle and presumed ovulation", *Linacre Q.,* vol. 79, no. 4, pp. 451-459, 2012.
[http://dx.doi.org/10.1179/002436312804827082] [PMID: 30082988]

[24] A.A. Shea, F. Wever, C. Ventola, J. Thornburg, and V.J. Vitzthum, "More than blood: app-tracking reveals variability in heavy menstrual bleeding construct", *BMC Womens Health,* vol. 23, no. 1, p. 170, 2023.
[http://dx.doi.org/10.1186/s12905-023-02312-4] [PMID: 37041503]

[25] K. Li, I. Urteaga, A. Shea, V.J. Vitzthum, C.H. Wiggins, and N. Elhadad, "A predictive model for next cycle start date that accounts for adherence in menstrual self-tracking", *J. Am. Med. Inform. Assoc.,* vol. 29, no. 1, pp. 3-11, 2021.
[http://dx.doi.org/10.1093/jamia/ocab182] [PMID: 34534312]

[26] K. Li, I. Urteaga, C.H. Wiggins, A. Druet, A. Shea, V.J. Vitzthum, and N. Elhadad, "Characterizing physiological and symptomatic variation in menstrual cycles using self-tracked mobile-health data", *NPJ Digit. Med.,* vol. 3, no. 1, p. 79, 2020.
[http://dx.doi.org/10.1038/s41746-020-0269-8] [PMID: 32509976]

[27] K. Fukaya, A. Kawamori, Y. Osada, M. Kitazawa, and M. Ishiguro, "The forecasting of menstruation based on a state-space modeling of basal body temperature time series", *Stat. Med.,* vol. 36, no. 21, pp. 3361-3379, 2017.
[http://dx.doi.org/10.1002/sim.7345] [PMID: 28543214]

[28] J.L. Yu, Y.F. Su, C. Zhang, L. Jin, X.H. Lin, L.T. Chen, H.F. Huang, and Y.T. Wu, "Tracking of menstrual cycles and prediction of the fertile window *via* measurements of basal body temperature and heart rate as well as machine-learning algorithms", *Reprod. Biol. Endocrinol.,* vol. 20, no. 1, p. 118, 2022.
[http://dx.doi.org/10.1186/s12958-022-00993-4] [PMID: 35964035]

[29] Logapriya E, Surendran R. Hybrid Recommendations System for Women Health Nutrition at Menstruation Cycle. In2023 International Conference on Innovation and Intelligence for Informatics, Computing, and Technologies (3ICT) 2023 Nov 20 (pp. 357-363).

[30] R.J. Fehring, M. Schneider, and K. Raviele, "Efficacy of an internet-based natural family planning system", *J. Obstet. Gynecol. Neonatal Nurs.,* vol. 35, no. 5, pp. 569-575, 2006. [http://dx.doi.org/10.1111/j.1552-6909.2006.00078.x]

[31] A. Padhan, A. Bhardwaj, and J. Sivaraman, *Effects of menstrual cycle on atrial ECG components. InProceedings of the International e-Conference on Intelligent Systems and Signal Processing: e-ISSP 2020.* Springer Singapore, 2022, pp. 219-227.

SUBJECT INDEX

A

Abnormal heart rhythm 189
Abnormalities 80
Absorption 27, 31
Accelerates drug discovery 101
Accelerometers 5, 41
Access control mechanisms 113
Accessibility and equity in mHealth adoption 185
Accountability 35, 58, 110, 197
Accurate menstrual cycle tracking 215
Acid-base balance 31
Adherence 15, 69, 82, 127, 136, 191, 194
ADME/T 30
Advanced cryptographic algorithms 102
Advanced imaging systems 80
Advanced wearable ECG 43
Adverse drug responses monitoring 32
AI-assisted clinical trials 98
AI-based diagnostic imaging tools 140
AI-powered diagnostics 22, 80
AI-powered virtual health assistants 202
AlphaFold 29
Alzheimer's disease 132
Ambulance robots 84
Amenorrhea 209, 217
Analytic hierarchy process (AHP) 141, 145, 146
Anovulation rates 218
Anticipatory treatment 23
Arrhythmias 40, 43, 45, 135
Artificial intelligence (AI) 6, 39, 99, 140, 149, 150, 172
Asthma management 9
Atrial fibrillation 45
Attribute-based encryption (ABE) 113
Authentication 107, 113
Automated external defibrillator (AED) 84, 85

B

Basal body temperature (BBT) 211, 219, 226
Behavioral factors 156
Big data and predictive analytics 136
Binding affinities 29
Bioavailability 31
Bioengineering 171
Bioinformatics 156, 168, 169, 172, 173
Biological clock 213
Biomarkers 43, 158, 159, 172
Biomaterials 171
Biometrics post-COVID 131
Biosensor patches 42
Biosensors 39, 41, 43, 135, 157
Biotransformation 27, 31
Blockchain integration 111, 113
Blockchain technology 64, 65, 68, 69, 114, 115
Blood pressure monitors 135, 188
Blood sugar 100, 190, 193
Body mass index (BMI) 216, 218
Bone morphogenetic proteins (BMPs) 160, 162
Bone regeneration 160

C

Cardiovascular parameters 127
Cartilage repair 161
Centralized authorities 106, 107
Cerebral palsy (CP) 85, 165
Charge-coupled device (CCD) 86
Chemoinformatics 31
Chronic condition management 179
Chronic disease management 1, 5, 9, 22, 40, 42, 47, 126, 131, 203
Clinical care 82, 83
Clinical decision support (CDS) 17, 18
Clinical practice 28, 44, 169, 171, 172, 173, 194

Arun Kumar Rana, Mandeep Kaur & Sumit Kumar Rana (Eds.)

Clinical trial management 62, 64, 65
Cloud computing 144, 179, 190, 191
Cognitive tasks 88
Collaborative filtering 220
Consistency index (CI) 146, 147
Consistency ratio (CR) 146, 147, 148, 149
Continuous glucose monitors (CGMs) 8, 13, 18, 40, 41, 42, 81, 127, 188
Convolutional neural networks (CNN) 28, 29
Cryptographic hash functions 106
Cyber-physical systems (CPS) 90
Cytochrome P450 31

D

Data encryption 102
Data fragmentation 56, 136
Data interoperability 102, 103
Data sovereignty 70
Deep learning (DL) 28, 29, 31, 132, 157, 172
Delegated proof-of-stake (DPoS) 116
Dental Public Health Bureau 165, 166
Dental pulp 160, 162, 172
Diagnostic imaging technologies 172
Digital Health Center of Excellence (DHCoE) 44
Digital health technologies 45, 124
Digital signatures 59, 107, 110
Digital twins 99, 100, 101
Distributed ledger technology (DLT) 104, 108, 110
Drug discovery industry 159
Drug supply chain security act 61

E

Early health issue detection 127
Effort expectancy (EE) 143, 149, 150
Electronic health record management 58
Electronic health records (EHRs) 6, 19, 21, 22, 51, 53, 54, 58, 96, 101, 102, 113, 136, 202, 203
Electrocardiogram (ECG) 131, 188, 226
Electroencephalograph (EEG) 131
Elliptic curve 110
Endometriosis 211
Epidemiology 155, 156, 171
European Medicines Agency (EMA) 44

F

Family Health Strategy (FHS) 164, 165
Feature selection 216
Federated learning 116
Food and Drug Administration (FDA) 17, 44, 67, 162, 198
Fuzzy analytic hierarchy process 139, 150

G

General Data Protection Regulation (GDPR) 15, 17, 54, 64, 65, 67, 96, 102, 104, 115, 116
Generative adversarial 29
Genetic markers 133
Genomic data analysis 111, 116, 133, 168, 169
Genomic medicine and bioinformatics 168
Geometric deep learning 29
Guided tissue regeneration (GTR) 160

H

Head and neck cancers (HNC) 159, 172
Health Insurance Portability and Accountability Act (HIPAA) 6, 15, 17, 54, 64, 67, 96, 102, 104, 115, 116, 196
Heart rate variability 42, 43, 45
Heavy menstrual bleeding (HMB) 218
Hidden Markov models (HMMs) 216, 220
Hidden semi-Markov models (HSMMs) 216, 220
Human-machine interface (HMI) 85
Hyperledger fabric 111

I

Identity-based encryption (IBE) 113
Immutability 52, 57, 59, 67, 94, 95, 108
Industrial Internet of Things (IIoT) 125
Inertial measurement unit (IMU) 213
International Medical Device Regulators Forum (IMDRF) 45
Internet of Medical Things (IoMT) 186, 202, 204
Interplanetary file system (IPFS) 109

K

K-nearest neighbors (KNN) 222, 224
Kolmogorov-Smirnov test 219, 221

L

Large language models (LLMs) 215, 227
Luteinizing hormone (LH) 218

M

Machine learning algorithms 132, 194, 214
Medical Device Regulation 44
Minimally invasive surgery (MIS) 87, 167
Mobile application rating scale (MARS) 217, 220
Multi-criterion decision-making (MCDM) 139, 141
Multidisciplinary collaboration 39, 155, 156, 172, 173

N

Nanomedicines 27, 33
Nanoparticle-modulated drug delivery 33
Natural language processing (NLP) 27, 28, 29, 30, 32, 99
Near field communications (NFCs) 98

O

Optical coherence tomography (OCT) 80

P

Performance expectancy (PE) 143, 144, 148, 149, 150
Personal health records (PHRs) 102, 114
Personal innovativeness (PI) 144, 148, 149, 150
Pharmacokinetics 27, 30, 31
Pharmacovigilance 33
Polycystic ovary syndrome (PCOS/PCOD) 210, 211, 213, 216, 217
Premarket approval (PMA) 44
Protein structure prediction 28, 29

R

Rapid eye movement (REM) 129
Reinforced adversarial neural computer (RANC) 30
Reinforcement learning for structural evolution (RLSE) 30
Remote patient monitoring (RPM) 2, 21, 68, 127, 130, 135
Retrieval-augmented generation (RAG) 222
Root mean square error (RMSE) 219

S

Secure hash algorithm (SHA-256) 106
Software as a medical device (SaMD) 44
Spinal cord injury (SCI) 85, 86
Support vector machines (SVM) 112, 224

T

Technology acceptance model (TAM) 143
Telemedicine and virtual care 6
Triangular fuzzy scale (TFS) 145, 148

U

User-incorrect data interpretation 136

V

Virtual reality (VR/AR) 21, 99, 100, 101, 202

www.ingramcontent.com/pod-product-compliance
Lightning Source LLC
LaVergne TN
LVHW070949210926
848482LV00002B/155
9798898815394